Bittersweet

BITTER

STUDIES IN SOCIAL MEDICINE

Allan M. Brandt & Larry R. Churchill, editors

The University of North Carolina Press

Chapel Hill & London

SWEET

Diabetes, Insulin, and the
Transformation of Illness

CHRIS FEUDTNER

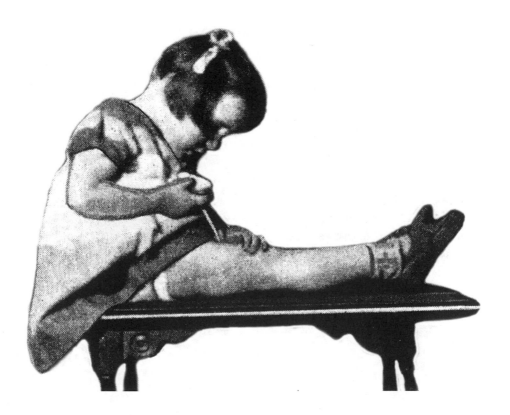

Set in New Baskerville and Didot types

by Tseng Information Systems, Inc.

The paper in this book meets the guidelines for permanence
and durability of the Committee on Production Guidelines
for Book Longevity of the Council on Library Resources.

Library of Congress Cataloging-in-Publication Data

Feudtner, John Christopher

Bittersweet : diabetes, insulin, and the transformation of
illness / Chris Feudtner

   p. cm. — (Studies in social medicine)

Includes bibliographical references and index.

ISBN 0-8078-2791-6 (cloth: alk. paper)

1. Diabetes—History—20th century. 2. Joslin Diabetes
Center. I. Title. II. Series. [DNLM: 1. Chronic Disease—
psychology—United States. 2. Diabetes Mellitus, Insulin-
Dependent—history—United States. 3. Diabetes Mellitus—
complications—United States. 4. Diabetes Mellitus—
therapy—United States. 5. History of Medicine, 20th Cent.—
United States. 6. Insulin—therapeutic use—United States.
WK810 F422B 2003]

RA645.D5F485 2003

616.4′62′009—dc21   2002151271

cloth   07 06 05 04 03   5 4 3 2 1

paper   07 06 05 04 03   5 4 3 2 1

To the diabetic patients whose experiences I have tried to chronicle,
to my family and friends who have urged me to feel as well as think,
to Lester Baker, who provided invaluable guidance and support,
and to Mary Steinmetz, who always wanted me to finish what
I started

CONTENTS

ILLUSTRATIONS

FIGURES

TABLES

PREFACE

LOOKING BACK AS A MEANS TO MOVE FORWARD

Eight o'clock in the morning. As occurs in many other hospitals across America, a team of physicians, nurses, pharmacists, and students is gathering. I am one of them. Our hospital caters to the needs of sick and injured children, and for the next hour or two, we will discuss each patient under our care. As the ward attending physician, I listen as team members present various aspects of each child's case. Not quite half of the children admitted to the hospital were healthy prior to this recent episode of illness, and if all goes well, they will return to full health shortly. The rest, constituting the majority, live with some form of chronic illness. For many patients, powerful new medications, available only in the past decade or so, can dramatically ameliorate the symptoms of their disease. For others, the most problematic aspects of their condition still elude our control: these children experience intractable seizures, progressive muscle degeneration, recurrent infections, or a slew of other ailments that wrack mind and body.

When we then visit these children and their parents, as a group we consider the current problems that brought them to the hospital and discuss not only what treatments are available but more generally the goals that will guide our care. What are these goals? Each child and family is different. For those patients who can reasonably expect full recovery, that is typically the goal. But for the rest, especially those with severe chronic conditions, clarifying the goals of care is difficult but of paramount importance. The underlying disease may block the path to a long and healthy life, compelling us to define another destination, building a new path as best we can. One conversation rarely suffices, as hopes and fears color our assessment of what are loving and feasible goals. Once these goals are clarified, though, we can then marshal the power of medical technology and the full capacity of our health care system to accomplish them.

This is good work that I enjoy, being a pediatrician who works with individual children and parents to secure a better quality of life. Away from the demands of day-to-day patient care, I also conduct research that strives to understand and improve the bigger system of what I've come to think of as "people care": all those activities that we engage in that aim to promote the well-being of individual people. Medical care is part of this encompassing "people care system," but so too are aspects of our social structure and cultural beliefs that lie outside the medical system. As I have oscillated between caring for individual patients and studying the overall people care system, I have come to realize how all aspects of this larger system play a role in shaping the formidable challenges we now confront.

Never has medical care offered more yet demanded so much. As we enter the twenty-first century, the catalog of marvels offered up by our health care system defies comprehension, spanning from minimally invasive surgery for malformed hearts to bone marrow transplants for cancers to an ever-widening menu of vaccines to stave off illness in the first place. At the same time, we are increasingly aware not only of the exorbitant sums of money spent on this care but also of how rising costs hinder efforts to improve access to and quality of medical care. Additionally, over the past few decades we have learned how technologically sophisticated health care, while prolonging life can—too often and quite ironically—dehumanize life, spawning an endless series of ethical dilemmas. Awed yet ambivalent, we embrace medical care while remaining wary of it, striving from birth to death to use this powerful force wisely. Our efforts, though, are hampered by how our culture has underconceptualized the tasks of medicine, ignoring large parts of our humanity. The dominant biomedical model, focusing on physiology and technology, narrows our perspective of health and hope and thereby limits what we see as possible and ultimately desirable.

I have attempted in this book to expand our vision and sense of purpose by examining one particular disease, emblematic of the triumphs and disappointments of twentieth-century medicine: Type 1 diabetes mellitus, which also has been known as juvenile-onset or insulin-dependent diabetes. The history of this disease in America is not one story but many: all the separate stories of patients young and old, of family members, and of health care workers who have lived with this disease. A tale of scientific medicine, complete with its loftiest lifesaving wonder and its most ironic and tragic failings, this history provides a strategic perspective from which to survey the modern terrain of health, illness, and life in general.

Central to this book is an argument about how we should think about the history of diabetes and the stories it comprises. To articulate this argument, the following chapters recount a small but central piece of this history, examining how the experiences of a group of people who became diabetic as youngsters were reshaped by medical intervention and cultural change. Through the stories of these individuals, they describe how so-called juvenile diabetes was transformed from an acutely lethal disease into a chronic entity, and explore what the bittersweet consequences of this transformation have been for patients and their families, physicians, and nurses, and others who provided care.

The impetus for this underlying argument began with a belief that over the years has grown into what I think of as my personal philosophy regarding disease, health, and the practice of medicine. Explaining how this philosophy (by which I simply, and humbly, mean the set of interconnecting thoughts that guide me as a physician) developed may help place this book and its argument into a broader context. In the mid-1980s, having enrolled in medical school, I laid plans to pursue both medical training and graduate work in the history of medicine, convinced—more with faith than evidence to guide me—that the study of medical science and of the humanities would complement each other, that the final result would be worth the time and effort. Little did I suspect how fascinating and frustrating it would be to turn that initial belief into the tangible reality of this account of diabetes history. Ever since those first heady moments, I have been on a journey of reconciliation, trying to span a troublesome divide in modern medicine between abstract knowledge and personal understanding, between laboratory science and the humanity of the bedside.

These days, medical understanding of disease prizes the reductive precision of scientific knowledge yet shies away from comprehending illness at a more individual and subjective level. As I came to appreciate after countless hours in darkened lecture halls, the biomedical view of disease looks piercingly through a patient toward some essential, objective, solid reality of biology—and yet in doing so it loses, like an X ray, almost any sense of flesh of the person. On the wards of the hospital, the contrast deepened between the individual we cared for and the image of the patient that we generated through tests and discussed on rounds—deepened and became more paradoxical, since both senses of the person seemed so important to providing good care. When I turned from my medical training and moved toward my historical work, the paradox inverted, as the current perspective of many historians tended to highlight aspects that biomedicine left darkened, yet ignored detail that science had clarified. Ultimately, I realized that the task for this piece of medical history was to incorporate the medical view of diabetes within a historical account, striving to put the flesh back upon particular women and men and painting a more sensitive portrait that restores human detail.

I chose to study the history of diabetes because I felt that it would permit, even demand, such a blending of medical science and humanistic sensibility. How could it not? The transformation of diabetes from an acute to a chronic ailment has profoundly affected the lives of countless people. Furthermore, while my interest in diabetes did not stem from personal experience (I am not diabetic, nor is anyone in my immediate family), I began to see similarities between diabetes and many other chronic diseases—such as cancers beaten back by chemotherapy, or heart ailments nursed along by surgery and medications— that have changed dramatically, for better and for worse, during the twentieth century. And I began to sense how, in writing a book on diabetes, I might learn things that practicing medicine could not otherwise teach me.

So I started my research and set about looking for some accounts of what diabetics had experienced during the twentieth century. I was hardly prepared for what I found. One afternoon in early October of 1991, at the suggestion of an epidemiologist at the Joslin Diabetes Center in Boston, I sat down in his office and opened a manila folder that held the medical chart of John Hansen (which is a pseudonym). John had first come to the clinic as a fifteen-year-old in 1940. Not surprisingly, the first dozen or so sheets of his record contained standard forms filled with terse and abbreviated medical jargon. But then followed a stack of letters written by John's mother when he was young and later by himself, complete with carbon copies of the replies that the clinic doctors had sent back. By the time I had finished reading those forty-odd letters, I knew that my project had been recast. It had to be. John's account of his illness (which appears in Chapter 7) challenged me— intellectually and emotionally—to recount the history of diabetes from the patient's perspective.

Fortunately and rather remarkably, the intimacy of John's chart was not unique. I have pored over a hundred similarly detailed and revelatory records. Collectively, they provide the center of gravity for this book. All aspects of the diabetic history that follow—whether they be scientific ideas, medical practices, or cultural influences—seek to understand these peoples' lives. The separate stories of juvenile patients emphasize a crucial aspect of their history: diabetic lives have differed. Although united to no small degree by their disease and its evolving transmuted course, people with juvenile diabetes otherwise have been as diverse as the general American population, reflecting its broad range of experience and life course. A single historical account can capture only a sample of this diversity. This book focuses on the experiences of a particular group of juvenile patients, composed almost entirely of white New England residents, each of whom was seen at a clinic staffed by several famous physicians in Boston. Such a homogeneous patient population limits the potential generalizability of any conclusions that might be drawn from their experiences. Still, I believe that this history of the transformation of diabetes is more than the sum of its parts. This is a case study that, through the interrogation of particular experiences, illuminates certain general themes.

I want to emphasize what I hope this book achieves. First, I want it to assist those who deal with diabetes and other chronic illnesses —patients, families, physicians, nurses, policy makers—to understand how medicine transforms disease and how patients and the health care system interact and adapt. Perhaps it will put into words what many already instinctively know, providing a language with which to express the experiences and dilemmas of living with transformed disease. I also hope that this work underscores modern medical practice's recurrent irony of solving one problem but creating new ones, and that a fuller appreciation of this irony focuses us on the often intractable realities of living with and treating chronic illness. For historians, this study ought to emphasize the value of a patient-oriented approach to understanding disease and broader cultural issues. But most important, I hope that by restoring the experiences of patients, we might remember the past more clearly, helping current patients and those who care for them to make better sense of the lives they live, assisting them in developing their own personal philosophy of disease, health, and medical care, enabling all of us by looking back to move forward with greater understanding and purpose.

A CURRENT VIEW OF DIABETES MELLITUS

While some readers already know a substantial amount about the current scientific views of diabetes mellitus, other readers are perhaps largely unaware of details about the disease and how it poses a formidable threat to health in the United States. For these readers, the following provides a brief overview. Be mindful, however, that present-day understanding of diabetes differs substantially from how doctors and patients in the early 1900s understood diabetes. As the century proceeded, these individuals sought not only to improve their knowledge but also to master the disease, to control its protean and often unpredictable effects on their lives.

Operating within a "patient-oriented" perspective, I focused the majority of this book on patient experience, largely ignoring scientific research. As I did so, I kept in mind a comment from Charles Best, co-discoverer of insulin, to a fellow research physician in 1965: "Progress in research is a wonderful thing, but it is becoming increasingly difficult for the clinician to decide what applies to his patient and what is still only of experimental interest."[1] In writing this history, the "thousands of new contributions to knowledge" that Best mentioned threatened to bury the experience of being diabetic under mounds of scientific facts and medical articles. To prevent this from occurring, I asked myself repeatedly, "Did this scientific discovery or theory have a significant impact on the patients presented on these pages?" If it did not—and most did not—I omitted it. Realizing, though, that some readers may want to know more about the theories and discoveries that I left out, I have suggested some further readings in the accompanying note[2] and offer here a synopsis of the major features of diabetes as understood today.

To begin with, the disease occurs in two different forms. Type 1 tends to occur in children and adolescents, when the pancreatic cells that make insulin are destroyed by a process that still is not well understood but probably is some form of an autoimmune reaction. Because Type 1 diabetes usually presents during childhood or early adulthood, it used to be called "juvenile diabetes," and because the people with Type 1 cannot make insulin in their pancreas and thus require insulin injections to stay alive, it also has been known as "insulin-dependent" diabetes. Type 2 occurs mainly in older adults and stems not from too little insulin but rather the body's inability to respond appropriately to the insulin signal (thus the names "adult-onset" or "non-insulin-dependent" diabetes). Approximately 0.3–0.4 percent of Americans have Type 1 diabetes, while at least 6 percent have Type 2 (with potentially many more people living undiagnosed with the milder symptoms of early Type 2 disease). The onset of new cases of Type 1 disease appears to be increasing throughout the Western world for reasons that remain unclear, while the incidence of Type 2 disease is also rising in parallel with the obesity epidemic in America.

The second level of information deals with how the disease causes its symptoms. Understanding the pattern of these connections is difficult because diabetes mellitus is an intricate metabolic disorder. In medical schools today, a student will typically learn about this complex disease half a dozen times or more—and subsequently forget most of the lessons. Physicians require years of study and clinical practice to learn how to care for diabetic patients. Even experts on diabetes disagree about details of its causes and consequences. For those readers who have little prior knowledge about diabetes, I hope that the following few pages will serve as a congenial introduction to the current theories about diabetes and will provide future reference and clarification. The key point to remember is that diabetes mellitus *is not* just about sugar.[3]

We first need to know how food is metabolized normally. Whenever a person eats a meal, the food is digested in the stomach and bowel into its components of fats (called lipids), proteins (amino acids), and carbohydrates (which include starches and sugars such as glucose). As these basic elements enter the bloodstream, certain organs detect their presence and determine how the foodstuffs will be used. Simply put, the components have four different fates: they are burned immediately as fuel, incorporated into the structure of the body, converted into other basic food elements, or stored away for later use. Between meals, the same organs direct the retrieval of the stored food.

The decision of how the digested or stored food will be used is, in a manner of speaking, determined by a committee, which we might call the Council of Food Utilization. This council consists of several organs—for example, the thyroid and adrenal glands, the pituitary and the liver, muscle and brain—and even specialized cells within organs, such as the pancreas's alpha (α) cells, beta (β) cells, and delta (δ) cells, which are located in small clusters called the islets of Langerhans. Some members of the council make their own decisions. The brain, for instance, has carte blanche to take as much glucose from the blood as it needs. Muscle tissue, while it is exercised, likewise gobbles up glucose without restraint. Most food-use decisions, however, are made by the committee working in concert, as organs communicate with each other via the language of hormones. Each organ makes its own stock of hormones, which are usually small proteins or steroids, and can send a particular message throughout the body by releasing a precise amount of a specific hormone. The council's continuous dialogue reflects the amount and type of food the body has eaten recently as well as the body's requirements for food energy. The rest of the body's tissues listen to this ongoing discussion and react to the overall pattern of hormonal messages. The food is then used—for burning, growing, converting, storing, or retrieving—as directed by the Food Utilization Council.

For our purposes, the major committee member is the pancreas and its β cells. The β cells monitor how much food energy the blood contains. If the digested food of a meal is flowing past, the β cells inform other tissues that the blood is rich with nutrient energy. The β cells do so by secreting the hormone messenger, insulin, into the bloodstream, where it mixes with additional hormones released by various members of the Food Utilization Council. As the body receives the messages conveyed by insulin and other hormones, the tissues begin to absorb the food from the blood and store it or turn it into energy. In particular, the liver and muscle stow away much of the glucose, fat cells warehouse the lipids, and virtually all organs gather up amino acids. In its broadest sense, then, insulin notifies the tissues that food is plentiful and encourages the body to grow.

Whenever the message that insulin normally conveys is missing or not heard loudly enough, diabetes mellitus results. This miscommunication can occur for several reasons. Sometimes other hormones, such as the steroids made by the adrenal glands or the growth hormone made by the pituitary gland, are secreted inappropriately due to various diseases; they might also be ingested as medicines. Disregarding these rarer forms of diabetes, the disease basically appears in two different types.

The first type arises when the β cells are destroyed by the body's immune system. This more severe form, called juvenile, or Type 1, diabetes, generally afflicts younger patients, usually around the onset of puberty, but ranging in some cases from birth to advanced age. Several theories offer different explanations of why the autoimmune destruction occurs, indicating a wide range of potential causes, from viruses to genetic predispositions to nursing on cow's milk. Regardless of what initiates the immune process, it results in the absence of a key member of the Food Utilization Council. Without the β cells that produce insulin, the body tissues never receive the message that the blood is laden with food, even after a sumptuous meal. Lacking any insulin, the well-fed metabolism behaves paradoxically, as though the body is being starved. This starvation metabolism fails to take the sugar that is in the blood and either burn it as fuel or store it away. Instead, the sugar accumulates in the circulation. The resulting high level of blood sugar can lead to all sorts of havoc, including the appearance of sugar in the urine. The overflow of blood sugar into the urine causes the patient to urinate copiously (polyuria), which in turn makes the patient extremely thirsty, creating an urge to drink excessively (polydipsia). In addition, without any insulin present, the metabolism also mishandles the storage of fats and proteins. All these effects leave the patient with a ravenous appetite (polyphagia) and, over the years, at great risk for various medical complications. More immediately ominous, the untreated starvation metabolism turns fats into toxic acids that can quickly poison the blood and induce coma, with its characteristic deep and rapid breathing, and death. These patients require insulin injections to stay alive.

The second and more common form of diabetes occurs when the body tissues no longer listen closely to the message carried by insulin. In these patients, who are typically forty years of age or older, and often overweight, the β cells actually make tremendous amounts of insulin whenever the person eats. The problem arises on the receiving end of the insulin hormonal message—the tissues have become, as I have suggested, somewhat "hard of hearing," resistant to the message that insulin normally communicates. For a time, the β cells can accommodate for this "hearing loss" by secreting more insulin, turning up the volume of the message. After a while, however, the beleaguered β cells can no longer produce enough insulin to accurately alert the tissues. The patients then manifest symptoms of so-called adult-onset, or Type 2, diabetes. In this more insidious form of the disease, the body has enough insulin to prevent starvation metabolism but not enough to entice the tissues to extract the circulating glucose and lipids from the blood. Consequently, these patients are not prone to coma, but like Type 1 diabetics, they do have high blood sugars (hyperglycemia), high blood lipids (hyperlipidemia), and sugar in their urine (glycosuria). They also often have the "polys"—polyuria, polydipsia, and polyphagia. Type 2 patients can manage their disease by curtailing the amount of food that they eat; by taking oral drugs that enable the body tissues to hear the insulin message with improved acuity; or by injecting more in-sulin to supplement what their β cells are already making.

To summarize, there are two major forms of diabetes mellitus. Type 1 usually begins during childhood or adolescence, destroying the pancre-atic islets of Langerhans and leaving these patients with no means to manufacture insulin on their own, and therefore is always treated with insulin, along with diet and exercise. Type 2 mostly afflicts older people, preventing their body tissues from "hearing" the message that insulin carries, and this type is treated with diet, drugs taken orally, and some-times with insulin. Both types affect the metabolism of carbohydrates (sugar and starch), proteins, fats, and other foodstuffs. Even though adult-onset, Type 2, often seems to be a milder version than juvenile, Type 1, diabetes, both types are deadly if left untreated, and patients with either form are susceptible to complications even if the disease is treated appropriately.

This vulnerability, persisting despite all the technological advances of the twentieth century, is the crux of the matter, around which the rest of this book revolves.

Life is an adventure in a world where nothing is static; where unpredictable and ill-understood events constitute dangers that must be overcome, often blindly and at great cost; where man himself, like the sorcerer's apprentice, has set in motion forces that are potentially destructive and may someday escape his control.

René Dubos, *Mirage of Health,* 1959

If a storyteller thinks enough of storytelling to regard it as a calling, unlike a historian he cannot turn from the suffering of his characters. A storyteller, unlike a historian, must follow compassion wherever it leads him.

Norman Maclean, *Young Men and Fire,* 1992

I
Disease
and
Medicine
Today

The medical art consists

in three things—the disease,

the patient, and the physician.

The physician is the servant

of the science, and the patient

must do what he can to fight

the disease with the assistance

of the physician.

Hippocratic *Epidemics,*

Book 1, Section 11

1

IRONY IN AN ERA
OF MEDICAL MARVELS:
DIABETES HISTORY
AS A STUDY OF HEALTH
AND HOPE

All changed, changed utterly:
A terrible beauty is born.
—W. B. Yeats, "Easter, 1916"

If today is like most days, approximately two dozen children across America will develop diabetes mellitus, joining a million other Americans who have so-called insulin-dependent, juvenile-onset, or Type 1, diabetes mellitus.[1] These girls and boys will present the symptoms and signs of the disease in a variety of ways: one might start to urinate prodigiously or wet the bed again at night; another may be mired by fatigue that has not lifted for weeks on end or by a cough and cold that will not release its grip; yet another may become gravely ill with diabetic acidosis, complete with heavy breathing and perhaps even coma or shock. No matter how their illness presents, the diagnosis of diabetes will for the most part be confirmed by finding an elevated blood sugar level. Other tests will be done, but the children will be started on therapy immediately, receiving their first dose—of a lifetime of doses—of insulin. Given either as a continuous infusion into a vein or as an injection just under the skin, this insulin will begin to save their lives. Over the next several days, these children and their families should receive careful and dedicated education about diabetes and how to care for this disease. For nearly all families, this will be a period of tremendous worry and stress. For many, during the months following their diagnosis they will settle into a life of living with diabetes. Perhaps they will read about the special summer camps for boys and girls with diabetes, or of famous athletes and actors who have diabetes, or even the possibilities of measuring blood sugar without having to poke through their skin and draw blood, or taking insulin by nasal spray instead of injection. For the most part, balancing trepidation with hope, they will start to look forward.

Why then—given the promise of future improvements in diabetes self-care—would any person with diabetes wish to look back? And why would anyone who doesn't have diabetes want to learn more about this ailment? These are reasonable questions, and this chapter introduces several answers that the remainder of the book elaborates. At the most specific level, examining the history of diabetic experience illustrates how people with diabetes have, over the years, faced particular challenges. Tracing the course of their struggles illuminates modern versions of these challenges. At the most general level, studying the history of a once acutely fatal condition transformed by medical intervention into a chronic illness reveals ironic dilemmas created by our prevailing views of illness and medicine, personal responsibility, and the pursuit of control over disease.

Typically, our understanding of both levels—of specific human illness experience and of philosophical questions about the role of medicine in our lives—is dominated by a "technological ethos." Since this ethos has fundamentally shaped how the history of diabetes has usually been recounted, we will begin our historical journey here with a brief but standard account of "diabetes history as the discovery of insulin" and consider how this account demonstrates precisely the problem of limited perspective that plagues us currently.

DIABETES AND THE TECHNOLOGY ETHOS

In the second century A.D. the Greek physician, Aretaeus of Cappadocia, declared, "Diabetes is a mysterious illness . . . [where] the flesh and limbs melt into urine." While earlier descriptions of diabetic-like symptoms appear in the *Papyrus Ebers* (an Egyptian medical text dating from the sixteenth century B.C.[2]), Aretaeus provides the oldest unambiguous depiction of diabetes, reporting how the disease made "life disgusting and painful; thirst unquenchable; . . . and one cannot stop them either from drinking or making water." A patient's condition was even more dire "if the constitution of the disease be completely established; for the melting is rapid, the death speedy." The term "diabetes" derived from the Greek word for "siphon," since ingested water appeared to run straight through the body and out of the bladder as urine, as though through a siphon. Although other physicians had used the term before Aretaeus wrote his tract, he applied it in a novel way. In his harrowing account, this triad of symptoms—never-ending thirst, copious urination, wasting of the body—signified a unique disease entity.[3]

In 1674 the Englishman Thomas Willis published "The Diabetes or Pissing Evil."[4] Like many physicians before him, Willis was greatly impressed by the volume of urine that people with diabetes produced, observing that "those laboring with this Disease, piss a great deal more than they drink, or take of any liquid aliment; and moreover they have always joined with it continual thirst, and a gentle, and as it were hectic Fever." Willis, however, disputed the claims made by other physicians that diabetics simply urinated whatever they drank, unchanged or "unconcocted." Willis asserted that all diabetic urine, "differing both from the drink taken in, and also from any humor that is wont to be begot in our Body, was wonderfully sweet as if it were imbued with Honey or Sugar."[5]

One hundred years later, the importance of Willis's observation of "honey" sweet urine was still being debated. Matthew Dobson, a physician practicing at the Liverpool Public Infirmary, summed up the medical dispute in an article published in 1776: "Some authors, especially the English, have remarked, that the urine in diabetes is sweet. Others, on the contrary, deny the existence of this quality, and consequently exclude it from being a characteristic of the disease." Entering the medical debate, Dobson reported studies he had conducted on a thirty-three-year-old former soldier. Peter Dickonson had been a healthy man until his diabetes began. "He first observed that he was very thirsty, that he drank large quantities of water, and made large quantities of urine." When Dickonson entered Liverpool's public hospital in October of 1772, "he was emaciated, weak, and dejected; his thirst was unquenchable; and his skin dry, hard, and harsh to the touch, like rough parchment." Dobson used a "gentle heat" to evaporate two quarts of Dickonson's urine. "There remained, after the evaporation, a white cake which . . . was granulated, and broke easily between the fingers; it smelled sweet like brown sugar, neither could it, by the taste, be distinguished from sugar." The sweet taste of the urine suggested to Dobson that "this saccharine matter was not formed in the [kidney], but previously existed in the serum of the blood." Dobson emphasized further that this observation "well explains [diabetes'] emaciating effects, from so large a proportion of the alimentary matter being drawn off by the kidneys, before it is perfectly assimilated, and applied to the purposes of nutrition."[6]

After Dobson's report there followed a succession of dietary therapies for diabetes—including John Rollo's prescription of an "animal diet" in 1797 that included "plain blood-puddings" and "fat and rancid old meats"[7]—each attempting to feed people with diabetes foods that their bodies could assimilate. Rollo's avoidance of sweet or vegetable foods evolved, by the early 1900s, into much more complicated dietary schemes of undernutrition. All the diets, however, were ultimately of minimal benefit in staving off death. Patients under ten years of age could hope to live no more than three years after they were diagnosed, while those aged sixty years or more lived about six years.[8] Diabetic patients who could afford the best medical care for their condition spent these terminal years living in a semistarved state that ended in either coma, infection, or starvation. By all accounts, diabetes was a deadly disease.

The prognosis for people with diabetes was forever rewritten in the summer of 1921 and the year that followed with the discovery and initial development of insulin by Frederick G. Banting, Charles H. Best, James B. Collip, John J. R. Macleod, and other researchers in Toronto. By the autumn of 1922, insulin was being made commercially. Among the initial medical reports on insulin, perhaps most compelling was Ralph H. Major's introduction to the readers of the *Journal of the American Medical Association* regarding the drug's miraculous effects, communicated with two contrasting photographs: "The boy shown in Figure 1 is an example of severe juvenile diabetes. At the time the picture was taken, Dec. 7, 1922, he had had diabetes for two years, and it had been impossible to render [his urine sugar-free] except on a diet of 5 per cent. vegetables [such as lettuce, cucumbers, water cress, broccoli, and the like], with days of complete starvation. His weight at this time was 15 pounds."[9]

Not quite three months after the first picture was taken, the unnamed child was photographed again on 26 February 1923. He had doubled his weight to thirty pounds and was consuming a diet of nearly 1,500 calories a day.

These two portraits were stunning. The boy's gain in weight alone was sufficient to impress even the most skeptical readers. Beyond this obvious improvement, other aspects of the photographs further intensified

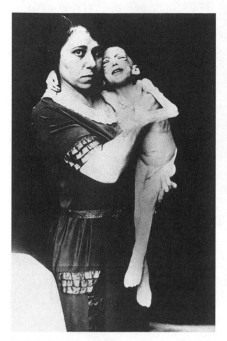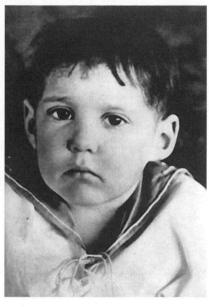

Ralph H. Major's patient, before starting insulin therapy (left) and after. Courtesy of the Clendening History of Medicine Library, The University of Kansas Medical Center.

their impact. Before insulin, emaciated and naked, the youngster clung to his mother, supported by her stout arms, his entire body on display; his closed eyes and fixed grimace, set alongside his mother's stoic gaze, heighten the sense of his suffering. After insulin, he was photographed sitting by himself, no longer dependent, peering at the camera, clothed in a sailor suit. Not only had his facial features filled out, the enlarged scale of the photograph made him look nearly twice as large. The message was clear and incontrovertible: insulin worked wonders.

Major was not alone in employing this powerful visual rhetoric. Several other physicians, whose pioneering accounts of treating diabetics with insulin appeared in the *Journal of Metabolic Research* during the late spring of 1923, also resorted to dramatic before-and-after pictures. Indeed, these images continue to appear to this day in texts on the history of diabetes and to be flashed upon the auditorium screen in medical lectures on diabetes.[10]

The discovery of the elusive pancreatic extract fired the imagination of laypeople and doctors alike. Early on, after the Toronto group of researchers and their American colleagues had miraculously "cured" sev-

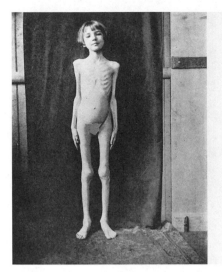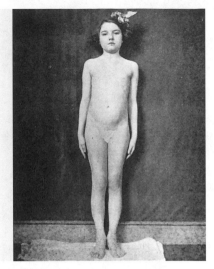

One of H. Rawle Geyelin's patients, before starting insulin therapy (left) and after. From Geyelin et al., "Uses of Insulin in Juvenile Diabetes."

eral emaciated, near-to-death patients with the pancreatic extract, the lay news media raved, awed at the power of a new scientific medicine. A May 1923 *New York Times* article, titled "Diabetes, Dread Disease, Yields to New Gland Cure," recounted how, "one by one, the implacable enemies of man, the diseases which seek his destruction, are overcome by science." Diabetes was "the latest to succumb. Its conquest is a feather in the cap of science."[11] A month later, insulin landed on the front page of the *New York Times,* which heralded the recoveries from severe diabetes of former secretary of state Robert Lansing and of Elizabeth Hughes, daughter of the then current secretary of state, Charles Evans Hughes. Lansing had not only "gained greatly in flesh and in strength, but his dietary restrictions have been completely removed, so that he is permitted to eat as much as he desires of all varieties of food." Elizabeth Hughes was "practically cured."[12]

The reaction of the medical community was no less enthusiastic. In 1923, Banting and Macleod shared the Nobel Prize for the discovery and initial development of insulin. By the mid-1920s the majority of articles appearing in general medical journals indicated that diabetes could be conquered by daily insulin injections. For example, in 1930 the diabetes expert Frederick M. Allen asserted in the *New England Journal of Medicine,* "Diabetes has been scientifically mastered. Theoretically, every patient can be expected to live out his full natural lifetime."[13] Allen echoed the sentiments of many physicians, who seemed to feel that even if insulin had not eradicated the disease, it had at least turned it into a problem that could be managed successfully.

To take a later example of such enthusiasm, a group of scientists in their book *The Story of Insulin: Forty Years of Success Against Diabetes* asserted, "Few stories of discovery carry more drama than that about Insulin. The leap from despair and death was so sudden." Writing in the early 1960s—at a time when countless diabetics were encountering the complications of blindness, kidney failure, and amputations—they went on to add, "Forty years after that discovery, the miracle of Insulin has an ever-growing significance; more and more people of all ages have had the moving experience of being drawn back from sickness and death into health and happiness."[14]

These photographs and verbal portraits of miraculous therapeutic success present a modern yet mythic account of diabetes history, accentuating the potency of insulin as a heroic wonder drug to rescue patients, vanquish disease, banish suffering, and finally secure an implied but unexamined "happily-ever-after" ending. Mythical storytelling elements such as these permeate much of our current appreciation of other medical technologies. When pharmaceutical companies launch promotional advertising campaigns showing pictures of bald yet smiling cancer survivors; or when proponents of the human genome project speculate how gene therapy will eliminate certain inborn diseases; or when former trauma patients testify how they were saved by the latest radiographic machines that swiftly provide remarkably precise body images; or even when the biotechnology industry shows film clips on television of children spared from blindness due to rice supplemented with vitamin A, these examples of scientific achievement are all presented in the mythical aura of an idealistic quest for a better world. As they tap into our fears and desires, these stories about medicine reflect a broad technology ethos in our culture, the American propensity to embrace more technology as the best solution to our problems.[15]

Perhaps no story of medical progress, though, has been more influenced by this technology ethos than the history of diabetes. Stories of insulin have served various needs while reinforcing deeply held beliefs of twentieth-century Americans. A parable of salvation, the tale of diabetic deliverance has spoken to the imagination of doctors and laypeople alike, serving as a potent and often cited symbol of scientific progress and the prospect of human mastery over disease. One of the most impressive stories about modern medical miracles, the tale of insulin saving diabetics has legitimated the prestige and power that Americans have invested in scientific medicine and its technical wizardry.

The mythically framed accounts of diabetes history, however, conceal more than they reveal. Focusing on a wonder drug, they distract from the human realities of living with diabetes—all the people involved in the mundane yet challenging realities of daily diabetic work and their personal struggles with illness that continued well after the discovery of insulin. Emphasizing a miraculous event, these accounts ignore the more sober legacy of this "miracle"—all the problems that remained, all the new problems created by the transmutation of diabetes into a chronic disease. Exulting in an unexamined belief in progress, they fail to grapple with the difficult task of weighing the mixed consequences of medical intervention—all the years of life added poised against all the ramifications of living with a chronic, often debilitating disease.

Simply put, we need to reappraise the happily-ever-after ending: diabetes still devastates lives. Approximately 1 million Americans currently have juvenile-onset, Type 1, diabetes mellitus, with perhaps another 10 million afflicted with the adult-onset, Type 2, form of the disease. Although much of the public believes that diabetes has been cured or at least tamed, the health statistics present a very different picture: Diabetes today is the primary cause of new-onset blindness in adults, accounts for a third of all cases of kidney failure, leads to half of all non-traumatic limb amputations, and overall stands as the seventh leading cause of death. Diabetics live with a substantial risk of heart attack, heart failure, and stroke. Infants born to diabetic mothers are more likely to have congenital abnormalities and to die either in utero or shortly after birth.[16] Even for those patients who do not develop complications, their lives are irrevocably altered by the diagnosis of diabetes, for they must monitor their diets and often either take oral medicine or inject or infuse insulin—and hope that they remain well. The "cure" of insulin has become the accomplice to a newly created disease of complications.

This contradictory legacy of insulin—of general triumph mixed with individual tragedies—challenges our views about technology and its impact on human health and hope. The most reasonable perspective seems to literally hang in the balance—the balance between acknowledging the remarkable benefits of technology and realizing the incompleteness and often ironic deleterious consequences of technological "solutions," the balance between questing for that better world and working to better the world that we have, the balance between the bitter and sweet emotions that suffuse the modern history of diabetes. Striking this balance requires that we move beyond the ready-made but incomplete answers to our health and health care problems offered up by the technology ethos.

In recounting the history of juvenile-onset diabetes in twentieth-century America, I have sought to strike such a balanced perspective. In so doing, I have been helped by a handful of authors who have examined particular aspects of this story. Their work has provided invaluable reference points that helped define what this study will and, as important, will not emphasize. For instance, Michael Bliss's *Discovery of Insulin* focuses on the labors of the Toronto group and the ensuing acrimonious battle among them for credit. Bliss vividly portrays the workings of medical research, strong personalities, and fame's allure. While Bliss brackets his superbly researched narrative with accounts of clinical diabetes preceding and following the hectic years of 1921 and 1922, he emphasizes the discovery and development of insulin that took place before and during this period.[17]

I have been more concerned, however, with the clinical realities and experiences of patients who sit at the periphery of Bliss's story. My focus has been on the changes that occurred throughout the twentieth century that affected people living with diabetes, changes that extended well beyond the discovery of insulin. Other historical studies have filled in some of the detail, focusing on famous specialists in diabetes[18] or a particular diabetic institution, such as the American Diabetes Association,[19] or chronicling the succession of medical ideas and technical developments.[20] These accounts are all a part of the broader story of diabetic patients, their families, and doctors—a collective history of biology and society, of therapeutics and technology, of medical culture and private experience, of scientific knowledge and human belief. I sought to synthesize these diverse elements, joining different yet complementary views and experiences of diabetes into one unified and coherent perspective: the human consequences of transformed disease.

The rest of this book refines this perspective, expanding its scope and enhancing its depth. In part, my efforts to understand diabetes have been guided by comparisons to conditions such as cancer, epilepsy, mental illness, sickle cell disease, tuberculosis, AIDS, and a variety of

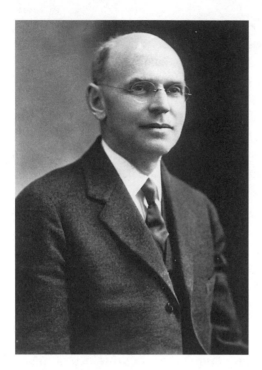

Elliott P. Joslin at sixty years of age.
Courtesy of the Joslin Diabetes Center
Historical Archive.

other conditions that have been the subject of fine historical studies.[21] But far more fundamental to the story told on the following pages have been primary historical documents: patient records and letters that have their origins over a hundred years ago in the office of Dr. Elliott P. Joslin of Boston, Massachusetts.

DR. JOSLIN'S RECORDS AND LETTERS

"*History of the Case.*—A. W., a boy of fifteen, became thirsty and tired in August, 1897." Although born with a slight paralysis of his left foot, Alvin Wilson's "mind had always been active and his health good." The onset of diabetes had shocked the family, none of whom had ever had the disease. Alvin lost twenty pounds in the following year, so that he weighed a mere ninety-two pounds when he arrived in Boston in August of 1898 to see Dr. Elliott Proctor Joslin.[22]

Alvin Wilson was the first juvenile diabetic that Joslin treated. The twenty-nine-year-old doctor, a man imbued with Protestant morals and socially progressive ideas, was in his first year of private practice, and this boy was his fourth patient. Joslin classified the young man's illness as a "severe type" and placed him on "the usual 'strict diabetic diet'

500 c.c. of cream, two oranges, 15 grammes of bread, and a little whiskey." "This diet was faithfully followed," Joslin later wrote in an article about the boy's case, "until the summer of 1900. At this time the patient clandestinely ate rather freely of carbohydrates." Soon thereafter, the patient succumbed to the grim metabolic logic of acid intoxication, manifested as diabetic coma and death.[23]

Alvin's entrance to and exit from Joslin's medical practice was soon repeated by other sick youngsters and anxious parents who visited Boston. The cases of these child diabetics who were stricken during the pre-insulin era all conformed to an inescapable plot that began with a symptom, followed with a diagnosis, and ended with their untimely demise. While some patients died almost immediately and others lived for a few years, diabetes ultimately made no exceptions in bringing the script to a grim conclusion. After the advent of insulin, the personal sagas of Joslin's juvenile patients suddenly stretched forward for decades. Whether their patient-physician relationship lasted a few days or fifty years, over the course of the first six decades of the twentieth century, until literally days before his death in 1962, Joslin compiled records about thousands of patients. These extraordinary medical records, thick with detail, are the bedrock upon which this book rests.[24] Although I have found and studied patient records and case notes depicting the clinical treatment of diabetes in New York, Cincinnati, Philadelphia, and Chicago,[25] the life histories presented in this book are drawn almost exclusively from the remarkable archive maintained by the Joslin Diabetes Center in Boston, Massachusetts.[26]

These charts reflect not only Joslin's penchant for precise and well-ordered recording of data and his interest in clinical research but also the state of medical technology and his style of communicating with patients. When Joslin began to practice medicine at the end of the nineteenth century, most laboratory tests of patients' urine or blood took several hours to a day or more to complete. Patients who he saw during his office hours would leave before the test results were known. A few days later, Joslin would mail patients their laboratory findings along with a brief summary of what they had talked about during the visit. He retained this habit of communicating by mail; even after the telephone was no longer a novelty, Joslin continued to write letters. Following the First World War, Joslin started to put carbon copies of his correspondence with patients into their files. He would typically begin his letters by mentioning any particular concerns that the patient had raised, then he would describe what the physical examination, laboratory tests, electrocardiogram, and X-ray studies had uncovered, and he concluded with a paragraph or two about the treatment plans Joslin and the patient had discussed.

Joslin also wrote letters to patients whom he had not seen in the preceding two or three years. Even if they had moved to another part of the country or had changed doctors, Joslin wanted to keep track of all of his patients and their health. He would write periodically, asking them to send him a note detailing the treatment regimen they were following and their general health and asking a few specific questions about matters such as weight or the health of their children. In response, patients or a family member (in the case of a child or disabled older patient) might provide only bare-bone answers, but more often they composed lengthy letters chronicling many areas of their lives. Joslin tabulated these follow-up statistics and presented them in many of his publications. Fortunately, he also tucked all the incoming letters into the patients' files.

Sometimes patients or parents would write Joslin on their own initiative. Usually, they had a problem: Would it be all right to substitute one kind of insulin for another? Was a change of diet needed? How could insulin reactions be averted? How should one treat a common cold? Joslin encouraged his patients to ask questions, and when he answered, these letters were also carbon copied to the files. At other times, patients wrote because a major medical problem had developed, or because they were especially happy or angry about some event in their lives. All of this was archived.

And so, during his career, Dr. Joslin, with the assistance of his patients, created tens of thousands of remarkable files. As he expanded his practice by bringing other doctors into the group, he enforced his letter-writing habit upon them as well. Consequently, many of the files at the Joslin Diabetes Center are filled with scores of letters exchanged between the patient and his or her doctors at the clinic, and between referring doctors and specialists as they discussed aspects of a patient's case. Even more valuable to the historian of a chronic disease, correspondence continued and the accompanying medical charts and notes were often kept up to date for several decades as the patient remained in contact with the clinic.

The power of the Joslin collection originates from this rich archive of stories and its many layers of storytelling. The letters, however, are not simple sources of unedited truth. The writers, be they patients or family members or physicians, all thought about what they should write and what face they wanted to present. Through their correspondence, they shaped their perceptions of themselves and projected images of how they wished to be seen. Independent? Compliant? Hard-working? Deserving? Trustworthy? Hardnosed? Authoritative? Compassionate? The letters reveal not only how diabetics wished to be perceived but also their concerns of how they might be perceived—concerns about their public image that shaped their experience with diabetes and their relationships with physicians.

At a more matter-of-fact level, the patient letters also provide a unique source of information about the kinds of lives that diabetics lived. They detail the daily rituals of eating and testing and injecting, as they also disclose how these routines did or did not fit into the patient's family and work life. They recounted the variety of problems that diabetics encountered, in voices of complaint or lamentation. The letters also were sometimes meditative, reflecting diabetics' thoughts on the disease, how it affected them, and how they hoped or feared it might progress.

The Joslin Diabetes Center, because of limited record-keeping space, has over the decades copied all the files of deceased patients onto microfiche records, subsequently destroying the original files and storing these microfiche records in a historical archive. In surveying this archive, I proceeded systematically, selecting files of patients who had juvenile-onset diabetes with a roughly even proportion of males and females. I targeted certain time periods, such as the pre-insulin era, the years immediately surrounding the discovery of insulin, and the ensuing decade. I also purposefully focused on female cases that I knew from other sources had at one point been pregnant. I also selected microfiche files that were thick, having learned that these thicker records typically contained more correspondence. In the end, I reviewed just over a hundred records in depth, stopping my survey when I found that additional cases were not adding substantially to my understanding of the history of diabetic experience. I then picked from all the cases a subset of patients whose experiences with diabetes raise recurring and fundamental issues. These illustrative patients will appear throughout the book. Even though all the diabetics who appear in the following pages died prior to the mid-1960s, I have sought to preserve their anonymity by referring to them (with few exceptions) by pseudonyms that reflect their gender and ethnicity, and also by changing minor details, such as hometown or precise occupation, to suitable alternatives. These measures, which are in accord with published guidelines on such matters, were reviewed and approved by the Joslin Diabetes Center when they granted me access to their archive of historical medical records.[27]

If the stories that follow are to be generalized at all, it must be done so circumspectly. We must be aware of their limitations yet attuned to the possibilities that such rich and circumstantial material provides. First, the Joslin Clinic was not typical within the larger diabetic world. Elliott Joslin and his staff had a particular philosophy about ideal diabetic care and a distinctive style of diabetic management. This approach tended to give each individual case a familiar cast. Sometimes, however, Joslin or the other doctors varied their approach, and other times certain patients steadfastly maintained their independence. This range of behaviors and attitudes permits some general themes to emerge. Second, the clinic was a major hub within the far-flung diabetic community. Patients and physicians visited from all over North and South America and Europe; meanwhile, Joslin and his colleagues were also engaged in clinical research and publication. The ensuing dialogues between the Joslin Clinic staff and patients or physicians with different philosophies or styles allow us again to see a range of possible views about diabetes and ideal diabetic care.

Finally, these individual patients do not represent all diabetics, nor do they furnish archetypal diabetic experiences. This book examines a cohort of juvenile patients, all of whom were white and most of whom lived in New England, who came to see a prominent physician in Boston. Such a restricted group of patients means that this history can say nothing directly about the experiences of adult-onset diabetic patients, African Americans, Latinos, Native Americans, or members of other minority groups with diabetes, or all those diabetic individuals who lived in other parts of America and saw different doctors. Those experiences doubtlessly differed—for age and race, cultural background and style of medical practice all influence the experience of illness potently. The clientele of the Joslin Clinic with juvenile-onset diabetes of long duration was, as a survey conducted in the 1950s documented, more likely than the general U.S. population to be engaged in professional or semiprofessional careers, yet it still included a sizable number of day laborers, farmers, and clerical workers.[28]

Although we must keep these caveats in mind, the detail and diver-

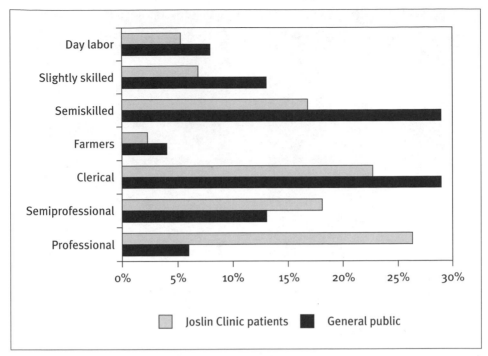

Figure 1.1. Occupations of 1,072 Twenty-Year-Duration Juvenile Diabetics Seen at the Joslin Clinic, 1898–1956. Source: *Adapted from Priscilla White, "Natural Course and Prognosis of Juvenile Diabetes,"* Diabetes 5 *(November 1956): 445–50.*

sity of the Joslin archive nevertheless enable the life histories chronicled on the following pages to illuminate problems that many diabetics have faced. These stories reconstruct a vivid collage of diabetic life before and after insulin, illustrating general concepts and themes through the investigation of particular experiences. One of the most significant concepts involves the changing nature of the disease itself, its transmutation from an acute to a chronic condition.

THE PARADIGM OF DISEASE TRANSMUTATION

By the time that insulin was discovered in 1921, Dr. Elliott Joslin had already been caring for diabetics—several thousands of them—for more than twenty years. When insulin arrived, Joslin stood at midcareer, having already made his mark as America's foremost expert on diabetic care. During much of the 1910s, this meticulous clinician had championed the use of stringent dietary regimens to eke out additional months and even years of life for young diabetics. Ever so gradually, the life

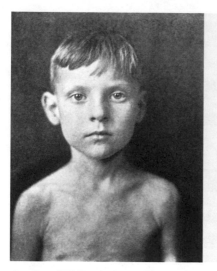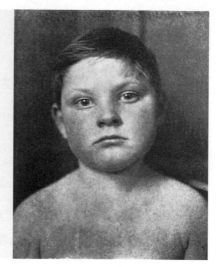

Another of H. Rawle Geyelin's patients, before starting insulin therapy (left) and after. From Geyelin et al., "Uses of Insulin in Juvenile Diabetes."

expectancy of juvenile patients under his care had improved. And the quality of life of his young patients was not quite as bleak as Dr. Major's photographs may suggest. These pictures displayed pre-insulin diabetic children who had suffered extreme emaciation, losing 23–50 percent of their initial body weight, but such weight loss was not typical. Looking at two samples of children who initially saw Joslin in the years 1909–10 and in 1915, the first group survived an average of thirty months and during that period lost essentially no weight, while the second group survived for forty-five months after diagnosis and lost an average of only 10 percent of their initial body weight. The typical experience of a child actually living with juvenile diabetes during the pre-insulin period, provided he did not die very quickly after developing diabetes, is probably more accurately conveyed by the less startling photographs of diabetic youngsters that were also published soon after insulin was first used.[29]

Nevertheless, insulin arrived like a thunderbolt. Joslin quickly perceived that his world had changed—changed utterly. Within a year after first administering insulin in 1922, Joslin declared, "A new race of diabetics has come upon the scene." Prior to the introduction of insulin, his patients had lived with the disease, on average, about three and a half years after diagnosis; by 1923, the average duration of illness had already been extended another two years by the pancreatic extract. Joslin drove home the profound nature of this prolongation of diabetic

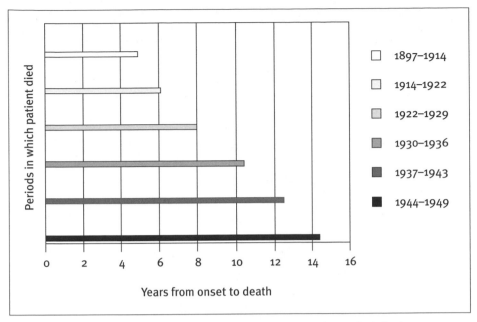

Figure 1.2. Average Duration of Illness at Time of Death in Successive Periods of Fatalities among Patients of the Joslin Clinic, 1897–1949. Source: *Elliott P. Joslin, "A Half-Century's Experience in Diabetes Mellitus,"* British Medical Journal *(1950): 1095–98.*

life by noting that, for clinicians who were caring for patients kept alive by insulin, their medical practice "this past year has been among the erstwhile dead."[30]

Despite the drama surrounding the introduction of insulin, the drug's arrival marked neither the beginning nor the end of astounding change. Joslin, throughout his sixty-year career, rode upon an upward wave of ever-lengthening diabetic life. Evidence of this long-term trend surrounded him. He was fond of pointing out how, if one examined the length of time from diagnosis to death among diabetic patients, one could see that this duration of illness kept getting longer with each passing decade.[31]

As Joslin himself realized, this prolongation of diabetic life was one aspect of a larger phenomenon, namely the aging of Americans that has reshaped the U.S. population during the twentieth century. "In North America," he noted presciently in 1924, "we are to dwell more and more with the old. A generation ago the average expectation of life was thirty-eight years and now it is fifty-seven." This aging, he predicted, would

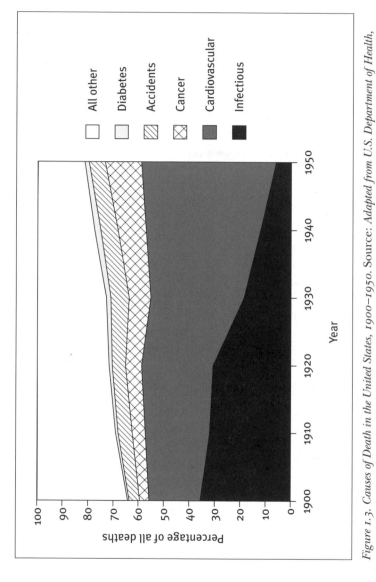

Figure 1.3. *Causes of Death in the United States, 1900–1950. Source: Adapted from U.S. Department of Health, Education, and Welfare, Vital Statistics 37, no. 11 (1950): 284.*

cause much social tension, for "although we as a nation want to live to be old, we do not want to be old too soon."[32]

Joslin turned out to be a true prophet regarding these matters. The life expectancy of Americans has risen substantially from 1900, and, consequently, older Americans have composed an increasing percentage of the U.S. population.[33] As Americans have survived illnesses that once would have killed them, the pattern of causes of death has changed dramatically. Instead of succumbing to the major killers of bygone eras —diarrhea, respiratory infections, tuberculosis—Americans increasingly die from chronic diseases such as heart failure, cancer, emphysema, dementia—and diabetes.

This transition, in which the leading causes of death shifted from acute infectious disease to more chronic ailments, is what we might think of as the *diminishment* and *substitution* of disease. In these reciprocal processes, the decline of one disease enables people to live longer, allowing another disease to rise to prominence, substituting for the diminished disease. Given that diabetes is more prevalent among older individuals, it was this model that Joslin evoked when he wrote that "diabetes ought, therefore, to be and is many times as frequent in the community today as heretofore, and with increasing longevity is destined to be more common." Similar arguments have been made about the rise of other chronic diseases.[34]

The processes of diminishment and substitution are only two of the patterns by which diseases afflicting Americans have changed (see Table 1.1). Demonstrating a third pattern, diseases such as cholera and influenza have also *relocated* from one part of the globe to another, altering world history in their wake.[35] A fourth pattern occurs when diseases *emerge de novo*. Lung cancer, for instance, was exceedingly rare until after the First World War, when many former soldiers had begun their habit of smoking tobacco while serving overseas;[36] similarly, the epidemic of AIDS, as well as outbreaks of other new infectious ailments, represent disease emergence.[37] A fifth pattern reflects the *reemergence* of diseases, such as tuberculosis, gonorrhea, syphilis, or measles through drug resistance and lapses of social policy.[38]

In the background, another process of disease change has gradually reshaped many of the illnesses that Americans encounter. The increasingly common process of disease *transmutation* has altered already existing diseases into essentially new entities—transmuted diseases. These transmuted diseases have been changed by medical therapeutics so that

TABLE 1.1. Patterns of Disease Change

Pattern	Examples
Eradicated	Small pox
Diminished	Typhoid, diphtheria, measles, rheumatic fever
Substituted	Atherosclerotic vascular disease, cancers
Relocated	Small pox, cholera, influenza, West Nile virus
	Diet-induced vascular disease, tobacco-induced cancers
Emerged de novo	Lung cancer, motor vehicle trauma
	AIDS, Hantavirus, *E. coli* O157:H7
Re-emerged	Tuberculosis, measles
	Syphilis, gonorrhea
	Antimicrobial resistant bacterial infections
Transmuted	
Patients dependent upon medicines	Asthma, hemophilia, enzyme deficiencies
Patients dependent upon machines	Cardiac pacemakers, renal dialysis, ventilator support
Patients treated for cancer	Leukemias or lymphomas with secondary tumors
	Breast, colon, prostate, thyroid cancer
Patients who survived . . .	Cardiac arrest with a consequent stroke
	Extreme premature birth with disabilities
	Major trauma with brain or spinal cord injuries
Patients aided by surgical interventions	Coronary artery bypass graft
	Transplantation of solid organs
Patients aided by psychiatric interventions	Schizophrenia
	War or trauma-related mental illness
Patients aided by medical interventions	Cystic fibrosis
	HIV-disease

they progress along a diverted course of either recovery or complications. This diversion suggests that the old notion of natural history does not accurately represent the realities of modern-day diabetes or of most other treated diseases; we now rarely allow a serious disease to follow its natural history. In each instance, medical therapy alters the fundamental biology of the disease, thereby warding off certain "natural" problems while allowing new problems to surface. The patient experiences an illness with a transmuted course.[39]

The difficulties that diabetic patients have encountered with their transmuted disease do not stem, for the most part, from medical, "man-made" errors; rather, transmuted diabetes presents novel challenges because medical therapy has enabled diabetics to live longer with their disease than the ailment's natural history once permitted. Indeed, this biological change from natural history to a transmuted course has been, overall, a godsend to patients. Unlike other diseases that have been turned from bad to worse by medical therapy—such as the tragedies wrought by thalidomide, diethylstilbestrol (DES), the artificial heart, or the program to immunize against swine flu[40]—diabetes is, by almost any criteria, an "improved" disease compared to what it was one hundred years ago. And diabetics are certainly better off now than in the past. Nevertheless, transmuted diabetes is not an immaculate good—for within this new disease lurks the possibility of debilitating complications.

Diabetics are not alone in confronting transmuted disease (see Table 1.1). From premature infants cared for in neonatal intensive care nurseries,[41] to children who have been cured of cancer,[42] to adults on dialysis for end-stage renal failure,[43] many patients now live with the ironic consequences of "successful" therapeutic interventions that have transmuted their underlying condition from an acute to a chronic ailment. In each of these cases, new therapies divert the disease away from its so-called natural history, as drugs and other medical interventions interrupt the pathological sequence of events so that the disease is shunted along a new and uncharted course.

For the past ninety years, this process of transmutation has reshaped the experience of being diabetic in a manner sometimes dramatically obvious, at other times elusively subtle. Examining how diabetics fared during the first ten years of their illness drives this point home. From the turn of the century through 1919, half of newly diagnosed diabetics were dead within two years, and fewer than 5 percent were still alive

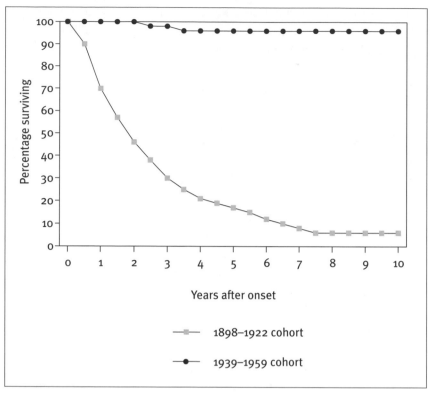

Figure 1.4. Changing Pattern of Survival of Two Cohorts of Patients Seen at the Joslin Clinic during the First Ten Years after They Developed Diabetes, 1898–1919 and 1939– 1959. Source: *Adapted from Andrzej S. Krolewski, James H. Warram, and A. Richard Christlieb, "Onset, Course, Complications, and Prognosis of Diabetes Mellitus," in* Joslin's Diabetes Mellitus, *12th ed., ed. Alexander Marble et al. (Philadelphia, Pa.: Lea and Febiger, 1985), 254.*

after ten years. Compare these dismal figures with the group of diabetics diagnosed between 1939 and 1959; in this later group, most survived their first ten years of living with diabetes.

Another way to gauge how much diabetes has changed during the twentieth century is to study the shifting pattern of lethal diabetic complications. In the early years, almost all diabetic patients who died did so in ketoacidotic coma; by 1950, fewer than one in ten fatal cases died comatose. But in place of coma, other menaces had emerged, such as cardiac arrest or nephritis and renal failure. Infections, which had been causing more death during the 1920s and 1930s, receded as sulfa antimicrobials became available in the late 1930s and penicillin arrived in the early 1940s. Not only was the length of diabetic life transformed but also the kind of life—and ultimately, the cause and kind of death.

While these summary snapshots provide a clear outline of broad changes wrought by the therapeutic transmutation of diabetes, they remain schematic and colorless. A more engaging picture, albeit suffused with ambiguity and irony, emerges from closer scrutiny of what it has been like for individual patients to live with their diabetes. This view underscores the second major concept illustrated by diabetic patients' stories: the transformation of the experience of being diabetic over the course of the twentieth century.

THE PHENOMENON OF TRANSFORMED ILLNESS

Insulin and other treatments not only transmuted diabetes into an evolving biological entity, they also radically altered what it meant to live with this transmuted disease. Emphasizing the nonbiological aspects of patient experience contrasts with standard histories of medicine that focus mostly on great doctors and intellectual understanding of diseases, describing medical theories through the ages yet neglecting to portray the lives of sick individuals. Beginning in the 1960s, some historians and advocates of what became known as "history from below" criticized the approach of conventional historical studies as elitist and divorced from the quotidian realities of the past. This criticism has culminated in a twofold movement toward patient-oriented accounts of illness experience and "behaviorist" studies of medical practice.[44] Parallel criticism has appeared in medical journals, where an articulate minority has urged its colleagues to expand the notion of disease beyond its reductive biomedical definition.[45] Both perspectives converge upon the credo: "No disease without people."

For people who have lived with diabetes, the meaning of disease has often transcended biology. While therapy-induced shifts in the ailment's physiology have been important, they have not been the only factors responsible for changing patients' experiences with the disease. People with diabetes are more than a compilation of biological mechanisms. Their encounters with the disease have been influenced by social and personal variables—such as access to medical care or family support—as well as physiological ones. As the disease itself has changed, so too have the lives of diabetics, their families, and health care workers, whose responses to new diabetic challenges have transformed the experience of living with this chronic illness.

The process of illness transformation for any particular patient has been linked to larger changes in the population of individuals with diabetes, to knowledge of the disease, to approaches to therapy and medical practice, and to cultural beliefs about the disorder and medicine. The overall pattern of these broader developments contains several motifs, the most visible of them being "progress" for diabetic patients with regard to understanding, treatment, and social standing. In 1900, diabetes mellitus was a single disease category; young patients might have been affected more severely than older patients, but medical opinion held that all people with diabetes had the same disease. The same view prevailed when insulin was first used in 1922. During the forty years that followed, however, this consensus was thoroughly revised. The drug set in motion a dialectic process—between novel treatments and the medical understanding of diabetes—that exemplifies the way in which much of modern clinical knowledge has emerged. Between 1922 and the 1960s, the medical community was confronted with an epidemic of newly created patients: chronic diabetics. Within this population, physicians distinguished several different subtypes of diabetes and developed a variety of models to explain the fundamental biological defects that they observed. Current views of diabetes (which are outlined in the book's preface) evolved largely in response to the advent of new therapies, as insulin and then the oral hypoglycemic agents prompted clinicians to make the distinction between juvenile- and adult-onset, insulin dependent or non-dependent, Type 1 or 2. The extension of life provided by insulin allowed the late complications of diabetes to emerge more clearly. Observations of patients who failed to respond to insulin guided researchers as they unraveled some of the relationships among the pituitary, thyroid, and adrenal glands, and the pancreas and liver. The development of an oral glucose tolerance test identified a whole population of pregnant women with subclinical gestational diabetes. In each instance, medical intervention revealed a previously unrecognized manifestation of disease, adding to clinical knowledge.

Treatment for diabetics has also progressed—or at least changed in cycles of therapeutic transformation. The advent of antimicrobials, longer-acting insulins, and the oral hypoglycemic agents constituted powerful additions to the pharmacopeia. Similarly, changes in the design of syringes and urine and blood glucose monitors helped patients and physicians manage the disease. Meanwhile, attitudes toward diabetes progressed as well. Over time, a diabetic individual's chance of facing discrimination in the workplace appears to have diminished. During the 1930s and 1940s, an alliance of doctors and life insurance companies launched sweeping public health campaigns to detect incipient diabetes and thereby begin treatment sooner. The news media and popular press reported favorably on these screening drives and recounted with admiration the stories of some prominent diabetics.[46]

Yet even after highlighting these many areas of upbeat progress, a contrasting motif in diabetic history—that of frustration—has been as prominent and powerful.[47] For despite therapeutic advances, physicians have been confronted by an ever-growing list of complications. By 1930, the *New England Journal of Medicine* began to carry major articles that detailed specific medical complications to which people with diabetes seemed prone, such as coronary artery disease, damage to the nerves, and elevated cholesterol levels in the blood of children.[48] With the description of characteristic kidney damage in 1936,[49] physicians increasingly realized that diabetes, far from being conquered, had been transformed insidiously from an acute to a chronic disease by insulin therapy. Much of the history of diabetes since the 1940s has been a struggle against complications—a struggle that, as patients and those around them have tried either to prevent complications or cope with them, has revealed differences not only in medical opinion but also in life experience and outlook.

The tensions between these two principal motifs—of progress and frustration—have been potent forces in reshaping the experiences of diabetics and those who cared for them. As diabetes has retained its tenacious grasp upon the bodies of those whom it afflicts, patients have had to cope with the ups and downs, the hopes and fears, of living with a chronic disease. Their stories speak powerfully about how much diabetes has changed—and at the same time, they reveal that the problems and dilemmas of chronic illness have remained the same for members of the diabetic world. This diabetic world was populated by all the people for whom the term "diabetes" was of more than passing interest: patients, parents, other family members, physicians, nurses, dietitians, laboratory workers, social workers, employers, life insurance agents. These people inhabited, worked, or played in many places that were designed, at least in part, with the tasks of diabetes in mind: the doctor's office, the hospital ward, the clinical laboratory, the home kitchen stocked with a pair of scales and diabetic food. Throughout the diabetic world, a complex and evolving system of beliefs about what diabetes meant and how it should be treated reverberated, creating fundamental tensions about the management of, control over, and responsibility for living with diabetes.[50]

Cases of specific patients clarify these tensions and how they changed over time by placing them in the context of both human relationships and physical bodies: they flesh out details of the diabetic world. In part, this case-based approach fits into the emerging genre of patient-oriented history, but it also tries to move in new directions, toward the introspective aims of novels and poetry.[51] Inspired by historical accounts that have demonstrated the analytic power and potential beauty of reconstructing history from the voices of past women and men from all walks of life,[52] I have sought to entwine the stories of these patients within a broader context, leading to a more meaningful understanding of what it has meant for people to live with disease, inhabitants of a historically shaped diabetic world.[53]

OVERVIEW

As I discussed in the preface, this book aims to help us refine our understanding and beliefs regarding health, disease, and medical care. Whether we are people living with diabetes or not, the central concepts of disease transmutation and illness transformation, and then their permutations in the themes of management, control, and responsibility, establish a perspective that can—I believe—be of use personally, in our own skirmishes with ill health, as well as collectively at the level of public health and health care policy. Accordingly, to keep the book focused on these concepts and themes, I have organized our historical tour of the modern American diabetic world like a series of walks through a huge museum, one that is far too large to examine in its entirety. Instead of marching from room to room, attending chronologically to successive time periods, I have chosen to make each chapter consider a specific concept or theme that cuts across time. The chapters are thus more like selective tours of the whole museum, striding through various galleries to highlight a variety of conceptually or thematically united events and issues, and then returning for another tour.

Within this conceptual and thematic architecture, the six central chapters all consequently draw on material from both the pre- and the post-insulin periods so as to demonstrate how these concepts and themes operated across time. Chapter 2 describes the concept of the biological transmutation of disease, and Chapter 3, the experiential transformation of illness, thereby providing us with some basic ideas about the "diabetic world" and a "language of living with diabetes" that are used subsequently in the book. Chapter 4 brings these ideas into sharper focus by studying how people managed the myriad tasks, ranging from physical labor to existential challenges, of living day by day with diabetes. Chapter 5 traces how the notion of control over the disease manifested itself in terms of the goals and behaviors of patients and providers. Chapter 6 then examines the medical care of pregnant women with diabetes and the personal consequence of this increasingly intensive care as culturally specific responses to the pursuit of control ideology. Chapter 7 takes the theme of alluring yet elusive control a step further, adding the theme of personal responsibility and exploring the dilemmas arising from the "predicament of dangerous safety," when medical care has a disease *mostly* under control. Finally, the concluding chapter considers implications of this history of diabetes for how we live—and hope—now and in the future.

As these chapters build a progressively more complicated view of what living with diabetes was like during the twentieth century, the primary lines of argument will cut in two directions. In one direction, the chapters will assert that changes in the diabetic experience arose from fundamental changes in this evolving diabetic world. Equally important will be the other direction of reasoning, which will contend that similarity of diabetic experience has been due to a deeper continuity within the diabetic world, spanning the pre- and post-insulin periods, regarding how people living with diabetes have grappled with the core issues of management, control, and responsibility. Viewed in this context, insulin can be seen in proper perspective—as a wondrous drug, but one that accounts for only a part of the bittersweet transformation of diabetes in twentieth-century America.

II

The Bittersweet Transformation of Diabetes

That adherence to treatment with diet, insulin and exercise finds ample justification in the good health, comfort and longevity of those who obey the rules as contrasted with the poor health, suffering and shortened lives of those who are careless.

Elliott P. Joslin,
Article Number Ten,
Diabetic Creed, 1946

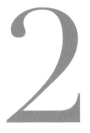

A DISEASE IN MOTION: THE CYCLES OF DIABETIC TRANSMUTATION

New medicines, and new methods of cure,
always work miracles for a while.
—William Heberden, *Commentaries on the*
History and Cure of Diseases, 1802

On a cloudy twenty-first of December, 1961, the temperature outside Elliott P. Joslin's window dangled just below freezing as he sat down to compose his annual Christmas missive to the diabetic patients and the staff of the Joslin Clinic. Just as he had for so many other hours during his seven decades of medical life in Boston, Joslin probably wrote at his rolltop secretary desk. Nearby stood the memorabilia of a career devoted to the care of diabetic patients, with pictures of heroes and friends hanging from the walls: paintings of the eighteenth-century surgeon and anatomist John Hunter and of the revered twentieth-century physician William Osler; photographs of a Joslin Clinic benefactor, George Baker, and of the co-discoverer of insulin, Charles Best.[1] Joslin may also have had, close at hand, copies of his numerous publications, from his initial article on diabetes composed in 1894 while a medical student at Harvard, to his textbook *The Treatment of Diabetes Mellitus* and his patient-oriented *Diabetic Manual for the Mutual Use of Doctor and Patient,* which were first published in 1916 and 1918, both running through many subsequent editions. Ninety-two years old and still active in the daily affairs of medical practice, Joslin penned his season's greetings from a unique position in the diabetic world, presiding as America's leading specialist in diabetes.[2]

No one could have predicted that the youthful Elliott would pursue a medical career so successfully. Born on the sixth of June 1869, Joslin had spent his boyhood years, along with his older half brother and sister, in the small Massachusetts town of Oxford, which combined a

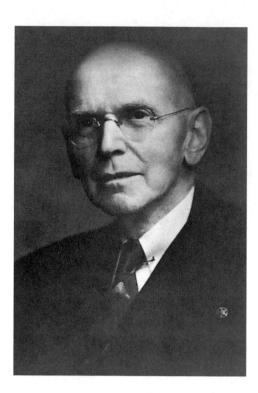

manufacturing base with a few farms scattered just north of the Connecticut border. His father, Allen, was a partner in the Joslin Shoe Factory, and his mother, Sarah Proctor, was related to the founders of the corporate giant Proctor and Gamble. No physicians in his family had served as role models; instead, Joslin credited his village doctor with sparking his interest in medicine. In Oxford, the young man developed an abiding fondness for the land and acquired a deep religious faith from the Congregationalist church. This childhood provided Joslin with fixed points of reference throughout his life. His education took him first to a boarding school, then to Yale College, and finally to Boston for medical school at Harvard and subsequently many years of practice, but he always maintained a second home at the family farm on Buffalo Hill in Oxford, returning often to the country and its fundamental verities.[3]

To those who met him, Joslin's physical features accentuated his personality. Half-rim wire spectacles intensified the determined gaze of his "keen blue eyes," while his spry body and tightly drawn face manifested a serene inner discipline and "stern New England conscience." He also impressed new acquaintances with his frugal habits. Rising early, eating

sparely himself, always immaculate in dress, he moved swiftly throughout the day from hospital to office and back again, eventually settling
down for an evening of reviewing records and dictating letters. His
notorious drive for medical work, Herculean in proportions, seemed
to emanate from devout motivation. Throughout his career, he combined his formal and gentlemanly manner with a showman's knack and
a preacher's zeal, always looking to spread his message of diabetic care.
He had long been a man with a mission.[4]

Sitting down that cold December day, Joslin may have reflected upon
his diverse accomplishments. He might have thought of the comprehensive care that he and his colleagues had provided to the nearly two thousand new patients who had entered the clinic that year—not to mention
the tens of thousands of returning patients. Or Joslin may have recalled
a few of the fifty-three thousand people he had cared for throughout his
career, some of whom were steady patients for as long as a half century.[5]
He could have surveyed in his mind the four-story Joslin Clinic, built
in 1956 according to his design and largely with money that he himself had raised. Or he might have considered how his clinic had grown
amidst one of the largest medical complexes in America, lodged next to
the New England Deaconess Hospital and down the street from Boston
Children's Hospital, the Peter Bent Brigham Hospital, and the Harvard
Medical School.

On another day, perhaps Joslin might have leaned back in his chair
and taken a broader view, meditating on the remarkable ninety years of
American history he had experienced. The pace and scope of change
must have been overwhelming. Born just four years after the American
Civil War had ended, he had lived to see two world wars followed by
an escalating arms race and then America's initial descent into a jungle
war. Around him, Americans had struggled through several economic
depressions yet also carried forward various reforms, securing the vote
for women and continuing the halting transition from Emancipation
toward equal civil rights. Witnessing the spectrum of political distance
between Reconstruction and the Cold War, Joslin had also traversed the
technological distance from telegraph to telephone to television. From
the clip-clop pace of horse-drawn carriages in 1869 Oxford to the high-
speed rush of trains and automobiles in 1961 Boston—with satellites
orbiting visibly overhead—time had shortened, space had contracted,
and the world had grown more complex.[6]

Many of these events were reflected in Joslin's life work as a medical reformer on behalf of diabetics, and he could have written about the social or political changes he observed over his years of practice. But Joslin instead focused his season's greetings on the dramatic events that had changed diabetes from a uniformly deadly disease into a manageable entity. "The status of diabetics before insulin was discovered," Dr. Joslin declaimed in his pious yet personal way, "makes me think of nothing better than the first ten verses of the 37th Chapter of Ezekiel and his description of the Valley of Dry Bones and [']behold there were very many in the Valley and they were very dry bones.[']" Joslin encouraged his readers to ponder those verses, "and then think of your share in helping to bring about the change which followed insulin: '[And I will lay sinews upon you, and will bring up flesh upon you, and cover you with skin] . . . and the breath came into them, and they lived, and stood up upon their feet, an exceeding great army.'* What a wonderful opportunity we have had in seeing this 'army' grow."[7]

A month later, after a full day's schedule—attending morning services at Old South Church and then corresponding with patients and friends—Joslin died at home in his sleep.[8]

DIABETES AND THE TRANSMUTATION OF DISEASE

Joslin witnessed, during his long career engaged in the lives of countless diabetics, an astounding metamorphosis—from bones to flesh, as he viewed it. The venerable doctor believed, along with most of his colleagues, that medicine, through the benefactions of science, had taken diabetes and reversed the order of nature: humans had conquered disease, not the other way around. His belief seemed warranted. When Joslin had begun practicing in 1898, the diagnosis of diabetes ushered feelings of hopelessness into the sickroom; by the time of his death in 1962, diabetes was thought by much of society to have been, if not cured, then vanquished.

Yet the diabetic situation after insulin was rather more complicated— a "terrible beauty" had been born. While the insulin developed by Banting, Best, Collip, and Macleod during 1921 and 1922 warded off coma and proved to be a tremendous boon to diabetics, the disease nevertheless remains a scourge, currently causing more renal failure, amputations of lower extremities, and blindness among adult Americans than any other disease.[9] Defying any simple synopsis, the metamorphosis of diabetes wrought by insulin, like a Greek myth of rebirth turned ironic and macabre, has led patients to fates both blessed and baleful.

TABLE 2.1. A Comparison of Natural History and Transmuted Course

Natural History	Transmuted Course
Stable disease entity	Dynamic and cyclic disease process
Biologic ontology	Biologic and social interactions
Preordained course	Human intervention
General and generic	Individual and specific
Complications	Substituted sequelae
Morally combative	Morally interactive
Stresses cure	Emphasizes care

To understand this contradictory history of diabetes in the twentieth century, we will need to reconstruct how the disease process of diabetes changed, and to do this we will need some new concepts about diseases and how they alter over time. Typically, Western medicine, from the seventeenth century onward, has conceptualized diseases as naturally occurring entities, like species of plants or animals, distinct from others and stable except for gradual evolutionary changes. Consisting entirely of biological processes, each disease is often said to have a natural history, meaning that the disease manifests itself with similar symptoms regardless of the individual afflicted and that these symptoms progress in a predictable manner that has not varied over centuries.

Throughout the twentieth century, however, few people living with diabetes followed the unadulterated natural course of the disease. Instead, medical and social interventions combined to divert individual patients' experiences with diabetes away from the path defined by the disease's natural history and toward what is more accurately called a transmuted course, which differs both in its direction and duration (see Table 2.1). Unlike the concept of a stable and preordained natural history, the notion of transmuted diseases stresses both the malleability of disease entities and the role of human choice: chronic diseases manifest themselves in a particular patient according to the combined effects of physiological processes and human interventions. Depending upon the therapeutic options available at the time, and the choices that a patient and physician made, each patient pursued an individually transmuted disease course: some sought strict control while others opted for free diets; some selected peritoneal or hemodialysis while others preferred a kidney transplant. Through varied medical treatment, the generic pat-

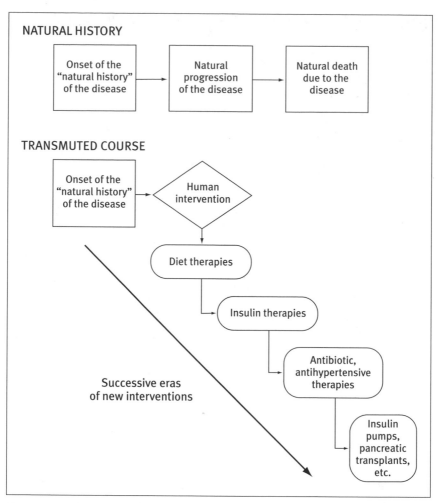

NATURAL HISTORY

Onset of the "natural history" of the disease → Natural progression of the disease → Natural death due to the disease

TRANSMUTED COURSE

Onset of the "natural history" of the disease → Human intervention

Diet therapies

Insulin therapies

Antibiotic, antihypertensive therapies

Insulin pumps, pancreatic transplants, etc.

Successive eras of new interventions

Figure 2.1. The Diversion of a Transmuted Disease Away from a Natural History

tern of a natural history has been diversified into separate courses of distinctly transmuted disease (see Figure 2.1).

Beyond this individual variability, as the years passed, Joslin and his patients participated in several cycles of diabetic transmutation (see Figure 2.2). Each dynamic and interactive cycle of disease change began with the advent of yet another novel therapeutic innovation, such as rigorous diets, insulin, or antibiotics. These medical interventions would ameliorate one set of problems but generate or reveal another set, effectively exchanging old concerns for new ones. Almost immediately, physicians and patients would recognize certain short-term consequences,

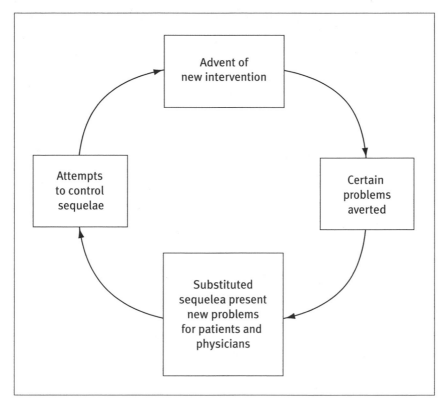

Figure 2.2. The Cyclic Process of Transmutation

positive and negative, of this exchange. For example, insulin could avert life-threatening conditions such as coma but at the price of several injections each day and the risk of causing hypoglycemic reactions. While these short-term consequences of the newly transmuted disease were readily apparent, the long-term sequelae emerged gradually, as more patients were treated and lived with the medically altered disease. From the late 1930s onward, patients and physicians strove to understand, prevent, and treat the long-term consequences of transmuted juvenile diabetes, sequelae such as obstructed blood vessels, failing vision, and damaged kidneys. As new sets of problems would appear, they would become the focus of subsequent efforts to develop additional interventions, which in turn would initiate another cycle.

Across the decades of the twentieth century, these cycles of therapeutically induced transmutation altered the biology of diabetes sufficiently to create variations of the disease over time (see Table 2.2).[10] Although we could choose different interventions or time points to demarcate these periods, the general scheme of eras or periods conveys how the disease itself has changed. Consider, for instance, the shifting pattern of causes of death that Joslin observed in the population of juvenile diabetics who attended his clinic between 1898 and 1950 (see Figure 2.3).[11] This evolving picture of diabetic morbidity and mortality has continued to the present day and shows no signs of slowing down.[12] Indeed, as diabetes has been diverted further and further away from its natural course, the very notion that this disease has an underlying natural history has become outmoded—clearly, a new paradigm of cyclic disease transmutation has taken hold.

This cycle emphasizes the interactive process of disease change—a process that cuts across distinctions typically made between the biological, psychological, social, and cultural realms. Life proceeds at all of these levels concurrently, integrating them into a dynamic system that, transcending any single level of relationship, we will call metabiosis. Just as symbiosis conveys the relationship between two organisms, metabiosis focuses on the comprehensive set of relationships among different aspects of human existence. The cycle of transmutation is one manifestation of metabiotic interaction. As human intervention engages with biological factors to recast diseases, patients' lives are altered, both at a physical level and at an experiential level. Until the twentieth century, the balance of power in the metabiotic interactions between pathological processes and human attempts at healing was tipped in favor of the physical, often infectious, processes. The development of potent pharmaceuticals, surgical procedures, and medical machines has reset this metabiotic balance. So, too, have social interventions, ranging from large public waterworks projects that protected against a host of contagious ailments, to the establishment of insurance funds that would pay for increasingly expensive medical care, enabling patients and physicians to finance hospital-based treatments that radically transmuted certain conditions, such as end-stage renal disease or extremely premature birth.

The shift in the balance of power has given us an unprecedented degree of choice in how diseases will affect our lives. The many difficult choices offered by the transmutation of a disease undermine any simple notion of progress. Medical advances have all been purchased at some cost. Often, these costs have not become clear until considerable time has passed; only then do the choices begin to take on their full

TABLE 2.2. Cyclic Periods of Diabetes Transmutation

Period	Therapies	Short-term Sequelae	Long-term Sequelae
Pre-1912	Diets Opium	Inexorable coma Infections Sense of hopelessness Relief of suffering	Few long-term survivors
1913–22	Low-calorie diet	Delay of coma Potential sense of failure Sense of some control	Starvation Infections
1922–29	Insulin	Prevention of coma Treatment of coma Decreased infections Immediate hypoglycemia	Suspected but unknown
1930–38	Modified insulins	Decreased injections Delayed hypoglycemia Infections remain problematic	Atherosclerosis Renal disease Retinopathy Neuropathy Pregnancy

1938–50	Antimicrobials
	Better laboratory
	  tests
		Many infections treated
		Better treatment of coma
		Sense of being at delayed
		  risk
			Renal failure
			Blindness
			Limb amputations
			Fetal mortality

1950–70	Dialysis Vascular surgery Renal transplant Antihypertensives	Renal function restored Amputations delayed Coronary disease diverted Hemorrhagic stoke averted	End-stage renal disease Immunosuppression Persistent fetal mortality

1970–2000	Retinal laser
	  surgery
	Insulin pump
	Pancreatic
	  transplant
		Retinopathy retarded
		Tighter control
			Cognitive effects of
			  hypoglycemia
			Immunosuppression

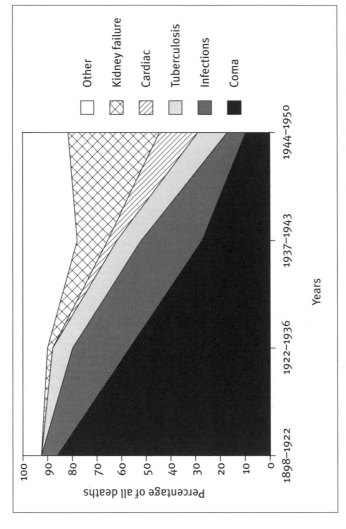

Figure 2.3. Cause of Death of Juvenile Patients with Diabetes, Joslin Clinic, 1898–1950. Source: Adapted from Elliott P. Joslin and James L. Wilson, "Lessons for Future Treatment . . . ," British Medical Journal (December 1950): 1293–96.

weight.[13] As diabetic patients have proceeded along their individually transmuted courses, they have encountered health challenges created by their transmuted disease, including debilitating sequelae of chronic diabetes. Calling these untoward health events sequelae underscores an important ramification of transmuted diseases. Currently, with a disease's natural history affixed in their minds, physicians often configure all untoward developments of a patient's health that run counter to the typical natural history as complications while hailing all therapeutically induced improvements in health as medical advancements. The transmuted course paradigm, on the other hand, views changes of the disease—beneficial and harmful—as sequelae of the transmutation, as medical intervention substitutes one set of risks and problems for another. This inevitable trade-off should give us reason to pause and reflect: just as the miraculous therapy of insulin has allowed long-term problems to emerge, other dreams of therapeutic success are also likely to find themselves mired in iatrogenic irony, with complete success proving to be complex and elusive.

This ironic view of medical progress raises a final issue relating to the transmutation of disease. During the twentieth and early twenty-first centuries, disease has typically been considered an enemy, existing as a natural threat to our well-being. Medicine, consequently, has been construed as a weapon in the battle against disease. This oppositional logic—based on the faulty premise that diseases exist as independent entities—misapprehends the interactive metabiotic relationships that develop between patients, physicians, and illnesses with each successive turn of the transmutation cycle. For better and worse, we have had a hand in making the diseases with which we struggle, thereby shaping the way we live and die.

FROM TRANSMUTED DISEASE TO
TRANSFORMED EXPERIENCE

The biological transmutation of diabetes, driven forward by medical interventions, altered the physiology of the disease, and thus the health problems and life expectancy of patients. These processes, however, do not fully explain changes in what patients experienced over the course of the twentieth century. In contrast to the biological transformation of disease, we will call these broader changes—arising from the combination of biological, psychological, social, and cultural processes—the transformation of illness experience. For people living with diabetes, the ways in which their experience has been transformed can be organized into three central themes. The first theme involves the never-ending work and effort that comprised the day-to-day management of this chronic illness. The second theme has been the governing strategy or rationale that patients and physicians developed to organize their daily efforts of managing. For many, control became a guiding principle that shaped the quality of lives they led. Lastly, as days lengthened to years, the daily issue of who was responsible for managing the illness emerged as a larger theme of ultimate responsibility—medically and morally—for the success or failure of controlling the disease.

These three life-structuring themes played out in many variations over the years as the diabetic experience was transformed from acute to chronic. Each patient handled them differently, while physicians had their own, often idiosyncratic view of how to deal with daily management, control, and responsibility. As the disease was diverted into a chronic condition, and as cultural beliefs about life changed, patients and doctors revised how they thought about these themes in their lives and practices. Still, these variations were not random; certain patterns of thinking and behaving do emerge from the medical records and letters.

The rest of this chapter will begin to explore the connections between disease transmutation and experiential transformation. We will focus on the medical life of Dr. Joslin and a few of his early patients, including the experience of James Dexter Havens, the first American to be "saved" by the introduction of insulin. Unlike most other patients appearing in this book, Havens appears with his real name, a fact that warrants explanation. Several years ago, I happened to meet Jim Havens's daughter, and she subsequently encouraged me to reveal her father's identity, which would have been difficult to conceal due to the singular role that he played in the history of diabetes in America. Through the lens of Joslin's and Havens's experiences, the many lines of the diabetic transformation—biological, cultural, personal—converge and project both inwardly to private lives and outwardly toward the public history of diabetes during the twentieth century.

DIABETES AT THE TURN OF THE CENTURY
Joslin graduated from Harvard Medical School in 1895 and then embarked for the great medical clinics of Germany and Austria, from Freiburg to Vienna and back to Berlin, following the well-worn path

of a generation of young and ambitious American physicians. Upon returning home in the summer of 1897, he served as an intern at the Massachusetts General Hospital for a year. Joslin then set up his private Boston practice in 1898, established ties with Harvard's Department of Physiological Chemistry, joined the staffs of the Boston City Hospital and the recently founded New England Deaconess Hospital, and worked part time in the Boston Dispensary.[14]

Joslin's interest in diabetes extended back to his undergraduate days at Yale, where a year spent conducting research as an assistant to the chemist Russell H. Chittenden had piqued his curiosity. As a medical student, he wrote his Boylston thesis on the pathology of diabetes mellitus and presented the case of his first diabetic patient in front of fellow students, a woman he had treated while working as a clinical clerk.[15] In the medical records of his clinic, Joslin enumerated this case report as "*Case no. 1.*"[16]

> Mary H—an unmarried woman, twenty-six years of age, came to the Out Patient Department of the Massachusetts General Hospital on August 2, 1893. She said her mouth was dry, that she was "drinking water all the time" and was compelled to rise three or four times each night to pass her urine. She felt "weak and tired." Her appetite was variable; the bowels constipated and she had a dizzy headache. Belching of gas, a tight feeling in the abdomen, and a "burning" in the stomach followed her meals. She was short of breath.

Mary Higgens was from County Cork, Ireland. She had immigrated to Boston five years earlier, working ever since as a domestic helper in the suburb of Somerville.

In Mary's case—which Joslin called "a severe form of diabetes mellitus"—he believed that "the dietetic treatment is of the first importance. The carbohydrates taken in the food are of no use to the body and must be removed by the kidneys thereby entailing polydipsia, polyuria, pruritus and renal disease." Accordingly, Mary was put on a "stringent" diet consisting only of protein and fat. Joslin observed that "the beneficial effects of this diet were seen at once." The sugar in Mary's urine decreased to half its former amount, and with the fall of urinary sugar, she was relieved of the pruritus and had to rise from bed only once a night to urinate. "She gained five or six pounds. She was advised to eat all the cream, butter and fatty food possible."

Beyond diet, the well-versed student also "most carefully considered" the "constitutional treatment" for Mary. In recommending a regimen that emphasized fresh air and exercise, Joslin reflected the importance that leading nineteenth-century physicians placed on managing what would now be called patient lifestyle. This was an era when infectious ailments such as tuberculosis seemed to prey upon the weak but even consumed hearty individuals, and the struggle with disease was viewed more as a personal trial than a technical problem. Accordingly, it was also an era in which strengthening one's constitution and cleansing one's air had different connotations than our current attempts to maintain or promote better health through low-fat diets, smoke-free rooms, and aerobic exercise. The treatment of diseases such as diabetes or consumption, both of which wasted the body, sensibly entailed fortifying regimens.[17]

Joslin also discussed the drugs that he could have used in Mary's case. "Codeia and opium," he asserted, "are undoubtedly the surest drugs to use in diabetes mellitus, but they were not employed in this case for the following reasons." His rationale for withholding the morphine painkillers was typical. For starters, "the great expense of codeia put it out of the question at once." As an ambulatory charity patient, Mary certainly could not afford to purchase the refined drug, which was more potent than opium, from her weekly wages. "Opium was not given 1) for fear of being obliged to increase the dose, 2) the danger of leaving it off having once begun, 3) the untoward effect it might have on the bowels, 4) the probability that the patient would be under the charge of different doctors." These customary concerns, especially the emphasis on addiction, were often focused on poorer patients.[18] Joslin also considered giving Mary extracts of "the pancreatic gland [which] has been recommended and tried in this form of diabetes (and will be further tested in this particular case). It has almost universally met with ill success, though in a few instances a slight amelioration in the condition of the patient has been produced."

Finally, Joslin mentioned the damage that the sugar in the urine was causing "the kidneys [which] are succumbing to the strain put upon them," as the urine showed "a trace of albumin," some renal cells, and "a few hyaline and fine granular casts"—all of which indicated that the intricate structures within the kidneys were being destroyed. Whatever finally happened to Mary (and her record does not tell), these early signs of kidney damage surely did not bode well for a woman already threatened by the immediate dangers of coma.

Four years after caring for Mary, Joslin undertook the care of his aunt in September of 1897. His record of Helen Joslin's case, like the records he kept on all of his patients for the first ten years of his practice, consisted of simple and terse notes jotted onto index cards. Joslin believed that her diabetes had developed seven years earlier, when she first became extremely thirsty. Since then, she had "lost much weight." When he examined his aunt, her "chief symptom [was] weakness . . . good appetite, but always is thinking, 'I can't have this—I can't have that.'"[19]

Joslin did not mention in the record what therapy he prescribed, and the next entry occurred a year and a half later. During this interval, though, the young physician had done more homework on diabetes. In addition to examining all the diabetic case records of the Massachusetts General Hospital, he had made a brief visit in the fall of 1898 to Dr. Bernard Naunyn, a renowned diabetologist living in Strassburg, Germany. When Joslin next documented his aunt's case, in March of 1899, she had a "slight sore throat" and was "weaker than usual." On the sixth of March, Aunt Helen had a "poor night—very weak." The following day, she was even "weaker." "Peculiar respirations began about 10 A.M.—continues and during P.M. out of head part of time. At 6 recognized me." Joslin, certainly aware that her condition was dire, prescribed as best he could, ordering "bathes. Rx. soda by mouth and rectum. Whiskey. Strychnine. Caffeine." These efforts were of no lasting avail. As the last entry, Joslin wrote: "Aunt Helen Joslin. At 10 P.M. was comatose and gradually failed and died at 8:48 A.M. March 8, 1899. *No Autopsy*."[20]

Less than three weeks later, Joslin's sixty-year-old mother, Sarah P. Joslin, became the eighth patient in her son's practice. Again, Joslin kept minimal notes, recording facts and figures and little else (a practice that would change radically later in his career). His mother had 5 percent sugar in her urine when it was first measured in June 1899—three months after her first visit. Joslin placed her on a "diabetic diet," and within five days she was sugar free. Like many of Joslin's subsequent patients, however, Mrs. Joslin and her diabetes proved difficult to control with any precision. Her initial weight of 165 pounds dropped to 160 pounds by August but then rose to the high 170s by the end of the year. By 1902, however, Mrs. Joslin's weight had come down to the low 150s, where it stayed for a decade until her final year, when it dropped to the low 140s. Repeated urinalyses made throughout her illness often showed sugar, sometimes 4 to 5 percent, usually 1 to 3 percent. When she died at seventy-four years of age in June of 1913, the autopsy Dr. Joslin ordered confirmed that she had suffered a stroke and then succumbed to pneumonia.[21]

Joslin's exacting style of medical practice began to take shape during this initial period of his career, spanning from his school days in the 1890s, through the early years of private practice, to 1913. Thereafter, a novel scientifically engineered diet not only would usher in a new cycle of diabetes transmutation but would also accentuate Joslin's drive for precision and control of the disease.

THE CYCLE OF RIGOROUS DIET

Over the years, Joslin's management of diabetic children was guided by his ideas of exactly what proved lethal for these youngsters. In keeping with the leading experts, Joslin believed that the diabetic's inability to metabolize sugar normally resulted in high levels of sugar in the blood and caused the body to produce substances that made the patient's blood acidic, eventually leading to coma and killing the patient. Doctors also realized that the urine of a young diabetic whose disease was dangerously out of control would contain both sugar and these acid compounds—acetone, diacetic acid, and β-oxybutyric acid— all of which were warning signs not to be dismissed.[22]

Joslin grounded his therapeutics in these theories and from 1914 onward, in their particular formulation by Frederick Madison Allen. Working as a fellow in the Preventive Medicine and Hygiene Laboratory at Harvard Medical School from 1909 to 1912, Allen had demonstrated that diabetic animals, when fed a diet with a radically reduced number of calories, seemed to revert to a more normal metabolism. Having moved to the Hospital of the Rockefeller Institute for Medical Research, he then applied these findings to patients in what quickly and notoriously became known as the "starvation therapy." Joslin, drawing on Allen's work as well as his own clinical observations and metabolic research, revised his initial "high fat, low carbohydrate" diet into an exacting diet of "low fat, medium carbohydrate, low calorie" foods.[23]

It was such a diet that Joslin prescribed for young Jim Havens. Born in early 1900 in Rochester, New York, the son of a prominent local lawyer who served in the U.S. House of Representatives, Jim had become diabetic around Thanksgiving of 1914. Looking poorly and developing polyuria, his urine was found to contain sugar shortly after New Year's, and by mid-January his hometown doctor, John R. Williams, had referred Jim to see Joslin in Boston.[24] After this visit, the young man—as he later recalled—would have every morsel of food that he ate meticulously weighed by his mother for the next seven years.[25] Williams remained his steady-handed physician (except for a period in 1917 spent under the supervision of Dr. Geyelin in New York City). "James D. Havens is still alive," his physician reported in a 1918 letter to Joslin, but "he was carrying a very high blood sugar . . . on a diet containing less than 1000 calories."[26] Three years later, the doctor wrote again. "You will remember the case of young James D. Havens. He is still alive and presents some very unusual features." On a diet of 1,020 calories, half of which were from fat, Jim's blood sugar was 28 percent, and his urine showed large amounts of both sugar and diacetic acid. His doctor maintained that he "feels remarkably well although he has very little endurance. In fact he seems to be better than he has been for a long time. . . . For more than a year the patient was on a diet containing practically no carbohydrate other than could be obtained from three water vegetables and for a time he did not have this." Summing up, he admitted, "The astonishing thing to me about the case is that he should survive such a long continued severe acidosis. I should be glad to have your opinion on this case."[27]

Two days later, Joslin replied. "Thank you very much for the copy of the note about James D. Havens. It is not unusual for a case with so much acid to live so long. . . . In the old days, before you were born, repeatedly I have seen patients do this and . . . live for years with severe acidosis." Joslin continued: "My suggestion is that when cases are going on in this condition in even a tolerable state their course should not be disturbed. If one tries to improve on the treatment one is apt to lose rather than gain."[28]

These notes were exchanged in October of 1921. In the months that followed, Jim's health began to deteriorate, his body slowly and inexorably wasting. Jim had already lived with his diabetes for nearly seven years, somehow managing to attend the University of Rochester, starting his apparently ill-fated career as a wood engraving print artist, surviving beyond reasonable hope. Discipline and the rigorous diet of Frederick Allen had done all that they could to check the disease's progress. Little did anyone suspect just how dramatically treatment was concurrently being improved in a Toronto medical laboratory and just how much would soon be gained.

The discovery and subsequent rapid development of insulin into a clinically effective drug has been honored by a Nobel Prize, celebrated in medical folklore, presented in a television miniseries, and retold thoughtfully by the historian Michael Bliss.[29] From the summer of 1921 to the end of 1922, Frederick Grant Banting, Charles Herbert Best, James Bertram Collip, and John James Rickard Macleod and several other scientists in Toronto wrote a remarkable chapter in medical history, and their ensuing internecine dispute over who deserved credit has provided a subtext of enduring controversy. More deserving of attention, though, was their collaborative efforts, which brought the quest for a pancreatic extract to a stunningly successful close.

The search had begun thirty years earlier. Until the last decade of the nineteenth century, conjecture as to the cause of diabetes focused on the kidneys, or on John Rollo's contention that the stomach's faulty digestion was to blame, or on Claude Bernard's experiments that implicated the liver and the nervous system.[30] Little attention was given the pancreas until April of 1889, when Joseph von Mering told Oscar Minkowski that it was impossible to surgically remove the entire pancreas from a dog and have the dog survive the operation. Minkowski thought he could. Later that day, working in Bernhard Naunyn's medical laboratory at the University of Strassburg, Minkowski operated with von Mering assisting. The dog survived the procedure. Several days later Minkowski made the now-famous observation that the dog—previously housebroken—was urinating everywhere. A well-trained clinician, Minkowski tested the urine and found sugar. The dog was diabetic.[31]

Although some physicians disputed the conclusion that the pancreas produced some substance that prevented diabetes, the "pancreatic theory" of diabetes thereafter formed a major research paradigm. A decade later, in 1901, the Johns Hopkins pathologist Eugene Opie reported that autopsies of diabetics revealed a specific abnormality of the pancreas. While most of the pancreas produces digestive juices that are excreted into the small intestine, certain small "islands" of cells are scattered throughout the organ. In diabetics, these cells—called the islets of Langerhans, after Paul Langerhans, who had first described them in 1869 while a medical student in Berlin—had been replaced by small deposits of scarlike tissue.[32]

The hunt for the substance that the islet cells produced intensified, driven by a therapeutic dream that, for another disease, had already become reality. Myxedema was an insidious illness that gradually robbed afflicted individuals of their physical vigor and mental acuity, rendering them dull, stuporous, comatose, and finally dead. Since many of these people also had goitrous thyroid glands, swollen at the front of their necks, doctors in the 1890s tried feeding ground thyroid gland to their patients with myxedema. This so-called organotherapy worked wonders (and, with some modification, continues to be the treatment mainstay for what is now known as hypothyroidism).[33]

Thinking by analogy, physicians searched for an organotherapy treatment for diabetes similar to processed thyroid gland for myxedema. In retrospect, a number of researchers came tantalizingly close to discovering insulin before 1922, the most prominent being Georg Ludwig Zuelzer in Germany, E. L. Scott in America, and Nicolas Paulesco in Romania. But none of them succeeded in making an extract of the pancreas that lowered the blood sugar consistently or that would not produce toxic reactions in the recipient.[34]

Then Frederick G. Banting arrived. Naive and energetic, the onetime orthopedic surgeon entered the field of diabetes research in 1921 with a simple idea of how to capture the vital pancreatic substance. After he had badgered and cajoled J. J. R. Macleod to give him laboratory space for the summer, Banting and the medical student Charlie Best began their work. By the middle of the summer, while Macleod was off in Scotland, they had produced an extract of the pancreas that managed to keep a depancreatized dog alive, seeming to reverse the dog's diabetes. For the next six months, the Toronto group worked furiously. Macleod returned and suggested new ways of isolating the pancreatic substance. He also recruited to the research team the young biochemist J. B. Collip, who worked on purifying the extract and quantifying its potency. On 11 January 1922, a junior physician at the Toronto General Hospital injected the extract for the first time into a diabetic patient, twelve-year-old Leonard Thompson. The boy's blood sugar decreased, but only modestly, and he seemed no better; the doctors caring for him decided against another injection. The Toronto workers persisted, however. Although problems with producing purified insulin plagued them through much of the early spring, by the summer their drug was being used in several leading diabetic clinics in America and Canada. At the same time, a few remarkably industrious physicians—such as Rollin T. Woodyatt of Chicago and William David Sansum in Santa Barbara—actually manufactured their own stock.[35]

The first patient in America to receive the wondrous insulin from Toronto was Jim Havens. During the final months of 1921, his health had spiraled downward rapidly; he was losing weight and failing in strength. When he had become diabetic as a fifteen-year-old, Jim had weighed ninety-seven pounds; by May of 1922, at twenty-two years of age, he was a meager "74 pounds, part of which was due to edema." As Williams reported in a subsequent publication, Jim "was a most pitiable spectacle. . . . For weeks the patient had suffered severely from pains in his legs, which made the constant use of codeine necessary. The edema and profound weakness confined him to bed and he was rapidly approaching death, when through the great kindness of Doctors Banting and Macleod, extract was supplied for his treatment." After the first injection of insulin on 17 May 1922, the subsequent gradual "restoration of this patient to his present state of health," according to the appropriately awestruck Williams, "is an achievement difficult to record in temperate language." Three hundred days into insulin treatment, Jim's metabolism of carbohydrates showed marked improvement. "The greatest improvement in the case," however, was in Jim's "appearance and general well-being. This cannot be measured in figures or well stated in words."[36]

Another vantage point on these early insulin events was supplied by Jim's father, who in a letter to a friend in August of 1922 told the story of how Jim's "condition grew worse and became desperate and just then we were able to get some of the pancreatic extract recently developed by Dr. Banting of Toronto and produced by the University of that City." According to his father, "at first the extract worked wonders and that continued as long as Jim was able to take it. He was able to take more food and he gained ten pounds in weight." Secretly smuggled across the border between Canada and the United States, the early batches of insulin produced by the Toronto group were fairly crude extracts. Relatively impotent (and therefore requiring each injected dose to consist of a large volume), this early insulin was loaded with salt residue from the extraction process and still laced with protein impurities, both of which greatly intensified the pain and local inflammation caused by the injections. This combination "after a few weeks began to produce so much pain that Jim could no longer take it in the doses required. One injection produced a big abscess which pulled him down terribly. Now he is taking it in half doses every other day and that is not enough to take care of sufficient food to keep him up." These adverse reactions to the pancreatic extract were not uncommon (and in fact had been one rea-son that investigators before Banting and his colleagues had given up). Jim was luckier, however, than all diabetics who had preceded him. Just as his body grew intolerant of the impurities, his family learned "that Eli Lilly & Company of Indianapolis, manufacturing chemists to whom the manufacture of the extract in this Country has been turned over, are able to produce the extract with greater potency so that it is less irritating." Jim was able to resume taking adequate doses of insulin.[37]

Suddenly, Jim and his family could look forward with newfound hope. The drug had created novel possibilities and untested expecta-tions. His father explained that insulin "suppl[ies] artificially the nor-mal secretion of the pancreas, which is almost entirely absent now in Jim's case." He then echoed the theories of many physicians, stating, "Whether it is possible that nature will restore the diseased pancreas when the strain is taken off [it] by administering this extract and while the other functions of the body and bodily strength is restored, is merely a hope. It may be possible. At any rate the Toronto discovery is almost the first advance in the treatment of this disease."[38]

Jim soon found out, though, that his difficulties with insulin were not over. Although the switch to insulin made by Lilly provided him with a purer and slightly more potent substance, this so-called Iletin form of insulin was made not from beef pancreas (as the Toronto ex-tract was) but rather pork. And Jim Havens was allergic to pork insulin. Immediately after one injection of pork insulin, Williams described a typical allergic reaction: "Three minutes later patient stated that upper lip felt stiff and swollen, followed rapidly by dry mouth. Small wheals then appeared on all parts of the body. The reaction increased in vio-lence for two hours, during which time the wheals became larger and coalesced. . . . Patient very weak and prostrated." Doses of adrenaline and atropine (used to treat bad allergic reactions) brought "slight relief. Twenty-four hours later patient had recovered from the reaction, but was very weak. The weakness and prostration persisted for four days. During this time much skin exfoliated from various parts of the body." Using specially prepared ultrapurified pork insulin led to similar un-toward reactions. Jim therefore went back onto the Toronto beef-based product from Connaught Laboratories, despite its impurities. Not until October, when Lilly began to supply Havens with beef insulin, was he able to take insulin without risking toxic reactions.[39]

For other diabetics during this first year of insulin's clinical use, the chief problem was an alarmingly limited supply of the precious substance. Some patients certainly died for lack of available insulin. The duty to produce mass quantities of the drug fell, among others, to the chief chemist at Lilly, George Walden. By the end of 1922, Walden had developed a novel method of obtaining insulin from pancreatic preparations by adjusting the pH of the solution precisely, causing the insulin to precipitate in a form purer than any previously obtained. With this method, scaled up for industrial production, insulin was in plentiful supply in North America by the early winter of 1923. Potency from one batch to the next was still quite variable (despite standardized rabbit testing of each batch's strength), leading to a greater risk of accidental overdoses with particularly potent batches of insulin. Thereafter, these inadvertent hypoglycemic reactions and the not-inconsiderable price of insulin—and surprisingly widespread suspicion in the general medical community about insulin's therapeutic value and lingering prejudice against the use of any medication requiring daily injection—were the chief problems that limited insulin's adoption and use.[40]

MANAGING NEW REGIMENS

"With the discovery of insulin in 1922 came the hope," wrote a social worker in the mid-1930s, "not only for added years of life, but also for happiness and normality in those added years." She realized that "for these benefits there was a definite price to pay which to most diabetic patients must have seemed small, the regular use of insulin and care in choosing the diet." Small or not, she wondered whether "the inescapable injections of insulin and constant weighing and selecting of food seem a terrific responsibility, and did the constant attention demanded prevent them from living as they formerly had lived."[41]

These questions that weighed benefits against costs and expectations against realities, while rarely raised in print, nonetheless permeated the letters of the diabetics who wrote to the Joslin Clinic. For these people, living with a constantly transforming disease meant never-ending work, managing their regimen of diet, exercise, and insulin while continuously adjusting their expectations for the future.

Frequently, diabetics' concerns focused on the details of their insulin schedules—a matter made more complicated over the years by changes in the drug itself. After 1922, the strength of the extract was standardized into fairly set "units" and two different levels of potency were marketed, one having forty units per cubic centimeter (U40), the other

having eighty (U80). This standardization enabled the diabetic to cal-
culate how much insulin to take (or the physician, how much to administer) once he knew whether he was holding a bottle of U40 or U80
insulin. Insulin was also modified, first as crystalline insulin (1926), and
then as protamine insulin (1935), protamine zinc insulin (1936), NPH
insulin (1950), and, finally, the Lente insulins (1950s). As these different
insulins entered the market, they each displayed their own virtues and
liabilities: some acted swiftly but only briefly, while others took longer
to act and affected the blood sugar level for many hours. Such variations
required them to be used differently, each requiring a distinct regimen.
Patients had to inject the short-acting crystalline insulin up to four times
a day, while with the long-acting protamine or NPH insulin they could
perhaps get by with only one daily shot.[42]

Jim, like many other diabetics, varied his insulin routine to accommodate the changing needs of his body and in order to benefit from
new insulin formulations that appeared on the market. In June of 1927,
he responded to a follow-up request from Joslin, informing the doctor
that he was taking U80 insulin, thirty units in the morning and twenty
at night. This regimen kept him sugar free. Five months later, he wrote
again. He was still on a high-fat diet totaling 1,800 calories, but he noted
that "this is only approximate as I do not weigh the food. From long
practice I think I am able to eat quite closely to a diet, and I figure that
a man cannot expect to live a normal life and keep himself constantly
under laboratory control. At least I seem to get along pretty well in this
way." He had decreased his two injections of insulin by five units each
to ward off "bad reactions" at night.[43] By the spring of 1929, he had
cut his insulin again, dividing it into three doses. "It seems difficult,"
he explained, "to maintain so careful a balance as to be sugar free and
still lead a normal life, in which constantly recurring insulin reactions
are certainly not desirable." Nevertheless, he let Joslin know that he felt
"exceptionally well all the time and enjoy life and my work."[44]

Jim started on protamine insulin in 1936, even before it was on the
market. When Joslin asked him in 1938 how he liked the longer-acting
insulin, he replied that it was a "great advantage to take one dose daily
instead of three—but difficult to prevent early morning shock—24
hours after taking."[45] A year later he wrote Joslin, "I haven't had any
thorough medical examination in some time. I'm taking 40 units of
Protamine insulin, Lilly 80-strength, daily, in one dose before breakfast.
Now and again I have a mild reaction, always about 24 hours after the

dose." Jim had recently increased his dosage from 30 to 40 himself when he began to get blurry vision and, checking his urine, found sugar.

"I eat rather freely but with the discretion of years. A touch of grippe just recently, but have kept very free from it by taking Lilly's ENTORAL, oral cold vaccine, this winter. The last two winters I took cold vaccine by needle, which also worked wonders." Although Jim had not sent a letter to Joslin informing him of his marriage several years earlier (perhaps he had told Joslin in person), the patient did proceed in this letter to tell his doctor of "another rather important development, which I expect you might like to keep track of, since you've followed my own career so long," namely, the birth of a red-haired daughter.[46]

By 1944, Jim was on yet another insulin schedule. "36 units," he told Joslin, "in one dose before breakfast of 80-strength Protamine-Zinc. But am now in process of trying the combination Regular + Protamine in same syringe at one dose." He monitored his diet "only approximately," measuring his food "seldom—if ever, lately." His urine tests were "Poor —in a recent test, showing 2% sugar much of the time. Hence above mentioned attempt to get better control."[47]

The last mention that Jim made of his insulin regimen came twelve years later, when he was taking one dose of regular and Lente insulin, mixed together, each morning. He had "recently substituted 'Lente' for the N.P.H. and it seems better, more even and less 'brittle' in effect."[48]

NEW EXPECTATIONS AND SOCIAL CHANGE

Juggling an ever-changing regimen of treatment was not the only task with which patients such as Jim had to contend after 1922. Diabetics and their doctors still had to grapple with tasks and problems that filled the lives of other Americans during the period, such as how to support themselves financially, how to conduct their personal relationships, and how to plan for the future. But more than that of virtually any other group, the private world of diabetics was particularly uncertain, having been radically diverted in course and extended in duration by insulin's discovery, deflected into uncharted territory.

No one was quite sure how long insulin could sustain a diabetic's life. Each year after 1922 new milestones were reached and, gradually, expectations rose. In 1927—the year he married—Jim wryly commented to Joslin that he had been "interested in your card of invitation to the reception in honor of one of your patients on her Tenth Diabetic Anniversary, and sorry that I was away and could not reply to it in time. Somebody will have to give me a party on my Thirteenth Anniversary the first of the year!"[49]

As diabetics began to live longer, the daily lives of diabetic health care specialists were also transformed. Few doctors at the turn of the century would have dreamed of specializing in diabetes—most dreaded the prospect of caring for diabetics with their invariable course toward death. During the 1910s, Joslin could count the number of colleagues who shared his clinical emphasis on diabetics. By the early twenty-first century, however, there were four thousand endocrinologists who spent much of their time with adult patients with diabetes, while another four hundred doctors treated diabetes exclusively, and another six hundred physicians focused on pediatric endocrinology.[50] In part, this expansion is due to the general growth of specialism within American medicine. Changes in the ailment's prognosis have also spurred the growth of diabetes as a specialty. More diabetics are alive today, and at least the early and middle phases of their illnesses, although still difficult for many, are not nearly so beset with disabilities as they once were. The job of being a diabetic doctor, while not free from frustration and heartache, is not as depressing as it once was.

This shift toward specialization reshaped the kind of care that diabetics were provided, as well as their expectations of what relationships they might have with their physicians. This reformulation of patient/ doctor relationships was further hastened by the rapid growth of the diabetic population. As the numbers of living diabetics rose dramatically, doctors had many patients to treat. The Joslin Clinic itself experienced exponential growth from 1920 to the 1960s, with only a dip in new patient enrollment during the Depression (see Figure 2.4).

Jim ran into the consequences of these developments when, in the early summer of 1933, he visited Boston and dropped in to see Dr. Joslin casually. At this point he was a highly regarded artist, creating prints mostly of natural scenes from wood-engraved blocks. Nevertheless, Havens was turned away after only a brief greeting from Joslin. A few days later, Jim wrote, "Of course I had no idea you were such a busy man—that it would be so difficult to have a little chat with you. After our correspondence covering so many and such trying diabetic years— and after the debt we diabetics have to you—I could not be in Boston without seeing you." Jim alluded to the financial constraints that the De-

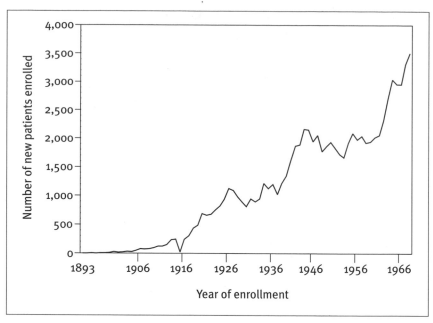

Figure 2.4. Enrollment of New Patients in the Joslin Clinic, 1893–1970.
Source: *Data from the ledger book of the Joslin Clinic, Joslin Diabetes Center Historical Archive, Boston, Mass.*

pression had imposed, explaining, "I had no idea of seeing you professionally—circumstances now are, indeed, such as to forbid it entirely." Still, he thought that Joslin "would want to see what I look like anyhow (it's unfortunate you cannot see the contrast with a few years back!)— and I'm glad to have been able to say Hello—and to have had you see Mrs. Havens. I couldn't take more of your time."[51]

Joslin replied to Jim's letter in the return post. He first tried to explain how "at the hospital with between 40 and 50 patients and often five doctors who have come there expressly to see me I cannot break straight in and take time off." Then Joslin told Jim that he really did "want to have a talk with you and if I set aside a time for you, then that would make it easy. You may have plans for the fourth of July. I expect to be here all day and that morning at the hospital of course I will be quite free because everyone will think I am taking a vacation. Nine or ten o'clock in the morning of the fourth will be all right for me." For Joslin, days of vacation were few—and, apparently, the doctor felt that the Fourth of July did not warrant a holiday, for himself or his patient.[52]

Diabetic lives were affected not only by changes in the medical world but also by broader social changes. These strong currents of history—from the conspicuous effects of the Depression and the Second World War to subtler shifts in how Americans' viewed themselves and authority figures—all worked to redirect the way that diabetics lived. For instance, on the back of a follow-up card dated 1944, Jim jotted a note to Joslin describing how he had been working on a voluntary basis "in a war plant as Chief Inspector in a small Parachute factory." The patient told his physician that he had "stood it fairly well for a time but got pretty tired, progressively more so, so that at last I was so tired every night that I couldn't keep at it. I worked 7–10 hrs. a day, 6 days, on feet much of the time." Jim explained that, "not liking the work, + being poorly equipped in training, and temperamentally, for it (I had to keep some thirty women inspectors in line!) are I believe as much factors in making me too tired as was the diabetes." Jim nevertheless realized the indirect consequences of being diabetic, in that he "was also inclined to eat too much for fear of having insulin shock while on the job, which may account for the current poor tests."[53]

Surrounding this exchange between Jim and his physicians was all the Sturm und Drang of the Second World War and the homefront war efforts in the United States. The war and its exigencies prompted diabetics—like other Americans—to adopt new roles, layered upon their preexisting roles within their families, communities, or workplaces. For many Americans, these new roles proved liberating, particularly for those women who entered the workplace in unprecedented numbers. For people such as Jim Havens, the war aroused sentiments that led them to volunteer their services, in whatever capacity, for the national cause. For others, however, the force of patriotic sentiment may well have contained coercive undercurrents (the draft being only the most blatant example); and when combined with a national call to service, some may have been pushed into ill-suited roles. Whereas most of these individuals remained silent, diabetics could maneuver their way out of the roles foisted upon others. Several diabetics who saw Joslin or one of his colleagues used the exclusionary license granted by their sick role to opt out of wartime service. In their candid discussions with physicians, diabetics—whether they were talking about the war or the Great Depression, or about trying to become mothers—revealed not only their own circumstances and how they related to historical developments in America but also the social and cultural circumstances that other Americans confronted. The history of diabetes—from the patient's perspective—has been embedded in American history.

The transmutation of disease has touched many lives in twentieth-century America—so many, and in so many different ways, that the process itself has almost become invisible. Even Joslin, in a personally immediate way, lived a transmuted life as he entered old age. "Thanksgiving really meant more than usual to me this year," the eighty-five-year-old doctor explained to a patient in 1953, "because four weeks ago I had an attack of appendicitis and was operated upon." Joslin had actually diagnosed the condition on his own, and after finishing the day seeing patients in his office, he ferried himself by taxicab to the New England Deaconess Hospital, where his longtime collaborating surgeon, Leland McKittrick, removed his appendix. "Fortunately, all went well," Joslin relayed, "and I am deeply indebted first to the Lord, and second to Doctor McKittrick, and third, to many others. As a matter of fact, although I had a red, hot appendix I was only in the Hospital eight days and came out to vote on the way home, and now have practically recovered."[54]

Just a few decades before, without the benefits of improved surgical and anesthetic techniques or of antibiotics and intravenous fluids, the octogenarian physician would probably have died. Instead, he lived another nine years—and worked the whole time, continuing to see patients and to oversee the operations of his clinic and its research projects. Those years were the result of the transmuted course of appendicitis, a course based on remedies that have come remarkably close to making circumstances universally favorable.

Not all pathological conditions have been so tractable. Diabetes, for one, has thwarted the hopes of clinicians and patients of finding that alluring fail-safe remedy. This is not to say that the variety of treatments developed in the past century have been useless. Far from it. With these therapies, and through his skill and judgment, Joslin kept countless diabetics on this side of favorable. Jim Havens was one such diabetic, his story being essentially one of successful navigation through the uncertain waters of his evolving disease and the social circumstances that surrounded him. When Jim eventually died of colon cancer just over a year before Joslin passed away in his sleep, both had followed the transmuted course of disease to a noteworthy end. Others, though, have experienced the transmutation of disease much less "successfully." To these diabetic patients and their predicaments of living with a transformed illness we now turn and focus our attention.

ILLNESS UNFOLDING: THE TRANSFORMED EXPERIENCE OF DIABETIC PATIENTS

*A man lives not only his personal life, as an
individual, but also, consciously or unconsciously,
the life of his epoch and his contemporaries.*
—Thomas Mann, *The Magic Mountain*, 1924

For most Americans, 1921 was a year of peace and of promise. Memories of the Great War were beginning to fade, a new president, Warren G. Harding, had taken office, and for the first time baseball was being broadcast live on the radio. As the Red Scare subsided and postwar inflation ebbed, the country looked forward—perhaps politically weary at home and wary abroad, but with an economy on the verge of a decade marked by unparalleled productivity and prosperity. American industry, society, and culture were about to turn *modern,* as automobiles rolled off assembly lines faster, Amelia Earhart flew farther, picture shows talked longer, and hemlines crept higher.[1]

For Sally M. Kramer and her family, however, this would be remembered as the year when she became diabetic. As the winter of 1921 was receding in the nine-year-old girl's northern Massachusetts hometown, the illness had crept up, gradually wasting away ten pounds and making her irritable. When sugar was discovered in her urine, she was fasted for three days, rendering her urine sugar-free. Her diet was then advanced to just above subsistence. Sally did well on this minimal regimen until six months later, when she again began to spill sugar. Her recently graduated doctor cut her diet repeatedly in what must have been seen as a dismally downward spiral. Then, in August of 1922, she was taken to see Dr. Joslin, who started her on insulin. Sally thus joined Jim Havens as one of the first American patients to receive the new "wonder drug."[2]

Sally would live for thirty more years. This chapter will consider her life history—marked by difficulty and disappointment—as it takes another step forward in the book's larger project of assembling a patient-oriented history of diabetes. Chapter 2 laid one cornerstone for this project, as its portrayal of Jim Havens detailed how therapeutic medical interventions had transmuted diabetes. A patient-oriented account of diabetes, however, cannot be constructed simply from stories of diets and drugs and medical devices, as they alone have not built the complete tale. A person's encounters with diabetes have varied by gender and across racial and ethnic groups, and have been affected by whether that patient was rich or poor, well educated or unschooled, socially sophisticated or naive, part of a supportive family or more isolated. Since forces beyond the changing technical capacity of medical care have influenced peoples' experiences with this disease, a patient-oriented history must be fashioned from a broader array of materials, seeking to understand how medical therapy combined with aspects of twentieth-century American social history and cultural values to transform the experience of chronically diabetic patients.

The stories of individuals can illuminate an epoch. In charting the course of Sally Kramer's life, we shall strive to use her individual experience to shed light on the more general social and cultural dimensions of living with an ever-changing chronic disease. Our method to recover some of these deeper aspects of diabetic history will be through a close reading of the letters that Sally and her mother exchanged with the Joslin Clinic physicians as part of a decades-long dialogue, focusing on what we will call the "language of living with diabetes." Such a language—so remarkably pervasive and potent in the lives of people with diabetes—points to major forces that have shaped the diabetic world and has itself been a prime influence in this world. Given its importance, we will digress briefly in order to examine this language in some detail before resuming Sally's narrative.

THE LANGUAGE OF LIVING WITH DIABETES

Much of the diabetic language has been built around the day-to-day practical problems of living with diabetes and, in turn, the difficult choices that confronted patients. As the letters of the Joslin Clinic attest, sickness disrupted the patterns of life that diabetic individuals and their families had established before the disease intruded. Diagnosis wrought change at several levels of living. Patients restructured their daily lives to abide by dietary rules and adhere to a schedule of insulin injections. Beyond this routine diligence, whenever a crisis occurred (such as an

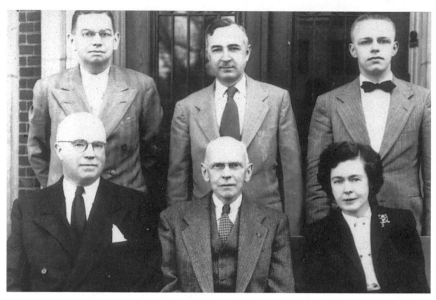

Physicians of the Joslin Clinic, circa 1950. Left to right, standing: Allen P. Joslin, Alexander Marble, Robert F. Bradley; sitting: Howard F. Root, Elliott P. Joslin, Priscilla White. Courtesy of the Joslin Diabetes Center Historical Archive.

infection, a bad hypoglycemic reaction, or the development of a new debilitating disease sequela) these efforts had to be redoubled. The rest of life—family, school, job—would be affected, prompting many people with diabetes to rethink their expectations for the future, even recasting their sense of self.

Diabetic patients and their family members typically couched their discussions about these experiences in a particular hybrid language that combined two other ways of talking about life. The first of these was a fundamentally moral language: the commonplace conversations that Americans have held among themselves about how to live, pondering the proper relationship between individuals and society, or the relationship of human choice and inscrutable fate. With the abiding concerns of work, self-control, and personal responsibility being so prominent in this diverse American conversation, discussions about the diabetic life appear as stylized versions of this broader cultural dialogue, tailored to living in a world of a particular illness.

The second language was medical. The technical terms and phrases used by doctors—diabetes mellitus, hypoglycemic reactions, ketoacidosis, Kussmaul respirations, proliferative retinopathy, insulin units per cubic centimeter, intravenous catheters—were one level of the medical language that diabetics encountered. For some patients, this jargon remained baffling and alienating; for others, mastery of this dialect became a point of pride.

At a level beneath this technical terminology, the medical language centered on three key terms: "management," "control," and "responsibility." With these words and the ideas they conveyed, the medical and cultural languages merged as patients and physicians tried to communicate their fundamental views about living with disease—not always clearly or amicably, and frequently with problematic implications for diabetic patients.

Each of these key terms, which appear in the language of living with other chronic diseases, has its own specific historical connections to the constantly changing diabetic life. For instance, doctors and patients have spoken of the "management" of diabetes for more than a century. During this time physicians, clinical investigators, nurses, and patients have developed a complex system to manage the disease. In the pre-insulin era, it revolved around diets and urine tests for sugar. Since then, not only have various insulins entered this management system, but so have sharper syringes, more frequent blood sugar tests, softer shoes, pressure dressings, oral hypoglycemic agents, and other drugs.

All of these methods to manage diabetes have entailed work—unremitting labor that has come in many forms for patients and family members alike, shaping their days and molding their interpersonal interactions.[3] Over the years, diabetics have also had to deal with a widening range of health care providers, extending beyond family practitioners to include diabetic specialists, educational nurses, and diagnostic laboratory workers, not to mention the outpatient clinic or hospital where these people work. Simply scheduling and keeping appointments, for many patients, have become time-consuming chores. In sum, diabetics have had to manage not only their disease but also the work that this management system has created for themselves and the effects of this self-care work on their relationships with others.[4]

"Control," another key term in the diabetic language, has also figured prominently as diabetes care has evolved. Beginning in 1900, this idea principally meant controlling a child's aberrant metabolism so as to prevent coma. From the 1930s onward, as delayed sequelae such as blindness or circulatory problems or kidney failure became more common, doctors retargeted their control efforts, seeking to prevent these additional problems or at least ameliorate their symptoms. Throughout the century, though, the idea of control has persistently implied that if diabetics could control their disease, they would remain healthy.

Just how diabetic control was put into practice, however, depended not only upon the therapeutics available at that time but also upon where the patient was treated and by whom. Patients have entered the medical world at different points—from rural general medical offices to urban tertiary care hospitals—and the practitioners at each site have had their distinct fund of knowledge, level of competence, and style of care. Accordingly, diabetics have received different treatment at the hands of a varied medical profession. Their doctors have also differed regarding how much control they thought was necessary or beneficial for patients' well-being. Physicians seem to have formed their opinions about control based not so much on scientific evidence as on their own beliefs about what constituted a good and healthy life. Their public debates about diabetic control were heated. Some physicians, such as Joslin and his colleagues, championed self-control as a virtue, medically and morally. Others, with more fatalistic or laissez-faire philosophies, countered that there was no hard evidence to elevate the ideal of diabetic self-control as the central dogma of therapy, suggesting that an undue emphasis on self-control bespoke a high-minded judgmental attitude.[5]

While doctors were debating, patients like Jim and Sally did not stand by idly. They had their own feelings about the value of control and their willingness to pursue it. When patients' desires and actions agreed with their physician's, praise abounded—and when not, the resulting discord typically raised one of the most interesting and profound aspects of living with a chronic illness—"responsibility."[6]

All the work of managing juvenile diabetes (and especially how the labor of this care has been divided among patient, parent, and physician) has made responsibility into a pivotal term in the language of living with this disease—even more so as diabetes has been transmuted into a chronic illness. Many of the tacit rules that have governed the sharing of responsibility between patient and doctor emerged from the practice of medicine in the treatment of acute illnesses.[7] Unlike these acute episodes, in which the physician and nurse briefly assumed much of the responsibility for providing care, in chronic cases the lines of responsibility have been less clearly drawn.[8] From the beginning of each relationship, patient and doctor have often tried to decide who was responsible for managing particular aspects of the illness that brought them together. The resulting negotiation has been sometimes overt and straightforward, sometimes subtle and ambiguous. Both parties have had to decide who is in charge of what—a judgment underwritten by beliefs about individual perseverance, personal accountability, and even moral character. These deliberations over who was responsible for particular aspects of care in turn often have been followed by implicit judgments about how well a patient or a physician had discharged his or her responsibilities, and ultimately by verdicts about who or what was responsible for therapeutic success or failure—the patient, the physician, or the obscure workings of the body.[9]

Much of the meaning of living with diabetes has resulted from the interplay of management, control, and responsibility—a meaning that, while composed of common terms, has been nonetheless distinct for every patient. Even if their key words were born out of the union of moral and medical languages, their individual way of speaking and thinking about the diabetic life soon has distinguished itself from the cultural and medical thought that conceived it. While patients have shared with physicians and other members of society some common notions of how to live with disease, diabetics have formed their own opinions regarding how to manage their disease, what represents good control, and how they are responsible for their condition. These opinions have resonated with the circumstances of that patient's life and developed as the patient grew older.

Indeed, the individual language of living with diabetes was closely tied to the patient's private life course, his or her own history of personal development.[10] How a nine-year-old diabetic patient such as Sally thought and spoke about her diabetes obviously changed as the youngster grew into adulthood and then aged, experiencing the multifaceted vicissitudes of family and work life. Above and beyond such "normal" variation, the life courses of male and female diabetics have been subjected to the unpredictable advances and setbacks of chronic illness and the hopes and frustrations of new medical therapies.[11]

The individual language of living with diabetes has bubbled up from this confluence, where the unpredictable course of life intersects an uncertain illness course. People with juvenile diabetes have lived with their chronic illness at this turbulent juncture—and it is here, in this highly individualized zone, that I shall try to recount Sally's life. My narration of her story mimics the development of her own experiences, proceeding neither smoothly nor logically but rather in fits and starts, the forward flow of daily routine punctuated by crises that seem to wind time backward, ultimately undermining any orderly sense of growing older. At the end of this chapter, we shall return to the tumultuous qualities of her story, for they reveal problems that are germane not only for the historian trying to describe another person's life, but also for patients, their families, and physicians as they try to create sense out of living with diabetes or other chronic conditions.[12]

LEARNING THE LANGUAGE OF DIABETIC LIFE

Three years after Sally became diabetic, her mother wrote to Joslin, "Sally has just recovered from a case of acid poisoning," which Mrs. Kramer believed was "due to the fact that we did not take her to the Dr. for two months or more." Sally had "seemed to be getting along fine, but in the meantime must have had more fats than she could take care of." A slight miscalculation, perhaps, in the preparation of Sally's diet—but for diabetics, small details could have critical repercussions.

Both doctors and parents sensed, in different ways, that young diabetics were chronically vulnerable and threatened. For these children, unlike their healthy friends and playmates, a hundred dangers lurked nearby. Much of the parent and physician concern focused on the precise management of diet and insulin, on efforts to strike a balance between excessive and inadequate blood sugar levels. Mrs. Kramer, for instance, paid close attention to how much insulin Sally received, making sure that the dose was not too large by having her daughter "show a little sugar at night as we have had trouble twice with her having reactions after going to sleep."[13]

Diabetics also seemed threatened by commonplace events, as otherwise normal occurrences could quickly become cause for alarm. A slight illness might precipitate acidosis and coma; a sore throat could lead to "blood poisoning"; a minor cut on the foot might develop into gangrene. The major bane of Sally's early diabetic life was her repeated bouts with "a hard cold." Like virtually every other child of that period, she had had her tonsils and adenoids removed as an eight-year-old in 1920, but the remnants of tissue left behind by the surgery continued to be a site of infection.[14] Her local doctor, concerned about Sally's increased need for more insulin whenever she was sick, wrote Joslin asking why her troublesome adenoids had not been completely removed when she had visited Boston in 1923. Joslin answered that "last spring we were not so enthusiastic as now, because we did not feel it as safe as we do now, to operate for such troubles."[15]

Joslin's comments reflected the shifts in medical judgment that were being wrought by insulin. "For years," an editorialist in the *Boston Medical and Surgical Journal* declared in 1925, "the diabetic has been taboo for the surgeon." As the author observed, people with diabetes in the pre-insulin era had been notoriously prone to life-threatening operative complications and so only the most desperate cases were taken to the surgical suite. "But however justifiable such a view may have been in the past," he concluded, "the advances in the treatment of diabetes are compelling its abandonment."[16] Gradually, from 1922 onward, insulin assuaged the elite Boston surgeons' fears of acidosis during the operation and coma or poor wound healing after the surgery. Joslin was willing to recommend that Sally return to Boston for possible surgical treatment.

But Sally's "troubles" extended beyond the realm of hormones, microbes, and operative risk. Several months elapsed before Joslin received another letter from her doctor, who had suggested to Sally's mother that the girl have her tonsils removed. He confided in Joslin, "To be truthful, every time I mentioned it they were undecided, and it has just come to me through a friend that they want to but have not the money, as it takes about all above expenses for the Insulin." After inquiring about the estimated expense of the operation, the doctor signed off: "Please do not consider this a begging letter but I wish you to know the facts."[17] Joslin replied that "if the family ought not to incur expense" he would treat her pro bono, the surgeon would charge a very modest fee, and the hospital board would run $3.75 a day for the one- to two-week stay.[18]

Four years later, Sally still had not had her tonsils removed. When Joslin wrote the family again in 1928, he informed them that a newly established fund at the New England Deaconess Hospital would cover one-third of the hospital board. Money, however, was still an issue. While Joslin was "more than glad to make no charge whatsoever" for his and his associates' services, he did ask Mrs. Kramer to "pay the one who operates upon Sally something because I have so many favors to ask for my patients that it is an embarrassment."[19]

Joslin's request reflected two particularly difficult aspects of medical billing in the first half of the twentieth century. First, throughout his career Joslin strove to maintain collegial relations with fellow physicians

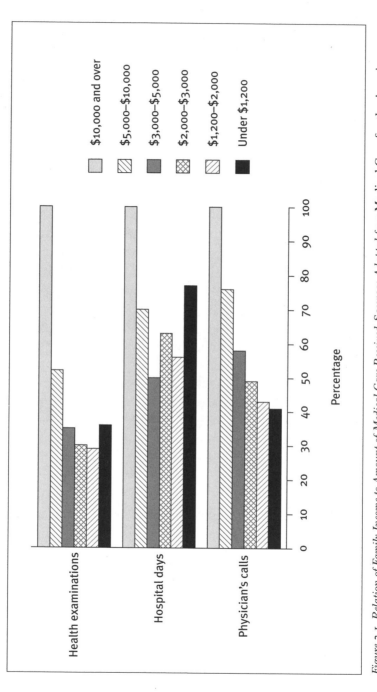

Figure 3.1. Relation of Family Income to Amount of Medical Care Received. Source: Adapted from Medical Care for the American People: The Final Report of the Committee on the Costs of Medical Care (Washington, D.C.: U.S. Department of Health, Education, and Welfare, 1932), 6, fig. 1.

by cautiously maneuvering through a professional environment that espoused charity yet demanded that the patient who could pay did so. This mix of paternalism and profit motive had a well-established history in American medicine. Through the closing decades of the nineteenth century, physicians had railed at what they called "dispensary abuse," when patients who could pay a local doctor's fees opted instead to attend a free medical dispensary. In most physicians' eyes, free health care turned patients into paupers and—more important—created unfair competition for hard-working solo practitioners. When the dispensary declined as a viable medical institution during the early years of the twentieth century, physicians identified the free medical care provided by hospitals as a new threat.[20]

Joslin's request for partial payment of the surgeon's bill also underscored a stark economic reality: Sally's family could not afford all the health care that Joslin prescribed. In this regard, Sally's case was hardly unique. In the late 1920s, a federal commission studied the medical care that white Americans received. They found that as a family's income level rose, the amount of health care that the family received increased. This trend had only a few exceptions, the major one being that the poorest families who were eligible for "charity care" at hospitals and medical clinics received slightly more health care than families perched just above poverty level (Figure 3.1). When the commission defined an appropriate dose of high-quality medical care, they found that no group of families—not even the most affluent—received an adequate amount of health care. The commission also uncovered that over the course of a year, nearly half of the poorest families had no medical, dental, or eye care. In this health care environment, the types of financially oriented medical decisions that Sally's family made were probably quite common.[21]

In the late 1920s, while Sally and her family repeatedly postponed her operation, few sources of funds were available to mitigate the financial burden of medical care. Health insurance, for example, did not exist in America, despite a handful of earlier attempts to establish it. From 1912 onward, debates over national health insurance flared periodically. Heralded first during the Progressive period, the call for "compulsory" insurance subsided during the First World War, was defamed during the Red Scare of 1919, and was scuttled by 1920, branded as "Un-American, Unsafe, Uneconomic, Unscientific, Unfair and Unscrupulous." A decade later, the Great Depression allied with steadily

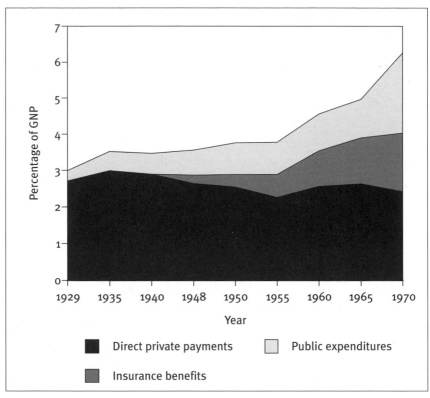

Figure 3.2. Personal Health Care Expenditures by Source of Funds, as Percentage of Gross National Product, 1929–1970. Source: *Adapted from U.S. Bureau of the Census,* Historical Statistics of the United States . . . Part 1 *(Washington, D.C.: GPO, 1975), 74.*

mounting personal health care expenditures (Figure 3.2), and health insurance returned to the national agenda. At the same time, group health insurance plans such as Blue Cross emerged, providing coverage for basic hospital care and surgical procedures to those who could afford to enroll. By the late 1940s, despite a vigorous national debate regarding possible public, state-sponsored insurance immediately after World War II, the explosive growth of the private health insurance industry established this system of insurance as the chief protection against medical care bills (Figure 3.3).[22]

The development of health insurance, however, did little for Sally and her monetary predicaments. Although health insurance generally became available during the later years of her life, she—like many other patients—found herself outside its protective net. She seems never to

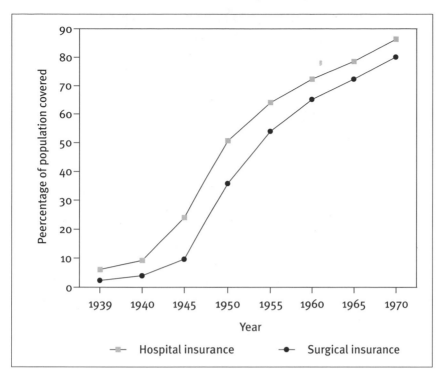

Figure 3.3. Percentage of U.S. Population with Hospital or Surgical Insurance, 1939–1970. Source: *Adapted from U.S. Bureau of the Census,* Historical Statistics of the United States . . . Part 1 *(Washington, D.C.: GPO, 1975), 82.*

have worked for an employer who offered insurance, nor was she able to purchase it on her own. Even in more favorable employment or financial circumstances, other diabetics often found that they were barred from health insurance schemes specifically because of their condition. For many of these diabetics, the price of health care remained a lifelong concern, shaping and constraining their medical options.

When Sally finally went to the hospital in late 1928 and had her adenoids and tonsils removed completely, this early chapter of her diabetic life closed—but its lessons could hardly have gone unnoticed. While many physicians such as Joslin taught diabetics and their parents to live in a state of perpetual vigilance and unrelenting control of the disease, Sally and her family had already learned of the disparity between what was held as ideal diabetic medical care and what they, given their financial circumstances, could achieve. And yet, after five years of inquiries and deliberations, her tonsils came out, extracted not merely by surgical wire but by her family's enduring desire to care for Sally, the persistent interest of her physicians, and a new hospital fund to defray medical costs. As we shall see, there were many other reasons that patients either did or did not follow medical advice—reasons and motivations that reflected and incorporated the language of management, control, and responsibility as patients grappled not only with their disease but also with other important aspects of their lives.

THE PUNCTUATION OF CRISES AND TRANSITIONS

Few lives unfurl without wrinkles. As men and women move through their life courses, the transitions from one stage to the next can be abrupt and the future direction remains uncertain. Plans change, new duties dominate, dreams are realized, dashed, or stowed silently away. For many diabetics, the course of their lives has been detoured even more unexpectedly by the effects of their disease. Life events that those without diabetes often took for granted, such as becoming a mother, could become points of crisis for diabetics.

In November 1929, Dr. Jones in northern Massachusetts wrote Joslin that one of their mutual patients, Sally, was two months pregnant. He was alarmed on two counts: first, he felt that "the fellow she went with is in no position to take care of her financially or morally." Second, he was concerned about the risks of pregnancy in a diabetic. He cited a textbook by Joseph B. DeLee (a Chicago obstetrician "in whom I have a great deal of respect"), which had "some startling statistics in regard to mortality and his treatment is a therapeutic abortion at this time." Jones noted that the fourth edition of this text "was out a little while after Insulin was used and he says reports are too small to judge any different. Anything you tell me in regard to the above would be greatly appreciated."[23]

Joslin must have been accustomed to reading this kind of note, as he received many similar appeals from other doctors who looked to the diabetes expert for advice. These letters reflected how widely physicians differed regarding what they knew, how they practiced, and the circumstances they confronted. In this case, the local general practitioner relied on a 1924 textbook for guidance in how to manage a clinical problem that was evolving rapidly. Indisputably, what the community of medical experts in Boston and other major research centers knew was not necessarily known everywhere. Knowledge took time to spread.[24]

Variation in knowledge was not the only feature that distinguished the doctors in Boston from those in outlying communities, for these two groups faced markedly different situations. Therapeutic failure did not weigh upon every pair of medical shoulders with the same weight. By the late 1920s, the specialists in Boston felt comfortable managing a diabetic woman through her pregnancy because they had acquired experience managing complex cases. As important, by being members of large and famous medical establishments, they possessed institutional and financial security that protected them if a particular patient took a turn for the worse. They could afford to take certain risks. Meanwhile, doctors in the community who rarely encountered pregnant diabetics were more exposed to public scrutiny and vulnerable to the economic and emotional repercussions of an unexpected death. Like his colleagues scattered about in other small towns, Dr. Jones, who was only in the tenth year of his medical practice, had to be much more concerned about the possibility that the mother might die.[25]

"I have your letter about that poor child," Joslin replied, reassuring Sally's doctor that several of his patients had recently "gone through labor successful. Practically all do well if under close observation."[26] Joslin recommended that Sally visit Boston to see "if she should be aborted."[27] Ten days later, Sally saw Joslin and his obstetrical collaborator, Raymond Titus, both at no charge. Titus, by means of a thorough physical examination, determined that she was not pregnant (no laboratory tests were recorded in the chart).[28]

For two and a half years, Sally's diabetic life seems to have settled down. Now nearly twenty years old, she married and began to write to Joslin herself, telling him in one note that she felt fine but did "not always stick to my diet as I should."[29] This relative calm—as a physician might have perceived it—came to a sudden end when Dr. Jones next wrote to Joslin. "I had not seen Sally Jackson, nee Kramer for some months until two days ago and to my surprise found her about six months pregnant, a temperature of 103 and pulse of 100 and not a thing to account for it." The doctor had examined her urine and found some sugar and acetone along with "pus cells." The morning that he wrote, the family had telephoned, alarmed that "she was shaking and shook for over an hour and her finger nails were blue."[30] Sally was rushed to the Deaconess Hospital, where she was diagnosed as having a severe case of pyelitis (a kidney infection). This required several weeks in the hospital, her temperature rising as high as 106 degrees, while "fluids were enforced," before the infection abated (the sulfur antimicrobial drugs were not available until the mid-1930s).[31]

After this scare, though, Sally did very well, "a shining example of what strict adherence to directions will do," according to one of the clinic doctors.[32] She kept her diabetes under tight control and was brought into the Deaconess Hospital well before her due date to assure a healthy outcome. But despite these efforts, Sally "had rather an unfortunate experience during labor," as Dr. Priscilla White (who was, as we shall learn, one of Joslin's closest colleagues) related to Sally's doctor back home. "She developed diabetic acidosis in the early morning of October 14. By two o'clock she was in typical diabetic coma. She thought that she had felt fetal motion during the preceding days, but she was delivered of a macerated fetus by high forceps." An autopsy of the child showed that "the baby must have been dead for at least 48 hours, White continued. "After labor, [Sally] recovered quickly from her coma."[33] The local doctor wrote back to White, thanking her "for informing me in regards to Sally and was sorry to hear that she had hard luck but I believe some One saw into the future."[34]

In March 1933, Sally's doctor again wrote Joslin, this time telling him beseechingly that Sally's mother was "in my office now and can hardly talk, crying and worried to death. Her daughter . . . has not menstruated for three months and her urine is very cloudy and [she] is afraid [of] a repetition of the past pregnancy. . . . She begged me to write you to see what could be done as she is miles away from medical care."[35] Sally was immediately seen by Joslin and White, who recommended that she abort the pregnancy. As White told Sally, this pregnancy had followed too quickly after the preceding one and the doctors were "afraid that the pyelitis will return and that at the present time you have not sufficient immunity to resist such an infection." White consoled the young woman, assuring her that "during a later pregnancy if money is a factor Dr. Joslin said he would make arrangements for you to return to the hospital for the last month of pregnancy and that you would have a caesarean section."[36] Sally had the abortion but never became pregnant again.

For many diabetic women such as Sally, pregnancy was a major event both in their lives as women and their lives as diabetics. A point of confluence, the diabetic pregnancy enveloped an otherwise normal life event into the ongoing saga of living with a chronic illness. Pregnancy was a poignant example of how the disease infiltrated the lives of these women and affected their thoughts of themselves and their physicians. These women attested in their letters to how much depended upon whether the child lived or died—a sense of personal worth, a vision of a happy and fulfilled future—and the experience of being guided through the pregnancy, successfully or not, by Dr. White often bonded these women firmly to their charismatic doctor.[37]

The experiences associated with the diabetic pregnancy, however, differed substantially from what patients and doctors typically encountered. The time during which a woman with diabetes was pregnant was an acute episode of an otherwise chronic condition. Because of its limited time span, the level of motivation and the rules for sharing responsibility changed. All parties appeared especially dedicated, and the physicians assumed more responsibility for managing the illness and the outcome of the pregnancy. Once the women moved beyond their pregnancies, their situations resumed their chronic patterns, where motivation waxed and waned, and they assumed a greater proportion of daily responsibility.

THE GRAMMAR OF ROUTINE

In striving to understand a life, which is more important: to examine dramatic decisions and turning points or to embrace the common drudgery of daily routine and quotidian choices? To the historian, the question is one of emphasis. Both levels of understanding deserve attention. Too often, however, the answer has favored drama and ignored the mundane. Just as military historians at one time scrutinized the judgment of generals on battlefields while ignoring the foot soldier's food and friendships in the billet or bivouac, medical historians previously have focused primarily on the discoveries of "great doctors" and their heroic battles with dreaded diseases. This preference of former scholars is understandable, not only in terms of what they found interesting but also in simply what they found. The historical record often effaced the routine of daily life. People of bygone times were more likely to document what they felt were major events, so it has been far easier to reconstruct these occurrences in detail than to reweave the fabric of everyday existence.[38]

Of late, this predilection for the dramatic has been curtailed. Equipped with new methods and new commitments, historians have cultivated, particularly since the 1960s, the expanding field of social history. Studies of labor and family history, for example, have surmounted the limitations of certain written sources by turning to other historical materials, such as business ledgers or census tract reports.[39] More recently, cultural studies have extended the historian's repertoire of explanatory approaches, stretching it from anthropology to literary criticism.[40]

What bearing do these developments have upon Sally's diabetic life? Our study of her case—and, more broadly, the history of patient experience—fits into this scholarly trend, both in its emphasis and in its materials. We can learn from these historical methods as we seek to uncover the daily lives of these ordinary but chronically ill people. In particular, these new approaches educate us to both the pitfalls and the promise of using medical charts and patient-doctor letters as historical sources.

For instance, we must realize that the medical record presents a composite point of view. In the Joslin records, the physicians' commentary appears on hospital and clinic forms and in their letters, while the patient and family member's perspective is conveyed in their letters. Both points of view, however, are distorted and incomplete. Since both doctors and patients realized that others would read their comments, they certainly considered their audience when deciding what to write and what to leave unsaid.

In Sally's case, her dossier of medical charts and letters neglected or omitted many aspects of her life. It says little about her family and virtually nothing about her husband. Nowhere does it mention her schooling as a child or the precise nature of her work as an adult. From this silence we obviously should not infer that these issues were unimportant to Sally or to her health—rather, they simply were not considered noteworthy or relevant by either patient or practitioner. On the other hand, her medical record accentuates other issues. In particular, the details of her daily regimen, such as how many calories she was ingesting or how much insulin she was injecting, are noted repeatedly both by the doctors and by Sally (which is hardly surprising, given that many of her letters were direct responses to questions that Joslin or other doctors had asked). The medical record also compiled much greater detail about the acute exacerbations of her illness than about the nonthreatening—and hence "normal"—periods of her life with chronic illness. Finally, many of the exchanges between Sally or her mother and the clinic physicians addressed tensions generated specifically by the Joslin Clinic's philosophy of diabetic control, such as pursuing expensive medical care. Her record, then, is in part a dialogue about the practical implications of the Joslin system of belief—but a dialogue conducted largely within what were deemed to be the rules of proper patient and doctor roles and relations.

In other words, the charts of diabetic patients such as Sally were a mélange of facts and perceptions, an assemblage of judgments and opinions. They therefore must be read carefully, scrutinized for what they say and what they neglect to say, taking account of their bias toward extreme events and against certain kinds of routine health behavior. Nevertheless, these files do offer clues to the daily structure of diabetic lives, to the oft-repeated tasks, mundane expectations, and unwritten rules that imbued them with meaning and a semblance of order.

For instance, Sally's chart indicates that she, like Jim Havens, tinkered with her insulin dosages. Several of her notes to the Joslin Clinic physicians refer in detail to when and how much insulin she injected and assert the independence of her judgment on these matters. "I am feeling fine and have felt so for a long time," she told Joslin in the autumn of 1936, shortly after the long-acting protamine insulin had been introduced to the market. She was still taking regular insulin, four times a day. "I haven't started to take the new Insulin. Thought it was just as well not to do so just yet as long as I am getting along all right."[41] Two and a half years later, she told White that she had "tried taking the Protamine Zinc but didn't seem to have much luck. At the end of a month's trial I was taking sixty units daily and then had to take forty units of the regular Insulin to clear up the sugar."[42] Writing again in the summer of 1941, Sally let White know that "I have been feeling fine for a long time. Had to reduce my [regular] Insulin because of reactions."[43] In response to these daily practical problems of diabetic life, Sally made these educated judgments based upon her personal experience and the tenets that Joslin had taught—and this is precisely how Joslin wanted his ideally knowledgeable patients to run their lives. Even as she exercised her autonomy in reaching these decisions on her own, she framed her choices, at least in her letters, in accordance with Joslin's principles of diabetic management.

Sally's case file also illustrates how she grappled in her daily life with the advent of new medical technologies and novel standards of care. Current notions of routine medical care are amalgams, combining much older ideas about healthy regimens with modern techniques of preventing or screening for disease. During the twentieth century, American physicians developed the practice of what we might call preventive medicine or health promotion, first with the well-baby visits advocated by pediatricians, followed by trips to the doctor for an ever-widening array of vaccinations and screening tests such as blood pressure measurements, pap smears, or mammograms.[44]

For Sally and other diabetics, the hidden disease that many doctors targeted during the 1930s and 1940s was early tuberculosis. In 1934, Joslin's younger colleague, Howard F. Root, published a series of articles in the *New England Journal of Medicine* on the perils that tuberculosis posed to diabetics: nearly three-fourths of the juvenile patients who attended the Joslin Clinic, by the time they were twenty, had signs of incipient pulmonary tuberculosis. Root stressed, among other things, that "the hope for the future of diabetic tuberculosis lies in earlier diagnosis." Like other aggressive public health activists who campaigned against the tubercular White Plague during the interwar years, he turned to a new medical technology that appeared to be a peerless surveillance tool and hence a potent weapon in the battle against tuberculosis. Root recommended in addition to tuberculin skin tests "more frequent examination of the lungs by x-ray," believing that "early tuberculous lesions may be discovered when adequate treatment will permit healing to occur."[45]

Root put his suggestions into practice for the Joslin Clinic patients. Although Sally had no symptoms of tuberculosis, he urged her to have a chest X ray. She declined: "To be very frank about it, I cannot come to Boston and don't feel I can afford to go to [our local hospital] for x-ray much as I would like to."[46] A month later, Root told Sally that he was "still very anxious to get that x-ray of your chest," suggesting that she could get it "done near your home in one of the state clinics and that would cost you nothing."[47] Although the chart does not record her motivations for wanting to get the X ray, by the end of July, Sally's local doctor had sent a copy of the chest radiograph to Root.[48] Even though the roentgenogram showed no disease, her decision to be screened for tuberculosis (once again influenced by financial concerns) had added another level of vigilance to her life.

Finally, Sally's frequently repeated statement—"I feel well most of the time"—expressed a common sentiment among diabetics who were in good health. As she went on to say in a letter written several months after the United States entered World War II, "Outside of the fact that I have to take Insulin I seem to feel as well as most normal people."[49] Her comment suggested motion in two allied but distinct directions: away from illness and toward a state of de facto normality. The first direction depended upon the state of her health and the strange disregard that many people develop for nondescript medical events that happen each and every day. Like any other daily ritual, the routine of diabetic self-care during prolonged periods of good health would often recede into the background of a patient's life.

The second direction, striving after the life of "normal people," represented more than simply a movement away from illness or a "take up thy bed" attitude that spurned the limitations of sickness: it was a movement toward an elusive vision of the twentieth-century American dream. In 1920 President Harding had urged the country to return to a state of "normalcy": a clarion call to pursue a cultural mirage. Nostalgia crossed with naïveté, normalcy was a search for simplicity and security. As the new technology of mass advertising subtly promoted a commercialized version of the archetypal normal life, many people—particularly those who were chronically ill—were progressively estranged from this prevailing vision of who ideal Americans were. Although we can not be certain what Sally meant by "feeling as well as most normal people," by the middle of the twentieth century she could have been referring not only to the lives of others around her but also to a wider cultural depiction of the normal life as portrayed in newspapers, magazines, radio, and, within a few years, television. With World War II destroying any sense of normalcy abroad or at home, she felt well and was grateful for that—but how did she feel being childless in a culture that revered domesticity and motherhood, or how would she react in years to come as her good health failed and she was increasingly economically dependent in a culture that prized independence and productivity? While Sally never openly lamented her exclusion from the "normal life" of American culture, other diabetics—as we shall see—did.[50]

"COMPLICATIONS" AND THE
DENOUEMENT OF DIABETIC LIFE

Many diabetics, in following the orderly rules of hygiene, sought to maintain their fragile status quo of health. Particularly during the latter stages of their lives, the disease would threaten their conception of themselves as competent individuals, capable of earning a living or raising a family. Their individual dramas, as they proceeded toward frequently ambiguous and unsettling conclusions, would often draw on family members to play supportive roles as the disease dissolved autonomy and disrupted time.

In the typical diabetic life course of the Joslin Clinic patients, mothers served as the advocates when their children were first diagnosed. The mother brought the youngster to the clinic and corresponded with the physicians. Then, sometime during the teen years or early twenties, the patient typically assumed the duty of communicating with the doctors, the mother's voice disappearing from the records for twenty or more years. If the patient stayed well, the mother never returned. But in several cases in which the adult child became ill, the mother suddenly resumed her previous role as liaison and advocate. The patient—as in Sally's case—would become eerily silent. Disease had reversed the life cycle. For both patient and parent, the final chapters of their experiences with diabetes became meditations upon stress and coping, as they attempted to pursue and maintain hope, come to grips with disappointment and mounting debility, and ultimately apportion responsibility for sickness between themselves and their doctors.

In 1948, twenty-seven years after being diagnosed with diabetes, Sally first wrote to Joslin that she had a "kidney condition" and high blood pressure and that "I am still working although I find it very difficult to do so. My appetite is not very good."[51] This news must have been no surprise to Joslin and his staff. By the middle of the 1940s, the prospect of renal damage and failure among diabetics was well known. In 1935, Paul Kimmelstiel and Clifford Wilson of Boston City Hospital had identified a specific lesion in the kidneys of diabetics, providing a pathological explanation for the occasional diabetic who developed renal failure. Thereafter, as the juvenile diabetics—a population that barely existed prior to 1922—began to age, progressive renal failure emerged as a menace (Figure 3.4). Perhaps most disturbing, this then-intractably-lethal process of kidney damage afflicted patients who were only middle-aged (Figure 3.5).

Sally appeared to follow this sad course. Shortly after receiving her letter regarding her "kidney condition," Joslin wrote to her offering his help, and then to her physician, inquiring whether there was "anything I can do for her through you: Would you want her to come down here? If finances are a problem, please tell me. We are very much interested in patients who have had diabetes for 27 years and will do everything possible to help them."[52] Two years later, Sally's condition further de-

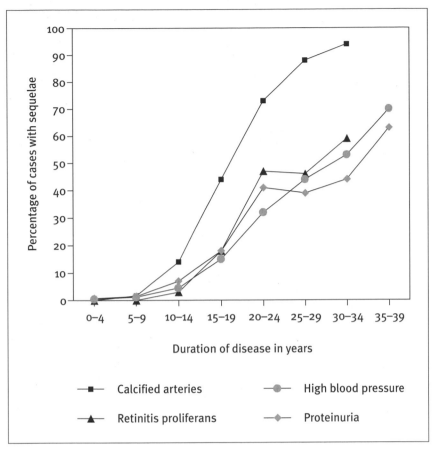

Figure 3.4. The Cumulative Incidence of Long-Term Sequelae of Juvenile Diabetes, by Duration of Diabetes, Joslin Clinic, 1898–1956. Source: *Adapted from Priscilla White, "Natural Course and Prognosis of Juvenile Diabetes,"* Diabetes *5 (November 1956): 445–50.*

teriorated when she had a left-sided stroke (another known complication of the transmuted disease) that rendered her unable to work. This prompted her, for the first time in eighteen years, to make the journey from southern New Hampshire to the Joslin Clinic, where the doctors detected retinopathy and early stages of renal failure. Dr. Beetham, the ophthalmologist affiliated with the Joslin group, told her "to take life as easy as possible."[53]

Half a year later, in early 1951, Sally's mother wrote to Dr. Robert Bradley, one of the young doctors at the Joslin Clinic. "Dear Sir: Would you be so kind as to try to answer one question—can anything be done

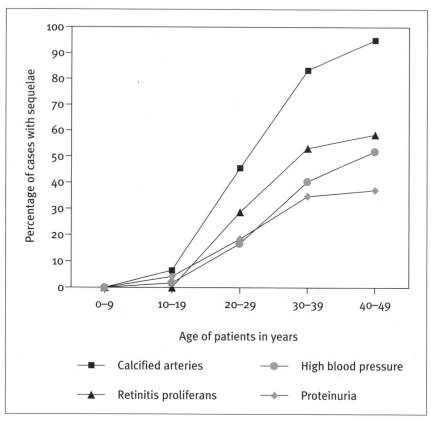

Figure 3.5. The Cumulative Incidence of Long-Term Sequelae of Juvenile Diabetes, by Age of Patient, Joslin Clinic, 1898–1956. Source: *Adapted from Priscilla White, "Natural Course and Prognosis of Juvenile Diabetes,"* Diabetes 5 *(November 1956): 445–50.*

to make Sally's kidneys function better, or can anything be done to make her feel better?" Apparently, shortly after Sally had returned home in August, her symptoms worsened. "She was very sick and she has never really recovered. She just drags around, has no strength or ambition, but she does want to get well and go back to work." Mrs. Kramer, who decades earlier had seen her "terminally ill" daughter rescued miraculously by insulin, still believed in medical science. "There seems to be so many new things being discovered all the while," she told Bradley, "and I am sure you would know if anything was discovered that would help her." Recently, her family had "read in the papers about the lady who had a kidney transplanted. Has this operation been a success? [Our local doctor] has not said so in so many words, but his attitude seems to say there is no help for her and it is awfully hard to take." Yet, as much as Mrs. Kramer yearned for a second miracle to rejuvenate her daughter, the seasoned mother looked to Bradley through the lens of years of dealing with doctors and hospitals: "Please don't ask her to come to Boston *unless you think you can help her* because money really is one draw back, and disappointment is another."[54]

Bradley responded that it was "all too true that very little hope can be extended for any improvement in the function of your daughter's kidneys." He dismissed the possibility of either transplantation or dialysis as unrealistic for a diabetic, explaining that these procedures, still experimental, were considered only when the renal failure was viewed as transient. "Unfortunately such is not the case with Sally." Bradley believed that she had extensive arteriosclerosis throughout her body and concluded that there was "only one possible course of action that might benefit in your daughter's case." He suggested she might gain some temporary relief from a strict rice and fruit diet, one with virtually no salt or protein. Although he warned that this diet was "a drastic program for anyone to follow," he felt she was "now desperate enough that such a program would be advisable." Since the severe diet produced a "considerable shift in body minerals and nitrogen," Sally would have to be hospitalized when she began it.[55]

Mrs. Kramer, upon receiving Bradley's letter, questioned him further. "Could you give us a general idea about the length of time she would be required to stay there, also what would be the approximate cost per week for Doctors and Hospital?" She also wanted to know whether Sally would have "to stay on this diet for the rest of her life (that is if it helped her)." Before closing her letter, Mrs. Kramer explained, "You see we are really trying to find out if the results would be worth the sacrifices we would be called upon to make."[56]

Sally decided to try the severe treatment and in March traveled back to the Deaconess Hospital. There, her doctors found that her renal failure was being exacerbated by a flare of pyelonephritis (a serious kidney infection) caused by bacteria that were resistant to penicillin but sensitive to other antibiotics. "Fortunately," when the appropriate antibiotics were given, her "pain and fever subsided very readily." Since Sally had "found the diet unpalatable," she was placed on a simpler salt-restricted diabetic diet.[57]

A month after her discharge, Sally's mother again wrote, informing Bradley that her daughter was now working three hours an afternoon, even though "she gets very nervous before going to work each day but after she gets there and goes to work she gets over it." Sally did not care for the salt-free diet, and so Mrs. Kramer asked whether her daughter could "have the new plastic drug that takes care of the sodium in the diet, when it comes on the market." She concluded that Sally "has been feeling better since she came back from Boston. I think her mind was relieved by things you told her—but I am not too sure about the work, if it is helping her or not—she does too much worrying about it."[58]

Mrs. Kramer next corresponded with Sally's doctors in January of 1953. "Sally is not very well," she informed Joslin. "Since Thanksgiving she has had infection in or around [her left] kidney three times. She is just getting over an attack now. It seems to bother her sight as well as her ability to walk." Mrs. Kramer reported that Sally was "very discouraged and wanted me to ask you if things have progressed so that any help for her was in sight?"[59]

Her forty-year-old daughter died two months later.

NARRATION AND CREATING MEANING IN LIFE

In the introduction, I compared this book metaphorically to a series of tours through a vast museum of diabetic history, each tour organized around a theme or concept. Another way to view the book is as a compilation of diabetic life stories. So far we have considered two, a narrative of Jim Havens's diabetic life set in the context of the cycles of diabetic transformation and now a story of Sally's life situated in her diabetic life course. As more follow, this collection of stories displays the wide range of patient experience and suggests that there are numerous perspectives from which to view the history of a chronic disease and its effect upon people.

This multiplicity of possible perspectives raises points worth pondering. If we wish to recount events—whether they transpired decades ago to others or are affecting us now—we have to choose which perspective to adopt and by so doing unavoidably set the tone of the narrative, shaping the meaning of the story. When a historian adopts a certain outlook or point of view, this decision has far-reaching implications, subsequently influencing the content and style of the final product. This book's patient-oriented perspective, for instance, guided how I made choices when I attempted to line up the stories of several people into a coherent narrative. Since the chronological story lines of their individual cases often splintered and diverged, I had to pick which story line to pursue. In Sally's narrative, people walked in and out of her life—from where? to where? What aspects of their lives matter? Should it concern us that Howard Root was a social worker before he became a physician? Or that Priscilla White never married? Or that throughout his life Elliott Joslin thought about the children who died before insulin was developed? And what of Mrs. Kramer, who figures so prominently in Sally's life yet appears in the medical chart only as the mother of a diabetic daughter? Or what of other family members? The narrative line of Sally's story—or the story of any other diabetic—would be further splintered if we tried to trace the developments in all the various areas of her life. Each context had, to a degree, its own history and chronology. While some choices I made regarding which among the many possible story lines to emphasize were based on limitations in the available historical sources, as frequently my decisions were based on my personal sense that the focus should be on Sally and the other patients: my choice of a patient-oriented perspective has had a profound influence on the tale I have told.[60]

Yet the problem of narrative perspective is not just the historian's problem. Lack of coherence often dominates patient experience, with illness disrupting both daily schedules and the larger sweep of what patients expect from their lives as they age, as flares of illness impose forms of dependency that seem to wind time backward toward childhood.[61] Medical accounts of chronic illness have dealt with these troubling features of patients' personal experiences largely by ignoring them. From the beginning of the twentieth century, the biomedical story of disease increasingly has commandeered a wide variety of stories about personal illness, reframing how our culture thinks about health problems with a few reductive questions: What caused this disease? Can it be treated? If so, how? While these focused questions serve a clear purpose with acute ailments, the resulting habits of common medical language and practice are too impoverished to capture the range of experience with chronic illness, and thus are too limited when physicians talk with patients about what has happened, what is likely to happen, and what they should do.

In contrast to the traditionally scientific way that medicine makes sense of disease as a single unified story, our emerging view of what living with diabetes has entailed needs to accommodate the diversity of stories told by patients about their experiences, especially since these stories have been one means for people to cope with a chronic illness that threatens life and potentially erodes its meanings.[62] Similar to the choices faced by a historian regarding which perspective to adopt when trying to retell a piece of history, choices made by those living with chronic illness or practicing medicine regarding how to view disease and its role in our lives have important implications. Patients and health care providers decide—usually implicitly but sometimes explicitly—what perspective they will adopt, choosing, for example, to view disease as an enemy that must be combated literally to the death, or as an unwanted yet dogged companion that must be tolerated and managed as best as possible, or some version in between. The characteristics of the disease (such as its likelihood of causing disability or death) and potential therapy (such as the likelihood of success or burden of side effects) are considerations that enter into the decision of which perspective to adopt, but so are the values, beliefs, and overall outlook on life of the patient or physician. Hybrids, then, of facts and values, these different illness perspectives influence how patients and physicians view themselves, the manner in which they conduct their relationship with each other, the nature of the health care choices that they make, and ultimately the experiences that patients have with their illnesses. The importance of what illness perspective is adopted cannot—in my view as a physician—be overemphasized. If this compilation of diabetic life stories enables us to become more self-conscious about the choice of perspective and to become more aware of its significance, then this history will be relevant not merely to our understanding of the past but also to our understanding of our future encounters with disease.

4

GETTING
THE POINT:
THE DAILY
WORK OF
DIABETES

Work shortens the day, but lengthens the life.
—Epigram from Joslin's *Diabetic Manual,* 1959

"I gave my first patient insulin," Joslin recalled years after the fact, "on August 7, 1922."[1] Elizabeth Mudge—her widely known true name—was a nurse who had become diabetic in July of 1917. She was thirty-seven years old. For the next two years, before coming under Joslin's care, she restricted her diet by omitting sugar and starches. Five feet five inches tall, Mudge lost forty pounds on this limited diet, dropping to one hundred and three pounds when Joslin weighed her in June of 1919. Her weight continued to plummet, so that by August of 1922—having survived several encounters with diabetic coma—she weighed a scant seventy-one pounds, living on a daily diet of just under 900 calories. The strict dietetic treatment, while allowing Mudge to live with her disease, had reduced the once-active nurse into a debilitated shut-in: she had ventured out of her Boston apartment only once during the previous months of 1922.[2]

A year earlier, in the late summer of 1921, Banting and Best had reveled in their first flush of experimental success: dogs whose pancreases had been removed and would otherwise have died swiftly of diabetes were kept alive by injections of a substance that had been extracted from the dogs' own pancreases. "Isletin," as they called the extract, appeared to lower the dogs' blood sugar to normal levels. After such heady results, the youthful investigators were hardly prepared for the nine months of difficulties that followed, as the development of purified insulin from this crude extract was fraught with technical difficulty and personal strife among the research group. Still, by January of 1922 the first diabetic patient had received an injection of insulin in Toronto. By the summer, the University of Toronto and Eli Lilly and Company (which was producing insulin commercially) had selected a group of esteemed diabetes specialists in America to test Iletin (the brand name) on their patients. By the sixth of August, a small batch of insulin had reached Joslin in Boston.[3]

And so, prior to lunchtime on the seventh of August, Mudge became the first diabetic in New England to receive insulin (Jim Havens having already been treated in upstate New York). Joslin's junior colleague, Howard F. Root, administered the dose. Having so little insulin on hand, and unsure of how potently the drug would act, Root injected only one-third of a cubic centimeter. This tiny amount seemed to do nothing. Mudge experienced no dramatic improvement in strength or vigor, and her blood sugar remained right were it had been, hovering above 0.30 percent. The next day, the doctors doubled the dose—still nothing. By the end of a week, they had increased the amount to four c.c., and at last the blood sugar fell below the 0.30 percent level. At the same time, Joslin was enlarging her diet. By the twentieth of August, he began to divide the four c.c. dose in half, establishing a pattern of giving 2 c.c. sometime in the morning and 2 c.c. in the late afternoon. Gradually, the wonder drug restored Mudge to a state of full vigor. Six weeks after that first dose, she was able "to walk with ease 4 miles daily," and by early 1923 she had "gained 10.5 pounds, and now cares for her invalid mother."[4] As she lived another quarter century with the drug's assistance, reaching the age of sixty-six years in good health before dying suddenly of a heart attack, Mudge certainly represented in the mind of Joslin and many others another success for insulin.[5]

By the beginning of 1923, Joslin had given the drug to another eighty-odd patients, ranging in age from two to seventy-seven years; thirty-three patients were twenty years old or younger. Many of the children recovered miraculously. Joslin was especially moved by insulin's effect on an eight-year-old named Frederic. Diabetic since the fall of 1919, "the little boy was so hungry that he would burn his hands taking food out of a hot oven, would get up at night when others were asleep to secure food." In November of 1922, his parents brought him "to the hospital saying, 'Dr. Joslin, do anything you want with Frederic, you can't make him any worse.' At that time he was carried in on a cushion, but about two weeks after his return home his mother reported that he was carrying a gun on his shoulder while marching with the other children." Similarly, five-year-old Dorothy had been unable to walk prior to insulin "but now 'walks up and down stairs, and dances with her brothers.'"

One can imagine Joslin and his colleagues staring in awe at these resurrected children, moving the physicians to exclaim that "nothing we can say based upon laboratory results can equal in importance statements of this character."[6]

Such pronouncements of wonder did not, however, do away with the realities—prosaic and profound—of living with a disease transformed by medical intervention, in particular the work that diabetes as a chronic illness entailed. This work—hidden in the repetitious routine of living with a chronic disorder—has been fundamental, constituting almost the fabric of history as lived by these patients. For similar reasons, though, these mundane daily tasks are difficult to depict and therefore have largely been neglected. Historical sagas of chronic illness, as a result, tend to "fast-forward" over the quotidian struggles and skip to acute exacerbations or other "interesting" events, essentially rendering the pace of the chronic condition as a more "exciting" acute disease. The work of diabetes has existed in many forms.[7] Each and every day of the twentieth century, diabetics and their families have had to manage the many challenges that the disease presents, from physiological abnormalities to social stigma. At a practical level, diabetics simply have to take care of themselves. Their lives have been marked by repetitious ritual: test the urine, inject the insulin, eat according to a prescribed schedule. To these necessities were added the intimate tasks that attend to the annoying or painful or dangerous complications of the disease: clip the toenails, inspect the feet, bathe in warm water for a flare of neuritis.

In these daily skirmishes with their ailments, people living with diabetes have looked for assistance, advice, and comfort from their doctors and nurses. During the twentieth century these patients and their families and health care providers had developed in the United States a complex system to manage the disease. In the pre-insulin era, it revolved around diets and urine tests for sugar. Since then, not only have various insulins entered this management system, but so have sharper syringes, more frequent blood sugar tests, softer shoes, pressure dressings, oral hypoglycemic agents, and other drugs. Diabetics also have to deal increasingly with many health care providers, extending beyond family practitioner to diabetic specialists, outpatient clinics, educational nurses, dietitians, social workers, and laboratory technicians. To no small degree, diabetics have had to manage the work that interacting with this management system has created.

For more than fifty years, patients young and old climbed the two steps leading into the house at 81 Bay State Road in the Back Bay section of Boston, opened the door, and entered the medical offices of Doctor Elliott P. Joslin and his associates. The doctor and his family had moved into the house in 1906, and there the clinic resided until 1956, when Joslin moved his burgeoning practice just a mile away to specially constructed quarters adjacent to the New England Deaconess Hospital. During the half century before this move, nearly fifty thousand patients crossed the threshold of the original Joslin Clinic, and whether they traveled alone or were accompanied by parents, spouses, or children, they all traversed those two steps.[8]

Many patients probably approached Joslin's clinic from downtown Boston. Walking into the Back Bay section along Bay State Road, they would have passed by several physicians' offices, housed in grand dwellings of lush red stone, before coming upon the plain brick front of number 81. Separated from the sidewalk by a narrow strip of lawn, the five-story building looked down upon the street through eleven windows, two on each floor, except for the three narrow windows of the attic. The door, bracketed by two simple columns, stood on the right, just above those two steps.

Up the steps and through the door, the patients—if they had heeded instructions and come prepared—left a bottle of their urine, neatly labeled, in the small laboratory room that was immediately to their left. Farther up the hall they came to the room where several secretaries kept the clinic in motion. After registering, the patients would ascend the next flight of stairs to the second floor and take a seat in the large hallway that served as the waiting room. At the front of this floor, looking over the street, the doctor had his private office, where he dictated letters and, in addition to his many articles, wrote his textbook on diabetes and his *Diabetic Manual for the Mutual Use of Doctor and Patient.* In the middle of the house were the examining room and a lavatory.[9]

Patients most likely did not know how the back of the second floor and the remainder of the house accommodated the Joslin family and their maids. Both the large dining room at the rear of the second floor and the living room overhead had a view of the adjacent Charles River, which in the early years of the twentieth century was often a malodorous tidal estuary. Immediately above Joslin's office in the front of the house was the master bedroom for the doctor and his wife, Elizabeth

Denny Joslin, whom he had married in 1902. In these rooms and others in the house, the Joslins raised their daughter, Mary, and sons, Allen and Elliott Jr.

Sitting in the hall, those patients who were devotees of Joslin's *Manual* may have thumbed through their personal notebooks, preparing to "show it to [their] physician at each visit." In these booklets, Joslin advised, "all questions about symptoms and diet which have arisen since the former visit should be neatly set down, with space left for an answer to each question." Such notebooks would eventually become individualized manuals for patients, fitting their particular needs and concerns. "It is a common error," in Joslin's opinion, "for patients to ask the same question many times, whereas if the answer is written down by the physician the question would thus be answered once for all time."[10]

Patients well-versed in the *Manual* might also have glanced at "a list" tucked between the pages of their notebooks "of what they ate in the preceding twenty-four hours," itemizing for each meal both the nature and quantity of foods they had eaten. This dietary account made the visit to the doctor even more efficient, freeing time for the head-to-toe physical examination that diabetic care required. "If thirty minutes are allowed for a visit to the physician's office," Joslin observed, "it is no exaggeration to say that unless this recording of the diet is neatly done, one-third to one-half of the visit is spent by the physician in learning what the patient has eaten."[11]

Regardless of whether they had arrived prepared with urine, notebook, and diet list—or whether they came with only their irksome symptoms—these patients sitting in the hall all did exactly that: sat and waited, mulling no doubt over their condition and those of the patients who sat next to them. Pervasive though this experience was in the lives of diabetics during the twentieth century, at 81 Bay State Road and countless other medical offices spread around the United States, few patients left any record of how they viewed the experience of making a visit to the doctor.

Fortunately, Guy Rainsford was one patient who did, and did so in his own inimitable style: Rainsford drew cartoons. Subtly observed and satirically pointed, these drawings offer a special chance to see how one man viewed the diabetic life. A traveling salesman from Maine, Rainsford (unlike the other patients who appear in this book) became diabetic in his midforties, learning that there was sugar in his urine after a routine physical examination in the spring of 1924. One year later

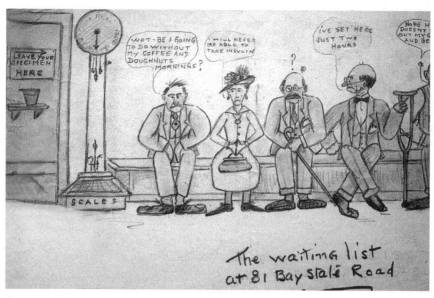

"*The Waiting List.*" *Guy Rainsford cartoon.*
Courtesy of the Joslin Diabetes Center Historical Archive.

he saw Joslin at 81 Bay State Road, beginning a relationship that lasted until Rainsford's death two decades later.[12]

During these twenty-odd years, Rainsford sent Joslin more than three dozen cartoons that depicted a variety of scenes from his own diabetic world, scenes such as "The waiting list at 81 Bay State Road, 2 to 5—any day." Seven disparate characters are pictured sitting on a bench, a weight scale to their right, a door into the "LABRATORY 'WEE WEE' DEPT." to their left. Each patient broods upon private thoughts. One middle-aged gentleman wonders, "Wot-be I going to do without my coffee and doughnuts mornings," while another thinks about his meeting with Joslin and "hope[s] he doesn't cut out my grog and beer," and a third man, looking peevish, complains, "I've set here just two hours." A slender lady with a frown on her face asserts, "I will never be able to take insulin," as a rotund lady at the end of the bench remarks, "Don't I hope I ain't got diabetis, hope he don't give me no physical examination, I am that shy." The boy perched next to her wistfully exclaims: "So long lolly pops." In Rainsford's estimation, such a rich dose of humanity, repeated every day, was "why doctors become slightly nutty at 50."

Rainsford's humorous and often ironic renderings of diabetic life offer a rare opportunity to explore an aspect of the diabetic world that warrants close attention—the ceaseless drudge of daily work.

MONITORING WORK

A nearly ubiquitous feature of current management of chronic illnesses such as diabetes (or disease such as cancer, heart disease, or depression) is some degree of ongoing monitoring. Doctors check whether a medication is working well, reducing symptoms or minimizing a health threat while not producing unacceptable side effects. Patients keep watch for changes in symptoms, or perhaps keep records of how their bodies respond to medication over time. The information gathered by these monitoring activities is used to guide future treatment and, it is hoped, to avoid therapeutic harm.

In diabetes care today, this monitoring has evolved to include periodic examinations of the eyes, feet, and skin, readings of the blood pressure, testing of sensation, and analysis of the urine for protein or other signs of kidney damage. Since introduced in the late 1970s, home blood glucose monitoring has also become commonplace, along with tracking of the level of glycosylated hemoglobin A1c (which indicates where the blood glucose level typically has been for the prior three months).

For most of the twentieth century, though, checking the urine for sugar was the mainstay of diabetic monitoring. With the development in 1911 by Stanley Benedict of a simple color-coded method of assessing the amount of sugar in the urine (with blue indicating no sugar, green a trace, and yellow, orange, or red increasing amounts of sugar),[13] most diabetic patients tested their urine with Benedict solution, up to several times a day. Joslin had a standard form for a "urine test report card" that had space to record results from tests done before breakfast, before the noon meal, before supper, and at bedtime. Each run of the test required the patient to obtain a fresh sample of urine, to add eight to ten drops of the urine to a teaspoon of the Benedict solution in a test tube, and then to heat this mixture to a boil for three minutes, allowing it to cool before examining the mixture's color. The time needed to perform the test four times in a day could add up. By the mid-1950s, simpler methods to test urine for sugar were being developed, including self-heating tablets and then test strips that were simply dipped into a sample of urine and watched for an almost immediate change in color. While these methods reduced the time required to test the urine for sugar, the daily work

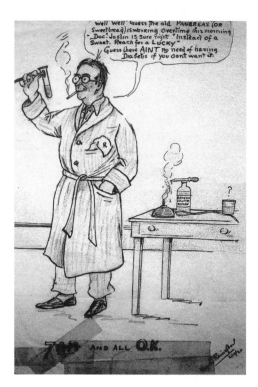

"*7 A.M. and All OK.*" *Guy Rainsford cartoon. Courtesy of the Joslin Diabetes Center Historical Archive.*

of monitoring was still considerable, especially since it had to fit into a schedule that accommodated the other work that patients had to do and since the information gathered through monitoring work was not always uplifting.

Rainsford illustrated both the time-consuming labor and the emotional implications of monitoring work. In one cartoon he announces to Joslin, "7 A.M. AND ALL O.K." Despite the hassle of testing the urine, his mood is bright. "Well well, guess the old 'PANCREAS' (or Sweetbread) is working overtime this morning. . . . Guess there AINT no need of having Diabetis if you don't want it." In another cartoon, however, Rainsford depicted himself "Giving the S.O.S. at 7 A.M." With Joslin's *Manual* tucked in the pocket of his bathrobe and a blood red Benedict test urine sample in his hand, he cries out to his wife: "Oh, Marion! Come quick for gosh sake—IT'S TERRIBLE 'WORSIN' I THOUGHT." Meanwhile, the artist personified his personal voice of self-recrimination in the form of a cat beneath the kitchen table who wisecracks: "What did he expect— eating pie-cake and ice cream. Probably taught him a lesson."

The cat's opinion was quite similar to Joslin's. While some physicians

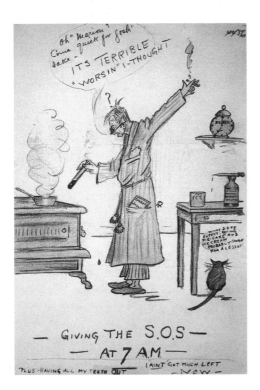

"Giving the S.O.S. at 7 A.M."
Guy Rainsford cartoon. Courtesy
of the Joslin Diabetes Center
Historical Archive.

believed that occasional lapses of diabetic control were entirely understandable, the venerable doctor from Boston viewed the matter differently. Lecturing to a British audience in 1955, Joslin noted, "The idea
has been raised [by other physicians] that a diabetic should not feel he
has done wrong if he has a poor Benedict test. I disagree. When I see
a red test, I know, if uncorrected, that patient is headed for destruction."[14] This view—combining as it did a conceivably objective prognosis
about future complications with implicit value-laden judgments about
the patient's conduct (a combination taken up in much greater detail
in Chapter 5)—cast the daily work of monitoring not simply as a system
that would provide feedback to enable corrective adjustments but as a
daily exercise that taught almost moral lessons in the struggle against
dietary temptation or self-care laxity.

DIET WORK

What to eat? People have long sought foods that would maintain or improve health, and dietary prescriptions have been a time-
honored component of medical practice.[15] As mentioned in earlier

chapters, during the century prior to insulin's discovery, physicians put forward a variety of diets as means to treat diabetes, from John Rollo's "animal diet" to Frederick Allen's "starvation diets." Increasingly, two rationales appear to have shaped the dietary advice. The first involved the "basic science" of food and metabolism, addressing the three fundamental food components (carbohydrate, protein, and fat), the calorie content of the diet, and some measure of the body's ability to metabolize the food appropriately. The second rationale focused on the ability and willingness of patients to follow the advice. Finding dietary schemes that met the objectives of each rationale was challenging.

Joslin responded to this challenge, characteristically, by imposing order. He applied this managerial strategy to all aspects of diabetic care, from nursing a patient in diabetic ketoacidosis back from the abyss to organizing efficiently the information in medical records.[16] To guide food choice, by the late 1910s Joslin had designed a five-day series of "test diets," each day providing fewer calories and carbohydrates than the preceding day.[17] An educator of patients and physicians alike, Joslin realized that the simpler his instructions, the better. Under his plan, a patient would proceed through the series until one of the test diets produced sugar-free urine. The diet on this day would indicate the diabetic's "tolerance" or capacity to metabolize food safely. The patient would then be switched to a "maintenance diet," which specified the amount of carbohydrate, protein, fat, and total calories.

To adhere to either the test or the maintenance diets, patients had to know—for any particular food they wished to eat—both the basic content of the food and the precise amount they intended to eat. Details mattered. In his *Diabetic Manual,* Joslin illustrated how eggs, potatoes, oranges, and grapefruit could differ in size, and thus differ in caloric content. He recommended that patients use a finely calibrated kitchen scale to weigh everything that they intended to eat in order to determine exactly how much protein, fat, and carbohydrate they were ingesting. To aid the patient in doing the necessary "diabetic arithmetic," Joslin even went so far as to print, on a pocket-sized 3-by-5 inch card, abbreviated guidelines for choosing foods that fit the total dietary prescription.

The daily chore of figuring out what to eat became less burdensome after 1950, when the U.S. Public Health Service, the American Diabetes Association, and the American Dietetic Association published a pamphlet titled *Exchanges Lists for Meal Planning.* This diet management

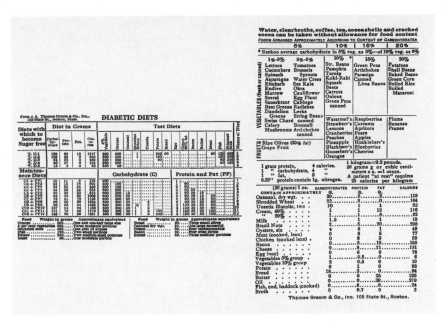

Food category pocket card, front and back. From author's private collection.

system (which has been revised extensively over the years) classified all foods into six groups based on their basic composition, provided a few basic meal menus, and then gave instructions on how to exchange single-portion servings of various food items within each class.[18]

Even though the process of choosing the right type and amount of food became simpler over the second half of the twentieth century, abiding by any set of dietary limits remained (and remains) a challenge. The typical complaint of menu monotony, lodged as far back as 1797 against Rollo's animal diet, has endured and can be heard today. Nonetheless, nutritional advice and dietary fads have proliferated endlessly in the United States, as Americans seeking better health have been willing to eat—at least for a time—other than as their appetite would dictate. Rainsford, for instance, had been encouraged by Joslin to eat so-called 5 percent vegetables (that is, vegetables with only a small amount of carbohydrate, such as lettuce, cucumbers, tomatoes, broccoli, or leeks). In a cartoon that he sent to Joslin wishing him a happy Easter, Rainsford conveyed his ambivalence to such a restricted diet. "If I keep up this lettuce and cabbage diet," he quipped, "I'll be hopping around like a rabbit. I look like one now." Yet moving beyond whimsy, he also added, "If lettuce and cabbage does this [that is, lead to a blue-colored urine

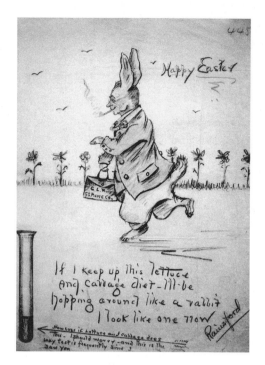

test result, indicating the absence of sugar]—I should worry [that you
will want to keep me on this diet]—and this is the way test is frequently
since I saw you." The common counterweight to any argument against
adhering to a preventive regimen, Rainsford's desire to stay well or his
anxiety over becoming ill, made the work of adhering to his severely
limited diet more palatable, motivating him and other patients to pursue all manner of medical interventions.

INSULIN WORK

"The million members of the Diabetic Club of America," wrote
Joslin and his colleagues in an article titled "Insulin in Hospital and
Home" that appeared in 1923, "occasionally spend a few days in their
various hospital club houses, but for the greater part of the time, like
most club members, they live at home. If insulin is to be of permanent
help in diabetes, it must be usable by diabetics in their own dwellings."[19]
Yet the sanctioned self-directed home use of a potent—and hence dangerous—medication by injection was unprecedented. Early after the
introduction of insulin, many doctors worried that patients placed in
charge at their homes with dosing the correct amount of drug and ad-

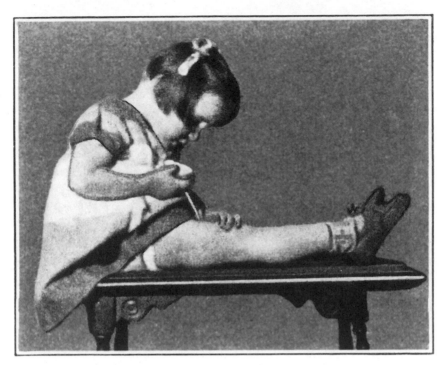

Young girl injecting insulin. From Joslin, Diabetic Manual, *6th ed., 122.*

ministering their own injections would make potentially lethal mistakes. Yet time and clinical experience taught physicians that most patients could master daily injections of insulin: as one physician stated in 1929, "It proved a simple matter to train patients to take insulin."[20] Joslin—quite the master of compelling visual rhetoric—made this point emphatically in his 1934 *Manual* by picturing a small girl injecting herself with insulin, holding her up as an inspiring example of proper training in action, of what today might be called an empowered patient.

When learning how to administer the injections, patients (or their parents) were given step-by-step instruction. First, the equipment necessary to inject the insulin had to be gathered and prepared. These supplies included not only a needle and the barrel and piston of the syringe but also—until the introduction of disposable needles and syringes in the late 1960s and early 1970s—some form of whetstone to keep the needlepoint sharp. To sterilize the equipment, the needle and syringe had to be either boiled or soaked in alcohol for three minutes. Patients then had to assemble the apparatus, taking care not to contaminate it.

Patients next determined what the appropriate dose of insulin would be, based on their recent diet, exercise, state of health, and urine (or, later, blood) glucose test results, as any of these factors could require them to take more or less insulin than what they typically injected. Retrieving the vial of insulin from the refrigerator or some other cold place, patients drew into the syringe the correct amount of the insulin-containing solution. In the early years of insulin therapy, this task—which has never been as simple as it might sound—was especially difficult. The insulin solutions where not well standardized, so that some batches of insulin were more potent than others. Even after 1930, by which point manufacturers such as Eli Lilly and Company in America and Novo Nordisk Pharmaceuticals in Denmark were making pure insulin solutions of consistent potency, some solutions were made so as to contain more units of insulin per milliliter than other solutions, causing confusion and calculation errors, and either under- or overdoses. Furthermore, the syringes were marked in a way that did not facilitate easy measurement. Not until the late 1940s would syringes with a standardized design for measuring insulin be put into production, and not until the 1970s would the now-uniform insulin concentration of 100 units per milliliter (U100) become widely adopted. Finally, patients quite often took two types of insulin, one fast acting and one slow acting, and so had to draw the insulin dose from two vials, making sure they had the right amount of each.

With the correct amount of insulin loaded into the syringe, patients next identified a suitable site on the body for the injection. Certain areas of the body were known to be more suitable sites for the subcutaneous injections that insulin dosing has required. Since injecting the same site repeatedly would damage nearby tissue, causing adjacent local fat cells to multiply into a so-called lipoma, patients were instructed to rotate the site of injection. Cleaning the overlying skin with a swab of cotton doused in alcohol and allowing it to dry briefly, patients then drove the needle through the upper layers of the skin into the subcutaneous tissue. After pulling back on the syringe (to make sure they had not pierced a blood vessel), they then injected the dose of insulin, pulling the needle out slightly as they did so as to deposit the insulin along a small tract under the skin. Withdrawing the needle completely from the skin and pressing the cotton swab lightly over the injection site, they finally had to clean the equipment in cold water, drying it and replacing a wire into the shaft of the needle.

How did this routine play out day after day for people living with dia-

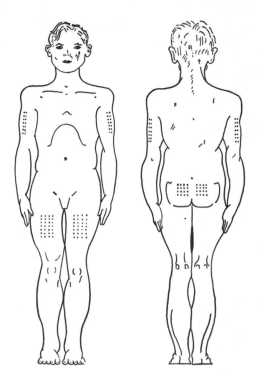

betes? When the process of injecting insulin was described in instructional books for patients with diabetes, illustrative photographs were often used.[21] These pictures had the aura of clinical cleanliness and order about them and typically featured only the disembodied hands of a faceless individual injecting into an arm or thigh. Such staged versions of daily diabetic practice, with the patient effectively kept off camera, contrast sharply with how Rainsford depicted his private injection ritual. He had first taken insulin to control his diabetes at "7 am Sat Sep. 23," capturing in a drawing the moment of "The first 'Jab'" as he injected into his thigh: "Here goes folks—WOW." No longer off-camera, the patient here commands center stage, but not like the small girl in her sanitized—almost saintly—portrait. Instead, Rainsford pictures himself striking quite a different pose, self-deprecating, caught literally with his pants down.

Many of Rainsford's cartoons revel in the tensions between ideals and realities, situating his daily labors in the context of the rest of his life, and casting all of this in the light of his idiosyncratic perspective, bringing out the humor and irony of his relentless skirmishes with his disease. In one portrait, he pictures himself in his pajamas, sitting on the edge

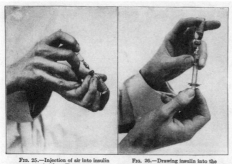

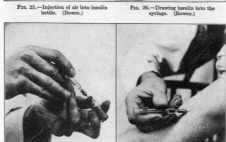

FIG. 25.—Injection of air into insulin bottle. (Bowen.)

FIG. 26.—Drawing insulin into the syringe. (Bowen.)

Disembodied hands injecting insulin. From Joslin, Diabetic Manual, *6th ed., 120.*

of his bed, surrounded not only by his coffee and hot-water bottle, but also his rubbing alcohol, milk of magnesia, and the "Lilly Set" of insulin supplies. "Nothing to do till tomorrow 8 A.M. program," the caption declares, underscoring the amount of work implied by the paraphernalia gathered in the scene. Rainsford seems to have recognized that his ability to self-administer insulin had empowered him to live yet also in part enslaved him in a ceaseless morass of self-care tasks.

SYMPTOM WORK

During the twentieth century, most Americans who lived with diabetes had, at one time or another, to deal with symptoms from their disease. Whether these were annoying chronic problems or acute critical threats to their health, managing symptoms for some patients constituted a large portion of their daily illness-oriented workload.

Episodes of hypoglycemia induced by an overdose of injected insulin—so-called insulin reactions or insulin shock—were (and remain[22]) a particularly worrisome symptom for patients, as well as those people around them who had to provide treatment. Documented in the earliest reports of the drug's use,[23] insulin reactions typically progressed

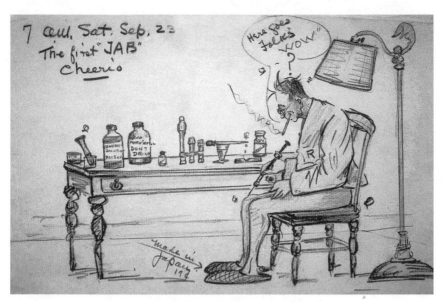

"First Jab." Guy Rainsford cartoon.
Courtesy of the Joslin Diabetes Center Historical Archive.

through stages as the patient's blood sugar level fell lower in response to the excess of insulin. A pamphlet titled *Treatment of Diabetes Mellitus,* published in 1926, described the progression of symptoms:

(1) Sudden and pronounced hunger.
  Sudden weakness or fatigue.
  A peculiar restlessness or nervousness, often described by the patient as a feeling of "inward trembling," or the "shakes."
  Pallor or flushing of the face; dilated pupils.
  Increased pulse rate (of diagnostic value in children).

These early symptoms may be made to disappear quickly and further danger avoided if the patient will immediately eat a little carbohydrate such as one or two lumps of sugar or candy, the juice of an orange, or a teaspoonful of syrup. If the overdose is sufficiently large and the above corrective measures are not adopted, then the following train of symptoms, all or in part, will follow:

(2) Sweating. (This is the most characteristic symptom.)
  Tremor and in-coordination of muscles.
  Anxiety, fear, apprehension, excitement and emotional disturbance.
  Vertigo.

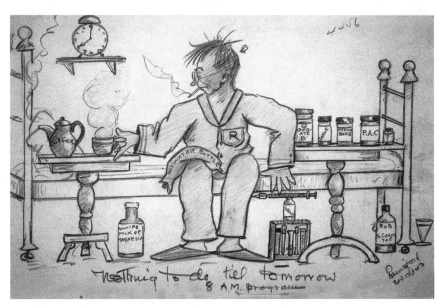

"Nothing to Do." Guy Rainsford cartoon.
Courtesy of the Joslin Diabetes Center Historical Archive.

Diplopia [double vision].
(3) Aphasia [inability to speak], disorientation, delirium, confusion.
(4) Convulsions, collapse.
Low blood pressure; low body temperature.
Unconsciousness.
(5) Exitus lethalis [death].[24]

If the patient's symptoms had worsened to the point where awareness of what was occurring was impaired, then family members, coworkers, or bystanders had to recognize the symptoms of hypoglycemia and basically force-feed the patient some form of sugar (which was difficult if the patient was uncooperative, as often was the case, or unconscious and thus unable to swallow anything safely). In 1961, six years after being isolated in a purified form, preparations of the hormone glucagon became commercially available.[25] A drug also given by injection, glucagon raises blood sugar quickly, counteracting the effect of insulin, and thereby providing another means to treat hypoglycemia regardless of the patient's state of consciousness.

Although insulin reactions during the daytime were, for many patients, socially embarrassing (because of the victims' disinhibited or incoherent behavior) or physically threatening (particularly because of the risk of injury while patients were driving or at work), nighttime bouts of hypoglycemia were viewed as extremely dangerous, as they could progress undetected until the patient began to have convulsions. Concern for nocturnal insulin reactions rose considerably when the longer-acting insulins—protamine, NPH, and the lente insulins—were first introduced in the 1930s, as a dose of these insulins would not have its peak effect in lower blood sugar until hours later, quite possibly in the middle of the night.

Managing insulin-induced hypoglycemia was further complicated by the overlap in symptoms—specifically, altered mental status ranging from irritability to somnolence to unresponsiveness—between insulin reactions and diabetic coma. Although patients experienced the onset of insulin reactions in a matter of minutes, while diabetic acidosis progressed to coma typically over the course of days, both processes culminated in stupor or unconsciousness. At this juncture, anyone happening upon the patient might be confused into thinking that the patient had slipped into acidotic coma instead of recognizing a sudden insulin reaction—or vice versa—and providing the wrong treatment. To guard against this unwitting mistake, Joslin advised that people with diabetes carry in their pockets an identification card, and he reported in the 1937 edition of his *Manual* that "one of my patients wears a bracelet upon the inside of which is inscribed, in addition to his name and address, the words—Coma or insulin shock. Which?"[26]

Rainsford, who frequently traveled away from home, staying in guesthouses and hotels, was keen to prevent a mishap involving either an insulin reaction or the onset of acidotic coma. He illustrated his tactic, picturing himself asleep in the quintessential hotel room, with instructions that he had written out perched on top of the dresser: "If I look as if I am dying or in a coma, please phone Dr. Joslin." Given the incapacitating nature of the threat posed by insulin reactions, this was his best way of "Playing Safe."

While insulin-induced hypoglycemia was a constant worry for people treated with insulin, and it might have constituted the majority of their symptoms early in the course of their experience with diabetes, ultimately the disease itself became the main troublemaker. Right from the start of the illness, the possible development of diabetic acidosis lurked in the shadows, an insidious bête noire. Joslin counseled that the "signs of the onset of acid poisoning are most indefinite. Consequently, it is

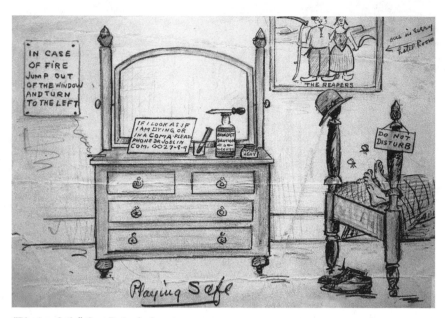

"Playing Safe." Guy Rainsford cartoon.
Courtesy of the Joslin Diabetes Center Historical Archive.

a good rule for any diabetic patient if he feels ill, and always if he has fever, to take for granted that he may have acid poisoning and adopt those measures which will prevent its becoming serious." In all versions of his *Manual,* he outlined some variation of the following:

Treatment of Acid Intoxication. Rules for the Patient.
1. Send for the doctor.
2. Go to bed.
3. Liquids. A cupful an hour. Hot water, tea, coffee, broths, water-oatmeal gruel, orange juice.
4. Take an enema. The enema clears the lower intestine so that salt solution, a teaspoon of salt to each pint of water, can be given later by the rectum in case liquids are not retained by mouth.
5. Keep warm: flannel nightclothes. Heaters, but put a blanket about the heater to avoid burns.
6. Secure a nurse or someone in the family who will spend her entire time caring for you until the doctor arrives.[27]

As greater skill in the medical management of acidosis and coma developed in the decade following insulin's discovery, and the incidence

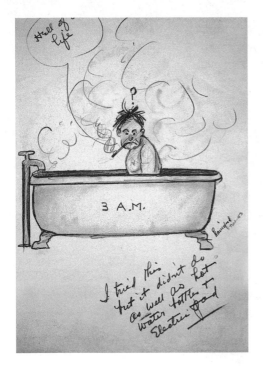

"3 A.M. Bath." Guy Rainsford cartoon. Courtesy of the Joslin Diabetes Center Historical Archive.

of death due to coma drastically declined, other problems came to the fore. Diabetes-induced damage to the blood vessels, especially those serving the legs, was a major source of morbidity. Poor blood supply would cause patients to experience pain when walking and make the feet exquisitely vulnerable to infections from even minor nicks in the skin. Diabetes also injured nerves over time, leading to numbness or pain in the feet, legs, hands, or practically any other part of the body. The combination of insufficient blood flow and numbness of the feet, along with an immune system impaired by diabetes, enabled infections of the legs to spread, leading all too often to gangrene that required an amputation of the affected limb.

Rainsford suffered the pains of nerve damage. In one of his drawings, Rainsford depicted himself sitting in a bathtub amidst a swirl of steam at 3 A.M., his disgruntled image looking directly out, muttering, "Hell of a life." In the caption, he explains that he had tried (presumably, on Joslin's recommendation) a hot bath for the pain of his neuritis, "but it didn't do as well as hot water bottle + electric pad." In another drawing for Joslin's benefit, Rainsford indicated exactly where he hurt. Mimicking the map of the body that showed where insulin could safely be in-

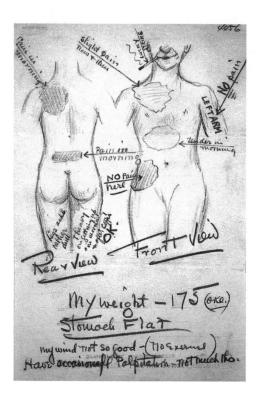

"Body Hurt Map." Guy Rainsford cartoon. Courtesy of the Joslin Diabetes Center Historical Archive.

jected, Rainsford provided a front and rear view of himself, complete with his omnipresent Lucky Strike cigarette dangling from his lips and areas of "pain in the morning" or "now and then" or "No pain here" clearly demarcated.

Various other symptoms also beset diabetic patients, ranging from the maddening itch associated with yeast infections in the groin region that were caused by sugar-laden urine, to the difficulty breathing due to congestive heart failure or the fatigue of chronic renal failure. Most harrowing for many patients, though, was the threat of blindness. By the mid-1930s damage of the retina from diabetes had been noted in the medical literature to be one of the major morbidities encountered by people who were living longer through the aid of insulin.[28] Patients came to fear this diabetic sequela even before any visual loss occurred, such that the anxiety of future impairment itself became a form of suffering. Again, Rainsford put the matter to Joslin starkly, sketching the stereotyped image of the blind man selling pencils on the street, observing simply: "I don't want this to happen."

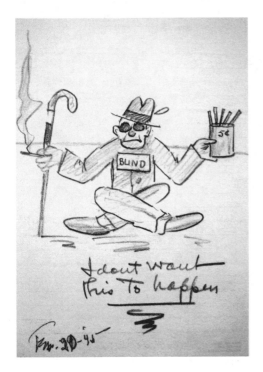

PATIENT-DOCTOR RELATIONSHIP WORK

Diabetes, transformed by insulin into a chronic illness, en-meshed patients in a complex set of ongoing relationships with care providers. The relationship between patient and doctor has been granted a privileged legal status and holds a rather sanctified place in the bioethical worldview, but for patients themselves, maintaining these relationships over many years clearly added another form of work to the illness experience. Indeed, Rainsford's cartoons themselves—and all the letters from other patients—can be seen as products of this ongoing relationship work, which often turned to several recurrent themes.

One such theme has grown out of the American health care system's underlying business model, and the need consequently for patients to pay for services rendered.[29] As discussed in Chapter 3, health insurance was a financial invention that did not take hold until the years following the Second World War, and then for coverage of hospital and surgical bills, not for routine doctor visits. Even when insurance for ambulatory care became more widely used in the 1960s, patients continued to pay considerable out-of-pocket expenses. These medical bills were a topic of many letters to Joslin and were addressed by Rainsford on several

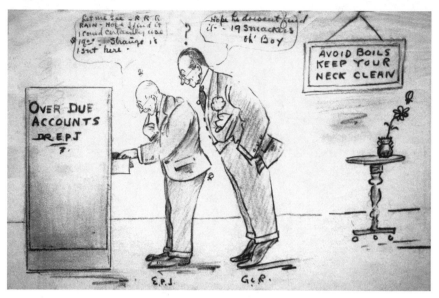

"Over Due Accounts." Guy Rainsford cartoon.
Courtesy of the Joslin Diabetes Center Historical Archive.

occasions. In one vignette, Joslin is seen peering over a drawer pulled out from a cabinet labeled "OVER DUE ACCOUNTS—DR EPJ," thinking to himself, "Let me see—R R R Rain. . . . Hope I find it. I could certainly use $19.00. Strange it isn't here." Meanwhile, Rainsford, perched over Joslin's shoulder, wishes just the opposite: "Hope he doesn't find it—19 smakers, oh Boy." In another message to his doctor, a nattily dressed Rainsford, immaculate from his fedora down to his spats, exclaims: "Well here I be—Folks. Better late than never with four Bucks."

A Rainsford drawing also touched on the issue of payment in the context of another aspect of relationship management, namely dealing with doctors who—in the estimation of this particular patient—were not competent. The "local medico," pictured with a box of pain pills atop his desk, pronounces, "You are not getting enough B-complex—You should eat more pie-cake + ice cream, this will stimulate your eyes, and take plenty of laxatives. Dr. Joslin is O.K., but I have my own ideas on diabetes. Take these pills daily + drop in + see me in 2 weeks. $2.00 please." In response, the skeptical Rainsford fumes, "No wonder the village is full of comas, reactions, & insulin shocks." More than just a humorous lampoon, the scene expressed an opinion shared by other patients who wrote to Joslin, namely that many doctors who they en-

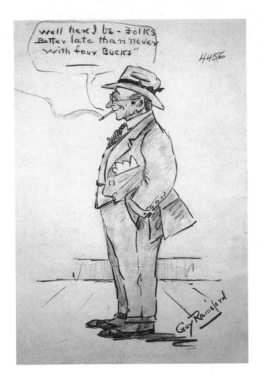

"Four Bucks." Guy Rainsford
cartoon. Courtesy of the Joslin
Diabetes Center Historical Archive.

countered were ignorant regarding diabetes and its proper treatment, and that these patients had to remain vigilant to protect themselves against improper advice or prescriptions.

Also quite common in the medical records were instances of patients explaining themselves to Joslin or one of his colleagues. In essence the flip side of passing judgment regarding the suspect knowledge or deficient skill of other doctors, here patients defended their own actions by supplying further information. Sometimes, the events in question were seemingly of no particular consequence, except perhaps that the occurrence might change how the physician thought of the patient. For example, Rainsford caught an image of himself once in the hospital, offering the nurse his "9.30 specimen" of urine, collected in a urinal. He stands with his buttocks exposed as his hospital gown (called a johnny) flaps open—a fact unbeknownst to him until the nurse replies, "Alright first put 4 drops in the rack + save the rest—and don't turn around until you've hooked up your Johnny." As he disclosed in the margin, "I landed at Deaconess [Hospital] without pajamas—so I landed in a 'Johnny'. No wonder I got balled out for making Indecent Exposures. Well how did I know."

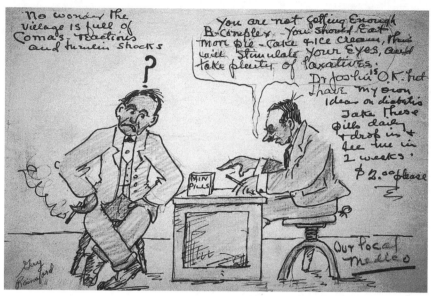

"Our Local Medico." Guy Rainsford cartoon.
Courtesy of the Joslin Diabetes Center Historical Archive.

Most instances of patients explaining themselves, as will become evident in subsequent chapters, were not handled as humorously, and appear to have been far more anxiety-riddled interactions for the patients. Whether the event warranting explanation was a laboratory test indicating poor control over the diabetes, or a behavior (such as missing an appointment or leaving the hospital without permission), or an ongoing refusal to follow a physician's recommendation, the subtext of any explanation was concern for the relationship between patient and doctor. Any occurrence that, in the eyes of the patient, threatened this relationship could prompt these efforts at repair, suggesting not only the importance of these relationships but also the work involved in maintaining them and the psychological risks involved in dissenting from doctor's orders.

·IDENTITY WORK

When the diagnosis of diabetes, along with all its consequences, intruded upon people's lives, they had to work to understand what this chronic disease meant regarding who they were and whom they would, over time, become. In other words, they had to forge a diabetic identity that fit into their encompassing sense of personal iden-

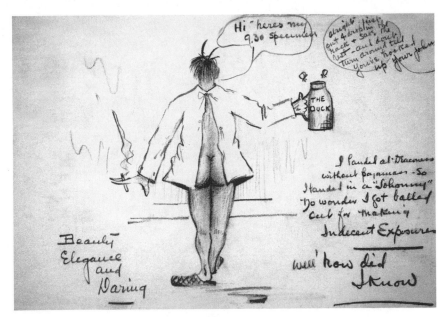

"Beauty, Elegance, and Daring." Guy Rainsford cartoon.
Courtesy of the Joslin Diabetes Center Historical Archive.

tity. This work invariably involved grappling with core values that distinguish good or worthy people and the related ideals of what people ought to believe and how they should behave. Joslin had no qualms about setting forth his idealized vision of the personal philosophy or lifestyle to which people with diabetes could aspire. Unequivocally and consistently throughout his entire career, Joslin encouraged his patients to adopt positive attitudes. In all editions of his *Manual,* he offered this Socratic exhortation: "QUESTION. What can a diabetic patient do for himself besides keeping his urine sugar-free? ANS. Be cheerful and also be thankful that his disease is not of a hopeless character, but a disease which his brains will help him to conquer."[30] He also used photographs as a medium for encouragement. Influenced no doubt by his own bucolic ideals of life on his country farm in Oxford, Massachusetts, Joslin inserted in the 1959 edition of his *Manual* a portrait of a family man, surrounded by his wife and children, embracing values that prioritized the duties and pleasures of marriage and fatherhood and living in a state of responsible disregard for the long-term implications of his disease.

Mr. Rainsford's vision of a normal diabetic life, as conveyed through his artistic eye, was more complex—and much more ribald. He did not

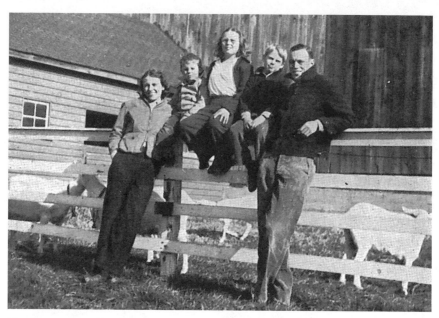

Family man, according to Joslin. From Joslin, Diabetic Manual, *10th ed., 24.*

shy away from potentially embarrassing or degrading aspects of being a patient but instead tackled them directly, transforming them with his humor. One of his illustrations makes this point quite clearly. Behind a screen that blocks all but the feet of a physician, the doctor requests: "Mr. Rainsford—will you oblige me by relaxing and drawing up your knees—*There*—atta boy! Guess the old prostate is OK. No obstruction." To which Rainsford replies, "That's swell, Doc. Glad I AIN'T got NO CANCER—Cheerio." The caption declares: "The perfect *Rectum*. About the only thing I have left to brag about."

Rainsford's full-bodied expression of the human condition was literally that: full of his body, the inescapable element in his life with chronic illness. In his unexpurgated cartoons, he conveyed the impact of diabetes—and the work of caring for his diabetes—upon his body, and hence upon his person. Yet at the same time, Rainsford's experience was not determined merely by what his body was experiencing: for all the physical manifestations of the disease, as well as the accoutrements of self-care, were transformed in his artistic representation by his personality, his wit and sense of irony. Poking fun was part of his identity work as he fashioned his own view of what life with diabetes was, what it meant, and what it held in store.

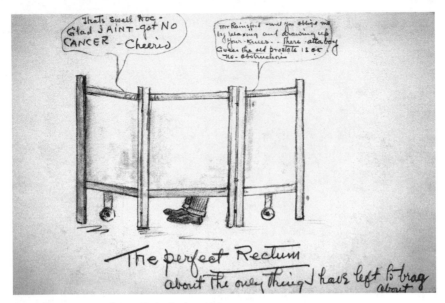

"The Perfect Rectum." Guy Rainsford cartoon.
Courtesy of the Joslin Diabetes Center Historical Archive.

In "The Rewards of a Misspent Life," Rainsford imagined himself at ninety-four years of age in a state of dapper decrepitude. Stooped, cane in hand, dressed in vest and coattails, his face reveals that the forces of gravity have been at work upon it for many years. Still, although seeming to totter, he exudes an air of spirited frailty. In his hand, he grasps his ever-present prop, a bottle of the copper-containing Benedict's solution, while on the table also rests a syringe filled with insulin and a copy of the *Diabetic Manual.* "Well Folks," he croaks, "I have won a hard battle—yes, Sir, got Old Man Diabetes on the run—I don't know what would have happened to the copper sulphate folks these hard times if it wasn't for me." On the floor near his feet stand two medals, replicas of the awards that Joslin had begun to hand out to people who had lived with diabetes for twenty-five or more years and remained in perfect health. (For more on these medals see Chapter 7.) Below these, in what is hard to interpret as anything but a parody of the moralizing ideology embodied in the medals, Rainsford wrote: "Any body mastering courage and self-control can look like this at 100 years old." Was this body, then, the rewards of a misspent life, much of it devoted to the self-care that he depicted in his other cartoons? No, there was more: "2 Medals and the Boston Post Walking Stick."

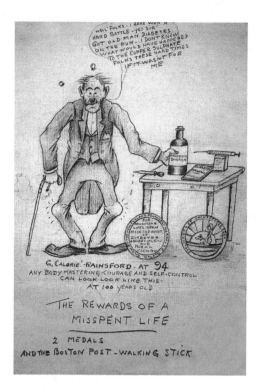

"Rewards of a Misspent Life."
Guy Rainsford cartoon. Courtesy
of the Joslin Diabetes Center
Historical Archive.

"WORK SHORTENS THE DAY, BUT LENGTHENS THE LIFE"

The irreverent and irascible Mr. Rainsford almost lived to see his seventieth birthday, but he never collected these rewards he had envisioned from a misspent life. He died shortly after World War II, having suffered a stroke and succumbing a few years later to renal failure. In many regards, his two decades of experience with diabetes—compared to other cases in this book—was atypical. He developed his illness in midlife, did not rush to use insulin until several years had passed, and survived to a much older age. And, beyond dispute, he certainly was idiosyncratic in his manner of communicating with his famous physician.

Yet despite these unusual features, Mr. Rainsford's drawings speak precisely and profoundly to the themes of this book and its aim to recount the twentieth-century history of diabetes from the patient's perspective. The cartoons get right to the point, literally illustrating fundamental aspects of life for almost all people who have lived with diabetes since the introduction of insulin—aspects so fundamental, in fact, that

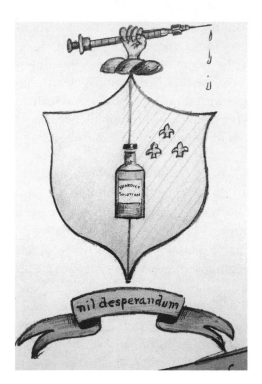

"Nil desperandum." Guy Rainsford cartoon. Courtesy of the Joslin Diabetes Center Historical Archive.

their ubiquity has rendered them virtually invisible to many doctors and historians of medicine alike. The daily toil of monitoring urine or blood glucose levels, eating in accord with dietary rules, administering insulin, managing symptoms: the vividness with which Rainsford captured his own interpretation of these recurring experiences greatly enhances our visual imagination of how a life with diabetes has been lived, both before and after 1922, enriching our understanding of the work that has long permeated the diabetic world.

Beyond aiding our visual imagination, Rainsford's cartoons help us to perceive more clearly certain intangible qualities of life with diabetes—the flux of emotions, the impact on body image, the delicate web of relationships between patient and physician—and through these perceptions to grasp subtle aspects of the transformation of diabetes into a chronic illness. The labor of coping with this disease has not been limited to performing physical tasks such as testing, measuring, and injecting, although these tasks have consumed a considerable amount of patients' time and energy. But, as the drawings suggest, diabetes-related work has also included dealing with inner states: reluctance, anxiety, fear, embarrassment, doubt, recrimination. These and other emotions and casts of mind certainly were common among patients before insulin was discovered, even though the nature of the threats was different. What changed over the course of the twentieth century, clearly, has been that patients have lived longer with these inner states, and with an ever-expanding range of choices regarding how to respond, because of relatively greater, but still far from absolute, medical control over the disease and its consequences.

The choice of how to respond, both to outward and inward challenges, has not been limited to just the selection of medications, equipment, or procedures (although these technological responses have been the chief drivers of the cycles of transmutation discussed in Chapter 2). Equally important has been the choice of outlook, perspective, philosophy, or whatever we call an individual's foundational system of belief and attitude, which has informed all other choices, small and large. For Elliott P. Joslin, his modus vivendi personified the Protestant work ethic, adorned in his case with a stethoscope, but true to the values of piety, thrift, and industry found across many generations of diverse individuals throughout New England. Every day for over sixty years of professional activity, Joslin operated within this system of belief. Rainsford embraced values similar to Joslin's, espousing them in his own inimitable style, although (as we shall see in subsequent chapters) this belief system created, as well as solved, problems for patients. To live without desperation—"nil desperandum," as the motto on his fanciful coat of arms declared—was Mr. Rainsford's choice, his statement of faith regarding how to best live with diabetes, his moral vision that imbued his drawings with a profound and at times disturbing sense of irony, and ultimately with humor and humanity.

5

THE WANT
OF CONTROL:
IDEAS AND IDEALS
IN THE MANAGEMENT
OF DIABETES

Better treatment of diabetes should be universal.
Diabetes should be controlled. The means are
at our door.
—Elliott P. Joslin, "A Renaissance of the
Control of Diabetes," 1954

In the early spring of 1927, four-year-old Arnold Burns arrived in Boston. A month previous, consumed by an unslakable thirst and a boundless appetite, he had begun to urinate frequently. His local doctor, upon finding sugar in Arnold's urine, immediately referred the boy and his mother, Ethel Burns, to the Joslin Clinic. After traveling the fifty miles from their Massachusetts home to Boston, Arnold was seen by Dr. Priscilla White, a twenty-seven-year-old member of the clinic staff who was in charge of juvenile cases. She noted that the child was frail and "drowsy," breathing deeply but otherwise "normal."[1] Once Arnold was admitted to the hospital, he and his mother spent a week learning about diabetes and how to control it through assiduous home management. Upon his departure from Boston, no longer healthy or carefree, he was required (with his mother's help) to inject three doses of insulin each day and follow a diet of precisely 960 calories.[2]

This rigorous style of managing diabetic life was exactly what Elliott Joslin envisioned as ideal care. Joslin believed in patient education and self-control even before he first administered insulin in 1922. Now, with the aid of the wondrous drug, he felt that disciplined diabetics could attain mastery over their disease. In this unabashedly assured spirit, Joslin wrote to the boy's local doctor a fortnight after Arnold was discharged. "Anything I can do to help you with that Burns case," he declared, "would be a pleasure. Of course you know that these diabetic children under ten years of age formerly died at an average duration of less than 1 [year] and 2 tenths, but now they appear to live indefinitely."[3] Like the majority of his medical colleagues, Joslin was confident that insulin had rewritten the future of the once swiftly fatal juvenile diabetes.

And so it had. Patients like Arnold survived well beyond childhood—but they certainly did not survive indefinitely. As insulin entered the clinical scene, no one suspected that the history of diabetes would become a story juxtaposing "success" and "failure" as a perceived medical victory evolved into an ambiguous and frustrating clinical reality. No one foresaw that many diabetic patients, while surviving longer, would be beset by painful or debilitating complications before succumbing to an unpleasant death. No one predicted the problems that transmuted diabetes would bring to the lives of patients.

The resulting intellectual and emotional dialectic—between triumphal and tragic outlooks—has long animated diabetic therapeutics, driving it almost obsessively toward the alluring yet elusive goal of controlling the course of disease.[4] Simply put, the modern medical management of diabetes mellitus has been shaped by four often contradictory ideals: complete cure, constant regulation, physician-control, and patient-control. These ideals, when put into practice, have generated tensions that have shaped the lives of diabetics, their families, and their doctors—who, importantly, have disagreed among themselves as to the health consequences of "tight" or "poor" diabetic control. Therefore, the human dimensions of the transformation of diabetes, spurred by a series of remarkable technical innovations, can best be understood by exploring how these ideals have been made manifest in thought and action.[5]

These shifts of biological process and therapeutic style have embedded the specific care of any given diabetic patient within a broader historical process, as prevailing ideas, innovations, and ideals have combined around the circumstances of a personal history, medical and otherwise. These components—specific individual experiences and general historical patterns—are inextricably connected and are best viewed as essentially complementary silhouettes of each other: the individual experiences compose the broader patterns, which in turn shape the individual experiences. Consequently, a historical overview of diabetic management must strive for a balance in its narrative account between this yin and yang, situating seemingly idiosyncratic occurrences and choices into the wider context of historical trends within a society and its cultural and social arrangements, using each aspect to explain the other.

This chapter examines the Joslin Clinic's distinctive style of patient management in the period after 1922—how it developed and the way that it enveloped and infiltrated the lives of patients and those around them. Contrasting the experiences of two specific patients and their families, we will explore both the public versions of how people with diabetes ought to conduct their lives (as expressed in medical articles and texts) and the private reality of diabetic control (as revealed in medical records and personal letters).[6] The first patient, William Ellis Hampden, received the best medical care that money could buy before dying at home just as insulin was being discovered; his history allows us to review what "control" meant—medically, socially, personally—before 1922. The second patient, Arnold Burns, became diabetic during the post-insulin period. His case reveals core aspects of what "control" meant after insulin, as his struggles with diabetes reflect certain typical and recurring conflicts. Arnold and his mother worked through their relationship with each other and with his physicians; they worried about money and employment; he sought to understand who he was as a diabetic; and finally the Burnses coped with medical complications and impending death: these were experiences both profoundly intimate and yet shared among diabetics of the twentieth century.

Arnold's case can almost be read as that of an unwitting protagonist placed center stage in a modern morality play—with therapeutic action and human choice unfolding as part of a larger struggle between the goodness that is health and the evilness of illness—surrounded by a cast of well-meaning supporting actors, physicians and family members who grappled with the tensions inherent in controlling disease. The play, with its specific characters and their particular difficulties, was shaped by a more generic plot that epitomized dilemmas so typical of twentieth-century American medicine—a plot that pitted patient autonomy against physician authority, posed present comfort against possible future health benefits, and interpreted clinical setbacks sometimes as intractable biological fate, other times as implied moral failing.

IDEAL CONTROL BEFORE INSULIN

I myself am a sufferer from this disease. I can get along very well without potatoes and pastry, but I must have bread, and if I do not get bread I become so weak I cannot work. I would rather have three per

cent. of sugar in my urine, and for the time-being feel strong, than
have only one per cent. or none and feel asthenic.
—A diabetic physician, 1896[7]

William Ellis Hampden became diabetic in July of 1916. The twelve-year-old boy had entered under Joslin's treatment in September of that year. After a two-week stay in the hospital had rendered William sugar free, he returned home and was promptly entrusted to the care of a private-duty nurse who prepared—and enforced—a strict diet. Two months later, the young patient was caught eating "a five-cent bag of salted peanuts." This act of insubordination led his father, a lawyer, to write Joslin about his son Ellis. Mr. Hampden bemoaned the fact that the boy possessed "an element of pleasure loving weakness in his makeup which we have not overcome." Since Ellis was "not keeping the faith" and would not "unless constantly watched," the father worried that his son would never recover.[8] Yet despite these early episodes of laxity, the boy soon reformed his ways. Six weeks after his father had written, the boy was sugar free and entered the new year of 1917 back on the straight and narrow path of diabetic self-discipline.[9]

At this point, six months into William's illness, the notion of controlling the young man's disease had already become a complex amalgam of technical and personal concerns. At one level, everyone involved in his care wanted to steer his diabetes clear of acidosis and coma, and they sought to accomplish this chiefly through the precise control of his diet. At a deeper level, when they were confronted by the daily challenge of enforcing a precise diet, their desire to manage his chronic disease turned into efforts to guide and enhance William's own self-control. For the remaining four and a half years of his life, these attempts at diet-control and self-control would shape his experience, combining toward the end of his illness in a final struggle to control the process of his dying.

The exacting control over William's dietary life appears most clearly in the letters sent to Joslin by the private-duty nurse. Her job consisted of attending to details, taking the dietary prescription and making it into a meal. On one occasion, she let Joslin know that her young patient "likes the Brazil nuts and the things we make with the sugar-free milk, which we have just been able to get." She and the boy's mother were curious to know "if Billy may have halibut. It is very hard to get clams here. We do get oysters and if we may give him scallops, we can get these easily." The nurse also apprised Joslin of her decision to "give up keeping the diet chart as the same mess is no longer interesting, but will keep on with the record of weight, volume of and sugar in the urine."[10]

The father's letters tended to address the questions of William Ellis's self-control and the parents' attempts to bolster it. In the spring of 1917, for instance, Mr. Hampden told Joslin that his son was "full of life and energy and exercises a great deal. We caution him against over exercise—but the caution is little heeded. He eats very rapidly and we seem unable to cure him of this habit."[11]

In December of that year, a concerned Mr. Hampden wrote again: "Ellis has shown sugar six or seven times in the last two or three weeks; once three days in succession. He had sugar yesterday, is free today. We are anxious and are trying to discover the cause." The father believed that his son "does not eat forbidden articles, but does eat too much of permitted articles. He seems always hungry, goes into the kitchen and eats between meals, does not weigh his food regularly. Day before yesterday he indulged in milk beyond the amount allowed." In addition to reporting these dietary excesses, Mr. Hampden also said he thought that the youngster engaged in imprudent physical activities. Ellis "seems strong," the father told Joslin, as the boy had "worked all day Friday ice cutting (a light part of the work!). This was done without any knowledge or consent and I was compelled to forbid him to return to ice cutting Saturday morning with temperature 7° below." The father's resolve seemed to waver, however, as he recounted this little episode; for Ellis's high-spirited activity and desire to work was also a source of paternal pride and happiness in the face of an otherwise debilitating illness. After having been "compelled" to "forbid" the boy's return to ice cutting, Mr. Hampden added wistfully: "He wanted to go."[12]

Billy, as he referred to himself in his own letters to Joslin, alluded to both the medical regimen and the management regimen that directed his life—all the while coping with a dire illness. "I am feeling fine," the fourteen-year-old boy exclaimed to Joslin in the fall of 1917, "and every body I meet says that I am looking fine also." He was testing his urine every day, and he weighed ninety nine pounds. "As a rule I will exercise by playing football one day, the next one or two days I will sort of loaf around doing not much of anything. As a rule I go to bed between 8:00 and 8:30 and get up between 6:30 and 6:45." Billy was considering, however, an amendment to these rules. He informed Joslin—who was a major authority on rules, diabetic and otherwise, in this boy's life—

that "I would like to join the Y.M.C.A." The youngster, reflecting perhaps his education and social station in life, petitioned the physician in a manner assured and seemingly autonomous. "I would like your advice as to whether I should. I would be able to go there and play billiards or pool and many other games, read and go in swimming."[13]

Although Joslin's reply was not filed in the medical record, the boy certainly found ways—sanctioned or not—to keep himself active despite his disease. In late December of 1917, just days before Mr. Hampden wrote about the ice-cutting incident, Billy informed Joslin, "I have had sugar [in my urine]." He was going to send a sample to Boston but maintained, "I have never felt better in all my life." Billy seemed only moderately concerned about the urinary sugar, eagerly reporting that "Sky Pond is frozen over so I go skating every day either in the morning or afternoon." Indeed, he seemed most concerned about his diet, detailing how he had "only a very little saccharin left. My father has tried all over Boston . . . but he cannot buy the kind which you prescribed to me, and I would like to know if I can use the other kind and if not could you send me some if possible." As a postscript, Billy provided a monitoring benchmark: "My weight has been between 99–100 right straight along."[14]

During 1918, Joslin was away from Boston, enrolled in the U.S. Army and stationed in Europe for part of that time. In his absence, Billy began to be treated by Dr. B. H. Ragle, one of Joslin's former assistant physicians, who continued to see the boy after Joslin returned. Under Ragle's care, Billy did well for another year. Indeed, during the first three and a half years of his illness, Billy had experienced mostly good health, and for much of this time he actually weighed a pound or two more than he had before his diabetes appeared in 1916.

This remarkable period of stable health had lasted until approximately February of 1919, at which point he began to lose weight and his health started to decline markedly. Thereafter, as the disease seemed to gain strength at the young man's expense, his physicians and parents thought less about controlling how Billy lived and more about controlling how he might die.

Ragle harbored no illusions about his patient's failing condition. "A year ago," he told Joslin in February of 1920, "Billy Hampden weighed one hundred pounds. Today he weighs between eighty and eighty-four." The doctor had no more room to cut the boy's diet, already restricted to a mere 700 to 900 calories a day. The time had come, in his opinion,

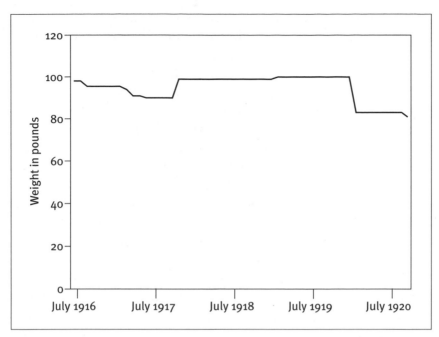

Figure 5.1. Weight of William Ellis Hampden, from Onset of Diabetes in July 1916 to Death in August 1921, with Last Recorded Weight in October 1920

to change therapeutic course. "It has always been my ambition," Ragle confided, "to let Billy live as long as he possibly could in comfort on this very meager diet and eventually feed him 1100 or 1200 calories" — a final concession to the disease but one that would allow the boy to savor a full stomach before dying. Ragle had not arrived at this plan himself but instead had "talked the whole situation out with Mr. Hampden. Of course he and Mrs. Hampden are completely reconciled to the situation and want [Billy] to have the maximum in comfort, even if it shortens his life a little."

The doctor attested, with a hint of vicarious pride, that "Billy has developed into an unusually intelligent little man, [and] has learned self control more than I ever thought possible." Pondering these admirable characteristics, Ragle carefully considered how his patient would react to the change of diet and its consequences. "When the time comes to increase his diet, and I feel that that time will be in the near future," he informed Joslin, "I shall tell him that the change of diet is to see if we cannot have him pick up a little strength." The nurse would be instructed to "test less frequently and if possible keep Billy from seeing the tests." With these rationalizations and shields from the truth in place, Ragle thought that they could "adopt the above regimen without causing him any great degree of apprehension. If he improves, as I have no doubt he will for a time, he will be satisfied."[15]

The approach that Ragle outlined, for the modern reader, raises several issues—especially truth-telling and quality of life—that have become central subjects of current ethical discussions about caring for terminally ill patients. Early in the twentieth century, physicians had publicly debated these aspects of medical care.[16] In Billy's case, the dilemmas and difficulties of his final stage of life were sorted through in the private dialogue between his physician and well-educated parents. While other patients clearly were not as lucky in these regards, Billy was fortunate to have such attentive, thoughtful treatment, and the financial resources to provide this end-of-life care.

Then as now, managing a terminally ill patient—and dealing with the uncertainty that surrounded such weighty choices—often prompted the attending physician to consult other doctors, soliciting advice about the best course to pursue. In this case, Ragle turned to Joslin, who also concerned himself with the quality of a patient's life. But Joslin had learned that many diabetic children felt better on a more stringent diet and that their quality of life was, somewhat paradoxically, improved by eating less. Through years of arduous clinical experience, Joslin had become wedded to a dogged strategy of steadfast treatment when facing medical adversity. His belief in incremental medical progress, along with his abiding religious faith, sustained him.

And so, within days of hearing from Ragle, Joslin had replied. While agreeing that, "of course, all of us wish him to live comfortably, even if his duration of life is somewhat shortened," the doctor argued for another course of therapeutic action. "Unless [William] is very unhappy now with his diet," Joslin advised Ragle, "I am inclined to postpone enlarging it for at least one month." His reasons were "twofold: first, the result of the work at the Carnegie Laboratory [with Francis Benedict on diabetic metabolism] is gradually coming to a head, and there may be a hint of something useful for William there, and I would like to see him get the benefit of what I have expended upon it." Second, Joslin had just received from a European colleague a new book on diabetes, "which probably sums up German treatment at the present time. In many ways it is pathetic and dreadfully behind what we believe advantageous here, yet it is possible I shall find something in the 400

TABLE 5.1. Hospital Course for William Ellis Hampden, October 1920

October	Urine Sugar	Blood Sugar	Diet
1	0.6%	0.238 mg/dl	approx. 900 calories
2–3	—	—	[Modified fast]
4	0.0%	—	[Advancing diet]
8	—	0.134 mg/dl	[Advancing diet]
12	—	0.189 mg/dl	1,038 calories
approx. 14	—	0.150 mg/dl	approx. 1,000 calories
18	Discharged		1,190 calories

Source: B. H. Ragle to Elliott P. Joslin, 18 October 1920, and B. H. Ragle to patient's mother, 18 October 1920, with Joslin's annotated calculations on the letter to the mother, Joslin Diabetes Center Historical Archive, Boston, Mass.

pages which would help William Hampden." Adding yet a final reason for delay, Joslin asked what Ragle would "think of Miss Pelley [Joslin's personally trained nurse] spending one or two days with [the Hampden's private-duty nurse]. Very likely she might have a few new ideas. She has fitted in very nicely doing this sort of work for short periods, and will be available shortly."[17]

Half a year passed. Perhaps Nurse Pelley had helped, or perhaps something that Joslin had learned provided a novel approach; the medical record is not clear. Regardless, the care that Billy received during these six months appears to have followed, more or less, the path that Joslin had prescribed, with the diet still restricted and the boy's health lingering just this side of precarious.

Then, in October of 1920, Billy entered the hospital under Ragle's care. The illness had not only affected the patient; the labor of caring for him had taken its toll on Mrs. Hampden as well. As Ragle explained to Joslin, the "main reason" for Billy's hospitalization "was that his mother needed a vacation, and she took advantage of the opportunity to have a few days of it." The patient's weight, at this stage, varied "between eighty and eighty-four pounds, stripped," and although the Benedict urine test was positive, "he did not know of the presence of sugar." Billy remained in the hospital for eighteen days, where a period of tight dietary control seemed—yet again—to re-establish a viable metabolic state.[18]

As Ragle prepared to send Billy home, he sat down to write the boy's mother. "The hospital permitted us," he noted resolutely, "to get him

sugar-free and to reduce his blood sugar to a figure that is not dangerous." Still, the road ahead was fraught with difficulty. For although Billy
"loses ground less rapidly than any young diabetic we know," he continued, ". . . I cannot feel that he is as well off as he was a year ago."
Ragle imagined "that we could feed Billy 900 calories, keep him quiet
most of the day so that he would lose very little weight and, barring
acute infections, have him go along without trouble for a year or two,
but I believe that Billy would be quite miserable and, frankly, I do not
think it is possible with him." Considering how best to manage the final
period of this particular boy's illness, the doctor asserted, "We must,
therefore, make up our minds for a rather long pull, and to keep him
happy as far as possible with the diet and his chosen activities."[19]

To keep track of the patient's condition during what he presumed to
be the terminal phase of illness, Ragle planned that Billy's "blood sugar
will be taken the first of each month" and so had scheduled an office
visit for the blood to be drawn. As for monitoring at home, the doctor
reported, he "told Billy that the [urine] testing was to be done twice a
week; therefore the saving [of twenty-four hours of urine] need be only
two days a week . . . and I requested that he do none of his own testing,
but that one of you should be responsible for it." Ragle—with one part
warning, one part reassurance—told the mother, "Should sugar appear
in the urine I believe it will be due to something that he gets between
meals rather than to the diet itself and yet he has determined not to
have anything at all between meals, and he is pretty tenacious."[20]

The "rather long pull" lasted almost a year. Late in August of 1921—
after Banting and Best had already performed the first successful experiments with their pancreatic extract—Billy Hampden died one mid-
night at home with a nurse in attendance. Ragle let Joslin know that the
young man had "kept up and about and really cheerful until Saturday
evening when he went to bed because of fatigue. As late as Saturday
afternoon he had insisted on going to Boston for his massage but was
completely done for [and exhausted] when he returned to [home]: went
into coma and died without waking up and perfectly peacefully."

Part of the physician's job in caring for a young dying patient, Ragle
seemed to believe, was to prognosticate when death would occur so that
the parents could be forewarned and prepare themselves. "I knew this
was coming," Ragle told Joslin. Since June, the boy had 1.3–3.3 percent
sugar and acetone in his urine; and then the doctor "had seen Billy early

the same week [of his death] and had written Mr. and Mrs. Hampden, telling them that it could not be long."

Billy Hampden's death affected Ragle, who revealed his feelings to Joslin through a personal testimony, shrouded in a veil of professional reserve. "I have never seen such courage and faith in anyone as he displayed throughout his illness and especially during the last year or two. It was always a pleasure to have him come to the office and instead of being an inspiration to him he was an inspiration to me." In his final adieu, Ragle admitted: "I became very much attached to Billy, as you know."[21]

IDEAL CONTROL INTENSIFIED

In the pre-insulin era, while children such as William Hampden lived and died with their diabetes, Joslin acquired more experience treating these young patients with aggressive dietary measures. As his faith in this regimen deepened, he incrementally redoubled his therapeutic pursuit of control. By 1922, this escalation had culminated in what one might call the "intensivist strategy" of diabetic management.

Joslin presented this strategy for control in his Shattuck Lecture, delivered before the Massachusetts Medical Society in the spring of 1922. He began by observing, "The average known duration of the fatal cases of diabetes in the city of Boston between 1895 and 1913 was 3.3 years; during 1915 it was 4.3 years, and in 1920 it was 5.3 years." He then asked, "Can this improvement go on? Can the present treatment, that is, particularly the dietetic, progress still further?" The rest of the lecture answered "yes," emphatically. Speaking about needless diabetic deaths, Joslin argued that coma, gangrene, and infection were all preventable. When a patient died of coma, the mishap could often "be traced to the advice of the laity or irregular practitioners, and often to the patients themselves. For all such deaths one feels regret, but not the keen concern excited by deaths under trained supervision, yet not quite free from errors of judgment." The doctors present were further cautioned: "Never allow one of your diabetic patients to develop gangrene ignorantly. Your warning and admonition should penetrate so deeply the souls of your cases that if such a catastrophe should ever occur the unhappy patient will feel compelled to say: 'Doctor, you warned me about injury to my feet, about the dangers in cutting corns, [and] toe nails, about blisters from new shoes or old shoes with poor linings, about nails in my shoes, flat foot plates and hot water bags. You are not to blame for my present condition.'" Joslin proceeded to outline his methods for placing a diabetic on a precise diet; he also advocated hospital admission for comprehensive education at the onset of the illness and periodically thereafter for regulation and routine annual medical examinations and the creation of diabetic centers to facilitate efficient continuing education and care. Then, at the end of his lecture, Joslin referred briefly to the recent announcements regarding insulin. Everything, it must have seemed to the speaker and his audience, was about to change: "It may take a decade or more before the treatment of diabetes is as simple as that of myxedema, but all will work more confidently now that . . . the promised land is plain in view."[22]

INSULIN AND CONTROL "AMONG THE ERSTWHILE DEAD"

The introduction of insulin in 1922 seemed to mark a sharp break with past therapeutic practices, providing physicians with a drug of unprecedented power and efficacy. Insulin also appeared to validate the "pancreatic theory" of diabetes. Based largely upon Minkowski and von Mering's creation of diabetes in dogs by resection of their pancreases and Opie's pathological studies of diabetic pancreases devoid of islets of Langerhans, the pancreatic theory located the cause of diabetes in this organ, spurring investigators to quest for the elusive internal pancreatic secretion.[23] Insulin's dramatic effects seemed unassailable proof that these ideas were essentially correct; the fundamental problem was too little insulin from the pancreas. Reasoning by analogy to the treatment of hypothyroidism (myxedema) with thyroid gland extract, many enthusiasts thought that insulin was about to convert treated diabetes into a benign entity. Even if insulin would not produce a radical cure, this form of organotherapy would prove nevertheless to be an extraordinarily effective specific treatment. •

But insulin did more than support medical theories and enable patients to metabolize food. This potent medical innovation and the surrounding network of ideas, in the mind of Joslin and many other physicians, subtly reconfigured therapeutic ideals. The conquest of all diabetic complications—a medical campaign that Joslin had mapped out in his Shattuck Lecture—became a new composite ideal. The aims of treatment began to move through the framework of constant and meticulous regulation (now aided by insulin) toward the complete cure of all untoward consequences of being diabetic. Two years after insulin was first put into use, Joslin enthused that "a new race of diabetics has come upon the scene." The Nobel Prize–winning discovery by Banting, Best, Collip, and Macleod had already extended the lives of diabetics by two years; "hospital practice, therefore," Joslin continued, "this past year has been among the erstwhile dead."[24] Not that Joslin viewed the extract as a panacea; "insulin does not cure diabetes," he stated repeatedly.[25] But, with insulin in hand to complement diet and exercise, he and his collaborators seemed to think that all manifestations of the disease (except the need to care constantly for oneself) could and should be eliminated.[26]

Patients such as Arnold Burns were the first generation after insulin to be indoctrinated in these values of intensive regulatory control. When Arnold was admitted to the Joslin Clinic and spent a week in the hospital, he and his mother, Ethel, learned about his disease and the proper use of diet and insulin. Such an experience was exactly what Joslin, from the pulpit of his self-styled diabetic care movement, had spelled out as ideal care, a high road to total mastery of the disease.

In Arnold's case, the early lessons of care and control were overseen at the Joslin Clinic by Dr. Priscilla White, who had joined Joslin's staff in 1924. White attended to juvenile patients and their parents throughout her distinguished career. She wrote a groundbreaking monograph, *Diabetes in Childhood and Adolescence* (1932), and was a pioneer in the field of prenatal care for pregnant diabetic women and their babies. Although herself a proselytizer of Joslin's doctrine of control, numerous sources (from journal articles and correspondence to anecdotes and testimonials) indicate that she delivered the message to patients in a distinct style, tempered with personal warmth, imbued with almost "charismatic attention" and concern. "No child," she believed, "can grow up without a scoop of ice cream once a week."[27]

Even Joslin—whose professional enthusiasm for diabetic control led some of his contemporaries to view him as an overly demanding zealot —also spoke to patients in more flexible and understanding registers, enunciating facts of diabetic life in soothing tones. In published works and private letters, Joslin often dwelled upon the mundane realities of living with diabetes. His therapeutics often consisted of simple advice, comprehensive in scope, delivered with the assured certainty of an experienced general practitioner who was comfortable managing many areas of patients' lives.

For example, after one of Arnold's visits to the clinic, Joslin conveyed to Mrs. Burns that young Arnold was developing normally both physically and mentally. He then went on to suggest that the boy's mildly protuberant abdomen might be helped by gentle exercises and that he should be "out in the sun as much as possible, should take cod liver oil, a teaspoonful daily, and eat liver twice a week in place of his usual meat."[28]

On another occasion, Ethel wrote Joslin that she was "taking advantage of the fact that you said I might write and ask you any question. I would like to know how to treat a cough? Arnold developed a cold and cough. . . . He has several coughs like this every winter and Arnold's father feels I have failed in my duty not to have asked you before now what to do." She had heard Joslin say that "codeine was the medicine a mother would give when you spoke over Radio about 2 yrs ago so I bought some Codeine . . . and it worked very well[;] now I would like to know if that was right? Arnold [is] fine now."[29] Joslin quickly replied that he thought the codeine unnecessary. "Upon just placing a child in bed," he advised, "with the quiet which that implies or either some tablet or even chewing gum, the cough should subside." Closing his note, he added: "We are always glad to answer questions."[30]

From bulging bellies to troublesome coughs to constipated bowels, Joslin had advice to dispense. Frequently, though, his patients presented more complex and often competing needs, many of which revolved around financial constraints that eroded patients' ability to control their disease. The medical records of his clinic are filled with references to money problems exacerbated by the burdens of buying insulin and other diabetic medical care.[31]

Arnold's mother referred frequently to money and costs. Once, she inquired about a bill that the clinic had sent for a pediatrician's examination that had taken place when she had last brought Arnold to the clinic. She explained, "It has puzzled me as to why [the pediatrician] was called in and nothing said until afterward. We are perfectly willing to do all that is necessary to help Arnold but we are not financially able to do anything that is not necessary and I am writing this so we'll understand each others['] ways." Having reasserted her prerogative to control how her family would spend money on Arnold's medical care, she closed by adding, "I hope you will understand the principle of this letter."[32] Three years later, she told Joslin that a year and a half had passed since she "last had Arnold to see you[;] since that time, owing to financial reasons, I have had to take 'a chance' with him that everything was alright."[33]

Things went from bad to worse for the Burns family when Arnold's father died suddenly from a stroke.[34] A month later, Ethel turned to Joslin for help. "Do you happen to have a woman patient," she wrote, "who would like to live in the country by any chance? I am desperate and must find a way to make a little money to help keep Arnold going as he should. . . . I would not bother to ask you if it were not that I must do something and am trying every way I can think of."[35] Although Arnold's medical file does not record what solution Ethel eventually found, clearly this case and similar ones impressed Joslin. Throughout his career, he solicited money to establish hospital charity funds and advocated medical care cost reform, and when confronted with a patient who could not pay, he frequently waived his fees and pressured his colleagues to do likewise.[36]

Money, however, was not the only factor shaping Arnold's health care. His insulin-transformed disease was still a lurking nemesis that physicians, now with emboldened expectations, sought to subdue through better control. Arnold lived as one of the "erstwhile dead," a young diabetic always threatened by lethal complications, particularly coma. In the late 1920s, Joslin had spearheaded a campaign to abolish diabetic coma. As he viewed it, "diabetes is a chronic disease, but diabetic coma is an acute disease. If this fact was recognized, deaths from diabetic coma should cease." The physician had to spot impending coma and treat it vigorously, while "the patient should be trained to avoid coma." A 1929 editorial in the *Journal of the American Medical Association* concurred, defining diabetic coma as "a medical state, possible to prevent, expensive, time consuming, and difficult to treat, recovery a miracle to all beholders, but death a lasting blot upon the reputation of the patient or his physician."[37]

Certainly, Joslin knew through his extensive network of correspondents how diabetics had languished or even perished because of poor medical care, such as treating coma with glucose or a host of other needless mishaps.[38] When Arnold was eleven years old, he nearly suffered a "lasting blot" upon what would have been his short-lived reputation, but he was resuscitated at the New England Deaconess Hospital, where his doctors followed an exacting protocol of treatment with large doses of insulin and intravenous fluids.[39] After this scare, Priscilla White wrote to Ethel, "Just why [Arnold] developed diabetic coma I am not certain. Children change very quickly." White went on,

> A safe program for you to follow on a day of illness would be to test the urine every 4 hours, to give 20 units of insulin if the [Benedict's] test is red, 15 if the test is orange, 10 units if the test is yellow, 5 units if yellow-green. If three consecutive specimens are red give him the same amount of insulin only give it every 2 hours instead of every 4 hours. During the day he could take 1½ quarts of milk, 60 grams of bread, 60 grams of potato, 30 grams of oatmeal, 200 grams of orange juice or gingerale.[40]

Diabetic coma and its grave consequences warranted this level of precision, since painstaking attention to detail could avert deaths.[41]

Nevertheless, intensive control applied to the daily management of diabetes was the Joslin Clinic's style—not a universal one. For example, the eminent Chicago medical chemist and diabetologist Rollin Turner Woodyatt, M.D., who was among the first American physicians to administer insulin, argued for a very different therapeutic strategy to a colleague in 1929. A canny researcher of meticulous habits, drawn more to his laboratory bench than his clinical practice, Woodyatt believed that "the object of treatment is . . . to keep the patient as well and strong as a normal individual with the least effort and with the lowest economic outlay possible, i.e., to make the patient as nearly normal as possible notwithstanding the existence of a nearly total diabetes."[42] Woodyatt, who had developed complex and rather daring dietetic formulas in the pre-insulin era,[43] was willing to concede sugar in diabetic patients' urine in order to avoid insulin reactions. Though Joslin and others were correct in protesting that the urine sugar test then became useless, the point for Woodyatt was moot since he instructed his patients to test their urine for acid and admonished them to stay acid free, not sugar free. In Woodyatt's opinion, the more liberal regimen (he advocated combining regular insulin doses so that there were only two injections a day) allowed a more normal life: "I think it is important with these youngsters in school or college to interfere as little as possible with their free physical, social and psychological development."[44]

But Arnold was a patient under the care of Joslin, not Woodyatt nor any other distinguished physician.[45] For Arnold, debates between experts mattered far less than practical urban-rural differences: living in a small town in rural Massachusetts posed its own problems. Medical knowledge has never been uniformly distributed,[46] and the heterogeneity of clinical experience and practice styles was a prominent aspect of many young diabetics' lives. While elite physicians in Boston felt comfortable dosing insulin and managing diabetic problems, local practitioners were often intimidated by the children's disease.

Ethel related one such incident to White. Shortly after seeing White, who had changed Arnold's diet and insulin, Arnold had broken out in a red rash, with a red throat. Initially, the local doctor had considered scarlet fever to be the cause, but the next day he changed his mind: "He decided it was a re-action to more insulin and different diet. Dr. came again yesterday to just look at throat and wanted me to write to you and tell you all about it and see what you thought, he says he never saw such a violent reaction. He is very interested. . . . Will you please tell me what to do?"[47] Alarmed, White dashed off a note. This might be, she said, a "toxic rash. I am quite worried about [Arnold] and the liberties he has taken with his diet and wish that you could let him come to the hospital for a week. I would be glad to have him come in on one of the funds. There will be no charge for medical care and no charge for the hospital."[48]

Arnold was hurried to the Deaconess Hospital, where the redness of his rash faded and his sore throat improved. White started him on the new, long-acting protamine insulin. Upon returning home, Ethel wrote White that Arnold was "delighted to only have insulin once a day and he is like a different young man he's so interested and bothers so much with his diet and tests. He also shows the good effects by stating he would have liked to have stayed in hospital longer, he was so interested and learning so much." She was pleased, too, that "his diet satisfies so much better and although he gets dizzy and shaky a little mornings he says not as shaky as he was, and straightens with lunch."[49]

STRIVING FOR CONTROL OF LIFE AND DEATH

It was the summer of 1938 and Arnold was fifteen years old. Ten years would pass before he contacted Joslin or White again. Like other young diabetics, Arnold was growing up, a member of a cohort of patients new to the world: juvenile-onset diabetics who lived well into adulthood. Many of these patients appeared to be uplifting portraits of therapeutic success; they engaged in competitive athletics, embarked on prestigious careers, bore children, raised families.[50] But for others, this portrait was beginning to be sketched in somber colors. In

1934, the *New England Journal of Medicine* ran an editorial that asked, "Of what shall diabetics die?" While coma and gangrene should no longer be permitted to kill patients, the *Journal* foresaw tuberculosis, pneumonia, stroke, and heart attack as the main causes of death.[51] Two years later, however, Paul Kimmelstiel and Clifford Wilson identified a specific pathologic lesion in the kidneys of diabetics, the first research finding heralding the emergence of renal failure as a major complication for many juvenile-onset diabetics.[52] By the middle of the 1950s, the Joslin Clinic was reporting that 50 percent of the young patients who died did so in renal failure, many when they were in their thirties.[53] This grim reality unfolded with bitter irony as the transmuted course of diabetes—the product of a singularly efficacious medical innovation—revealed one distressing complication after another.

Arnold reestablished his correspondence with Joslin in the midst of these ominous developments in the early spring of 1948. He was twenty-five years old and now spoke for himself, having assumed the responsibilities of work with much pride, his sense of self seemingly tied to his mastery of this chronic ailment. "I have been Working for the past six months as an automobile mechanic," he informed Joslin, "and have lost no time due to my diabetes." Then, although it violated one of Joslin's central tenets of ideal routine diabetic care, Arnold declared, "I have been to no doctor in connection to my diabetes since 1939 [nine years ago]."[54] Arnold's mother also recognized her son's pride in his work and his attendance, telling Joslin, "Arnold is getting along very well, . . . and works hard and steady as an auto mechanic, in fact he keeps up with the others not giving in days when I know he'd like to take it easy."[55]

Two years later, Arnold was asked to partake in a clinical study that Howard Root (a senior member of Joslin's staff) and another doctor at the Joslin Clinic were conducting. When Arnold agreed, trouble began to appear, albeit only in abnormal test results. Sugar was spilling into his urine and he had mildly elevated blood pressure, but more ominously, Arnold's eyes showed signs of substantial retinopathy and his kidneys were starting to struggle, with albumin appearing in his urine and an elevated urea level in his blood.[56]

A year and a half passed before these findings manifested themselves clinically. Ethel informed Joslin that she was "writing for Arnold. . . . He is working but acts so very weary, I would like to know what tonic he could take."[57] Several days later, Arnold himself wrote to tell Joslin that, while his diabetes was not causing him any difficulty, the vision in his right eye was poor and his right shoulder stiff.[58] Joslin responded separately to each note, telling Mrs. Burns that control of Arnold's diabetes was the best possible tonic and suggesting to Arnold that X-ray therapy for bursitis of shoulder, which had aided many other patients, might help. As always, Joslin also offered to see Arnold.[59]

Then, within a week, trouble turned into tragedy. Arnold explained in a neatly written letter to Root that he had recently switched jobs and was working in another garage.

> The second day there my right eye went blind so [that I can] only see light and dark. It was easier then to see with the left eye, [until] last Sunday [when] the left eye broke so I can hardly see news print. The garage people were afraid I'd get hurt so laid me off for a month to see if [my vision] will improve. . . . I called you last Monday afternoon but you were away. I called . . . [the ophthalmologist] and he said time was the only thing for the eye and advised no lifting or pulling.
>
> I know you see people who if [they] stub their toe run to a doctor. I don't do that but what am I supposed to do? What can I expect? If I can't work how can I live? Please tell me what to do.[60]

At the end of this letter, just underneath Arnold's signature, were the initials "E. B.": his mother had transcribed the letter. Perhaps even Root—who had been on the front line of the battle against coma and was now embroiled in a new struggle to control the disease's delayed complications—began to feel a constricting, claustrophobic sensation as Arnold's world started to collapse around him.

Half a year later, Arnold spent a week in the Deaconess Hospital. He had a "hacking cough," and his ankles were greatly swollen. As the test results came back, the picture grew bleaker. His kidneys were now putting out massive amounts of albumin into the urine. An EKG of his heart showed that Arnold had had a silent heart attack, and now he was in a state of congestive heart failure. Root wrote to the young man's hometown doctor, "Arnold represents a typical case of the diabetic triopathy. I venture to enclose a reprint summarizing 155 of our patients who have this condition. . . . I see nothing for Arnold to do more than to carry on his diabetic treatment as carefully as possible."[61]

The article that Root referred to, published in 1954, framed the syndrome of diabetic triopathy (nerve, eye, and kidney damage) as both a clinical observation and a pointed therapeutic indictment. After showing that these complications often clustered together, Root and his coauthors argued that the eye and kidney problems were the result of poor diabetic control. They stratified their patients into four classes of diabetic control—excellent, good, fair, and poor—based upon criteria that incorporated medical parameters (for excellent control, "patient must never have been in coma") and measures of adherence to a strict diet and doctors' orders ("diet must have been weighed at least 80% of the time," daily urine tests "with a conscientious attempt to have the urine sugar free," and "regular physical examinations and laboratory tests"). The tacit moral of the paper was simple: those patients who had poor control ("medical advice neglected") suffered the consequences of higher rates of complications.[62] With this linkage of lax patient compliance to inadequate control and thence to complications, Arnold—once so proud of his independence from medical doctors and the restrictions of his disease—was in poor standing, medically and morally.

A month later, Arnold managed to write a note to Root, his handwriting frail and tremulous. He wanted to thank Root "for making the arrangements to get me in [to the hospital]. I want to thank you, Elliott Joslin, Priscilla White, and the others for the past service in getting the swelling out of my ankles and making it so I can lay down and get some sleep. And for keeping my expenses at a minimum."[63] The same day, Arnold started another letter to Root.

> Dear Howard Root, I have a few questions I would like to ask.
> 1. What is suppose to be wrong with me?
> 2. Why do I get out of breath when I try do anything besides just sit around or walk slow? I used to be able to Work—Work hard anywhere from 8–16 hours a day. Now I am not good for ½ hours, feel like I am going to pass out.
> 3. They gave me some pills when I left the hospital. There were some big Red ones[,] the Bottle said to take 4 a day[,] the[y']re all gone, should I get more or not, don't feel any different with out them.
> 4. What did [you] think about my Left eye or do you think it will stay like it is or blow apart again? never mind this one [—] found out for my self—this is another day[,] got coughing last night[,] got up[,] lot of junk floating around in the left eye[,] have to keep moving my head around so I can see this page.
> 5. What makes my legs go numb when I sit or lay down?

Arnold concluded by stressing, "These are questions not complain[t]s. As I had 15 years w[h]ere I didn't have to take a back seat for any one[.]

But since last Nov. I been riding under the back of a dump cart with all the other junk."[64]

Arnold was losing control not only over his health but over his conception of himself as independent, self-sustaining, and hard working. A diabetic for as long as he probably could remember, who grew into adulthood proud of his ability to manage his ailment, he now confronted not only a grave medical condition but also an equally dire existential situation, as complications slowly eroded his self-image.[65] Root, who had anticipated this protracted deterioration,[66] wrote back to tell Arnold that he was "sorry to say that the trouble with you was the failure of your heart and . . . that means the heart muscle has lost some of its strength. Unfortunately, the diabetes spots in your eyes are the cause of the loss of vision." Then, in an avuncular way, Root tried to redirect Arnold's efforts toward coping. "I know it is very hard for you to take the back seat and take it slowly now, but I am afraid you will have to limit yourself in order to conserve the energy and protect yourself."[67]

· In the middle of autumn three months later, thirty-two-year-old Arnold wrote again: "My ankles have started to swell[;] they are about the size they were last spring. [T]he swelling goes part way up the legs and the legs are like two cakes of ice. I am starting to cough hard again and to cough in the night. I guess I sleep 2 or 3 hours a night. . . . I try not to be a pest with the questions. [B]ut if some thing happened, some people could say I didn't try to find out. . . . What do we do now?"[68]

By that winter, Arnold had suffered a stroke that paralyzed his right side. Two months later, he was hospitalized with a chief complaint of "Pain Right Leg." The leg was gangrenous, and so late that night, attempting to check his demise with a desperate intervention, the doctors amputated Arnold's leg at midthigh. The next morning the resident wrote, "Looks poorly—Cheyne Stokes respiration. [Then again, later that day] began to vomit coffee-ground material @ 6:30 pm. [Doctors] attempted to pass Levine Tube but [patient] appeared to aspirate vomitus and expired despite attempts to suction. Pronounced dead at 7:40 pm."[69] Arnold was thirty-three years old.

As was more customary then, Ethel permitted an autopsy, which reported "the major pathological findings":

Healed infarcts of the myocardium.
Mural thrombus of the left ventricle.
Hypertrophy and dilatation of the left ventricle.

Hypertrophy of the right ventricle.

Dilatation of the pulmonary conus.

Atherosclerosis of the coronary arteries.

General arteriosclerosis.

Recent infarct of the brain (left parietal lobe).

Infarcts of the spleen and kidneys.

Probable embolus in the right iliac artery.

Right mid-thigh amputation.

Bilateral pleural effusion, more marked at right.

Collapse of the right lung.

Marked congestion and edema of the left lung.

Acute ulcers of the duodenum.

Cholesterolosis of the gall bladder.

Acute hemorrhagic cystitis.

Slight edema of the left leg.

Diabetes mellitus (clinical).

The cause of death, based on these findings, is due to respiratory failure.[70]

If the postmortem had probed beyond this litany of pathologies and sought out the human circumstances of this man who had been so ravaged by long-term diabetic complications, it might have produced a more concise and revealing report: the circumstances of Arnold's death, like his twenty-nine years of prolonged diabetic life, had been shaped by medical intervention.

Shortly after Arnold's death, the operating surgeon wrote to Allen Joslin (Elliott's son, who had been the attending physician), "Just a note to tell you how sorry I am that we could not do more for your patient, Mr. Arnold Burns. I think the amputation that was done probably did get ahead of his gas gangrene but there were too many other problems to expect to get away with this in a man so sick. It is certainly a tragedy to see this condition in a patient who is so young."[71]

Allen Joslin sent condolences to Ethel, observing, "Arnold, was a most faithful patient as you know. . . . Your son did much better than all our diabetic children to date. We regret that some of our patients with over 30 years of insulin have complications. . . . His problems at the time of his passing were many."[72] Since Ethel had requested the autopsy findings, she also received a copy and an offer to answer any questions. A week later, she thanked Allen Joslin for the report, adding that she was "trying to straighten his financial affairs, I will be slow but will take care of them." Then, summing up not only the last letter she wrote to the clinic but, essentially, a whole dimension of Arnold's life, she went on to say: "I would like to take this time to thank all of the Joslin Clinic who were so kind to Arnold and also the nurses, Doctors, and all at the Deaconess, you know he called it his second home down there and felt it belonged to him."[73]

THE WANT OF CONTROL

Looking back in 1954, Elliott Joslin recalled "the ideas of the leading apostles in diabetes in the last century," all of whom believed adamantly in the virtue of control and sought to achieve it through diet. Then "insulin arrived and diabetics lived rather than died. . . . Patients treated with insulin did so much better than ever before that a relaxation in the management of the disease seemed harmless." Joslin continued, his rhetorical tone rising, to note how "the warning statistics of doctors schooled in the treatment of diabetes were decried. . . . Against this background of apostasy, therefore, it is heartening now to read of the advocacy of control of the disease by those who have witnessed the results of the lack of it."[74]

For Joslin and other American practitioners throughout the twentieth century, the central ambition of diabetic management—and its chief frustration—has been the want of control. The eagerness with which physicians have pursued this elusive objective, and in what directions, have distinguished various styles of managing the disease. Joslin may have declared partial victory at midcentury, but the advance of an alternative clinical style, which was less stringent regarding control and more concerned that patients live "normal" lives, would put his beliefs on the defensive for several decades. Since the 1950s, physicians have debated whether control could prevent long-term complications, and if so, how effectively. In 1993, the published results of a large clinical trial argued that Joslin was essentially right; patients placed on tight-control regimens, compared with those under normal diabetic care, lowered their risk of delayed complications markedly.[75] But this reduction of risk, important though it is, does not settle a more fundamental argument: even if the means of better diabetic control are now "at our door," the questions of what measures should we take to pursue control, and at what personal consequence to patients' lives, remain open, beyond the dictates of statistical data.

In many ways, what has compelled physicians to align themselves on one side or another of the control issue has never been a simple assessment of physiological efficacy but rather a complex set of ideas and ideals. The Joslin group structured their diabetic management around the ideal of seizing control of the disease, preventing all complications, and extending life at virtually any cost. Their collective commitment to this ideal of complete control was entrenched so deeply that it became a sacred ideal, beyond criticism, connected to other fundamental dichotomies, natural and moral[76]: control versus laxity; health versus sickness; life versus death; virtue versus sin. In one sense, Arnold owed his life to the uncompromising commitment that underwrote this scheme, as these values had propelled innovators such as Joslin forward as they pushed back the boundaries of what was medically possible, adding years to diabetic lives.

And yet, as Arnold's case illustrates so poignantly, these same values often imposed stern judgments and harsh trade-offs. When his complications first emerged, and then as his medical problems mounted, Arnold carried the burden not simply of his failing health but also of the medical attitudes that construed complications as the result of poor patient compliance and control—"medical advice neglected." Finally, near the end of Arnold's life, when gangrene was poised to cause his death, his doctors' aggressive interventions sacrificed his final hours in an uncompromising pursuit of medical control over death.

Arnold's experience encompassed all these paradoxes and dilemmas of medical practice and its connected ideals. Viewed from this perspective, his experience with diabetes transcends the inexorable course of an aberrant metabolism, becoming a powerful commentary on the often contradictory aims built into modern medicine. Arnold's case exhibits the bittersweet irony of an illness transformed by a therapeutic style of relentless control, tracing the mortal arc from a life saved, from the moment of clinical salvation through to the end of that life. What medicine had given to Arnold, it had—in an untoward alliance with the disease—taken away.

The twists and turns in this latter-day morality play remind us that the complex world of therapeutic options and decisions rarely admits to perfect solutions. Instead, clinicians and patients have long struggled with the inescapable trade-offs posed when limited knowledge and capacity to heal confront human disease and mortality. The choices that these players have made reflected the circumstances and temper of their times as well as idiosyncratic preference. Joslin embodied an ethos widely prevalent in twentieth-century American medicine and society: the desire to control disease and death. His achievements as both architect and spokesman for intensive diabetic management paralleled treatment strategies developed by other physicians in other specialties, evident from intensive care units to high-risk obstetrical practices to trauma surgical services. These endeavors express values that patients and physicians alike have promulgated, almost to the point where medical control has become a fetish, to be viewed as selfless or high-minded or even self-protective, providing some assurance in the face of capricious and seemingly cruel diseases.[77] And, no doubt, the exhaustive attention and increasingly sophisticated interventions of this therapeutic approach has benefited many patients, diabetic and otherwise, and will continue to do so in the future as more diseases are transmuted from acute to chronic forms.

From this point of view, the story of Arnold, his mother, Ethel, and the doctors who treated him emphasizes the central role that ideals of controlling disease have played in shaping patient care. Joslin, who combined remarkable dedication and integrity in his quest for a better diabetic world, was but one physician who espoused such ideals—ideals that together with brave new ideas and innovations have forged the predominant style of modern American medical therapeutics.

From another perspective, however, Arnold's case stresses a countervailing yet nonetheless fundamental force in the experience of illness, as it stands in sharp contrast with the history of Billy Hampden—disturbingly so. For the two cases, when placed side by side, accentuate the importance not only of medical technology but of social circumstances as well. Arnold accrued the benefits of insulin but died alone in the hospital; Billy wanted for insulin but instead received several years of attentive care from a personal nurse and the thoughtful treatment of his private physician before he eventually died at home. Of course, two different patients might not show the influence of money and quality of care so starkly—but Billy and Arnold do. Their experiences insist that, when we tell the story of how powerful medical technologies have affected human lives, we must attend to more than just new drugs, scientific ideas, and even therapeutic ideals. We must follow patients as they have experienced their illness and its treatment, and be willing to see that wonder drugs are only a part of the story.

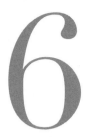

6 PREGNANT LONGINGS: MOUNTING MEDICAL INTENSITY IN THE PURSUIT OF MOTHERHOOD

The forty thousand potentially child-bearing diabetic women of the United States are concerned with the following problems: their chances (a) for conception, (b) for surviving pregnancy, (c) for reproducing living children and (d) for transmitting the tendency to develop diabetes.

—Priscilla White, "Pregnancy Complicating Diabetes," 1948

In the late 1960s, thirty years after the birth of her daughter, Ellen Nielson wrote to Dr. Priscilla White: "Perhaps you might be interested to know what I have been doing since our daughter was born at Faulkner Hospital. . . . As you may remember, Barbara Lynn was 'one of your babies.'" The letter recounted Ellen's busily successful life and her marriage of "31 wonderful years together." Now in her midfifties, she enclosed two photos of her and her husband with their young grandchildren on their knees. "I have always been grateful," Ellen went on to say, "for the help that Dr. Joslin, you, and Dr. Marble—as well as many others—have given me. The diabetes has been easy to control, and I have never had to treat myself in any 'special' way. Perhaps the age of 20 is a good time to start with diabetes—I have been most fortunate."[1]

The pursuit of motherhood has been an important element in the life stories of many women who lived with diabetes after the discovery of insulin. For some women, such as Ellen, this pursuit ended happily with the birth of a healthy child. For other women, like Sally Kramer in Chapter 3, the longing for a successful pregnancy resulted in frustration or grief. Be they joyous or sorrowful, these stories have unfolded in the decades since 1921 in an ever-shifting context, as diabetes mellitus was progressively transmuted into a chronic condition. In particular, the once-dreaded combination of pregnancy complicated by diabetes has become a clinical commonplace, requiring skill and tenacity but no longer an outright miracle to end with a healthy mother and child.[2]

The dramatic twentieth-century history of the diabetic pregnancy warrants particular attention in this book because it illustrates several important themes that resonate in the broader history of twentieth-century diabetes, and indeed throughout much of modern medical practice. These themes—a migrating focus of clinical concern, the mounting intensity of care, an expanding horizon of medical management, and the constant reconfiguring of relationships and responsibilities between patients and providers—represent four "historical motifs" or distinctive patterns of historical change that have recurred over the past several decades. Focusing on these motifs provides not so much a chronological timeline but rather a means to reconsider how the past shapes our present and informs us of what the future might hold (see Table 6.1).

Inextricably, these themes and stories of diabetes and pregnancy were interwoven into a backdrop of broader medical and social change regarding birthing and motherhood in America. The decline of maternal death rates in the first half of the twentieth century, along with the even more substantial reduction of neonatal mortality rates, recast labor and delivery from an often life-threatening trial to an occasion that can be managed safely and relatively comfortably (see Figure 6.1). Although less well documented, during the same interval, the most common birth location migrated from home to the hospital, and the attendants during labor switched from predominantly female midwives to male physicians, with a reversal of these trends occurring only during the later decades of the twentieth century.[3] Meanwhile, the cultural link between successful motherhood and fulfilling womanhood—although scrutinized by recent feminist critiques—has long created for most women an intensely felt belief that childbearing and -rearing are fundamental aspects of feminine identity. Even though the so-called cult of true womanhood, fixated on the maternal role as the raison d'être for woman, may now seem as dated as its early-nineteenth-century origins, the associated values, images, and judgments continued to greatly influence how women experienced their lives throughout the twentieth century.[4]

Keeping this social and cultural backdrop in mind enriches the context of the following four motifs, which have appeared in slight variation throughout the history of modern American medicine, arising when

TABLE 6.1. Evolving Medical Management of Diabetes and Pregnancy

FOUR HISTORICAL MOTIFS OF MODERN MEDICAL CARE

Period	Migrating Focus of Clinical Concern	Mounting Intensity of Care	Expanding Horizon of Medical Management	Reconfiguring Relationships and Responsibilities
Pre-1922	Maternal ketoacidosis Maternal infections Fetuses and newborns rarely viable	Pregnancy prevention Therapeutic abortion Diet	Immediate	Mother Father
1922–30	Less maternal ketoacidosis Still maternal infections Persistent late fetal demise	Regular insulin Close clinic or hospital-based observation	Late pregnancy through postpartum	Mother Father General physician or obstetrician
1931–70	Late fetal demise Neonatal demise due to respiratory distress, hypoglycemia, and congenital anomalies	Longer-acting insulins Elective cesarean delivery Hormone therapy	Mid-pregnancy through postpartum	Mother and father Rise of diabetes "specialists" and the interdisciplinary "medical team" approach
1970–90	Preventing fetal malformations Preventing macrosomia Postpartum newborn care	Meticulous glycemic control: blood glucose meters, insulin pumps Antepartum fetal testing: lung maturity, peripartum monitoring	Preconception through postpartum	Mother and father General and specialist physicians Proliferation of medical teams
Present	Maternal vasculopathy Long-term outcomes for child	Kidney-pancreas transplantation	Long-term maternal health Long-term health of the child Comprehensive "disease management" services	Mother and father Medical team Managed care organizations
Future	Greater emphasis on outcome measures, including satisfaction and quality of life Concurrent emphasis on costs and cost-effectiveness	Transcutaneous blood glucose monitors Inhaled insulin Encapsulated islets B-cell transplants Artificial pancreas	Preconception counseling of risk based on gene testing Efforts to prevent diabetes mellitus	Greater external influence on medical relationships and provision of services External monitoring of quality of care and patient satisfaction

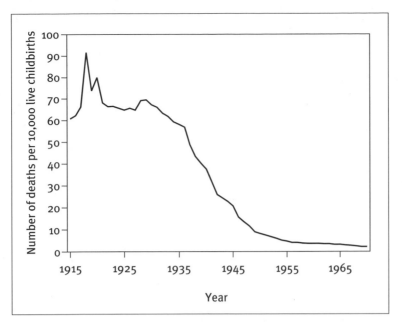

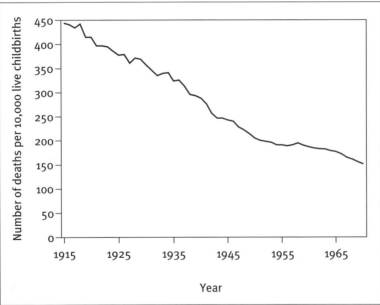

Figure 6.1. Maternal (top) and Neonatal Mortality Rates in the United States, 1915–1970. Source: *Data is from "Chapter B: Vital Statistics and Health and Medical Care, Series B 136—147. Fetal Death Ratio; Neonatal, Infant, and Maternal Mortality Rates, by Race: 1915 to 1970," in U.S. Bureau of the Census,* Historical Statistics of the United States, Colonial Times to 1970, *electronic edition edited by Susan B. Carter et al. (New York: Cambridge University Press, 1997).*

a goal as socially valued as the pursuit of motherhood intersects with an obstacle as complicated and threatening as diabetes mellitus. We will examine these motifs through the experiences of four women: Janice, Susan Thompson, Robin Jenner, and Bernadette Dane. Taking each motif separately, we will compose a collage that attempts to convey the history of diabetes and pregnancy, a complex and evolving ecology of desire and care.

MIGRATING FOCUS OF CLINICAL CONCERN

Before insulin became available in 1922, diabetic women did not frequently become pregnant: they either died too quickly or held onto life through a self-imposed starvation that left their bodies weak and infertile. When a diabetic woman did manage to conceive, pregnancy in the setting of diabetes was seen as a deadly combination. In 1882 Matthews Duncan of London published one of the first articles on the subject, reporting that of twenty-two pregnancies in sixteen mothers, four mothers died during labor, another seven died within two years, and nearly half the children were born dead or died shortly thereafter.[5] J. Whitridge Williams's report in 1909 was equally somber, finding that half the women died during the pregnancy and, among the remainder, nearly half of the fetuses or neonates died.[6] Joseph DeLee recommended in his obstetrical textbook, published in 1913, that all diabetic pregnancies be terminated with a therapeutic abortion as soon as the diagnosis was made: "The attempt to carry the patient up to term or even to viability of the child is too perilous—either the shock of delivery brings on coma, or some other nervous shock does it, or the disease aggravates dangerously, and, too often, the child dies in utero."[7] Until the late 1920s, this gloomy assessment preoccupied the minds of most physicians, who feared for the mother's life, either from ketoacidosis and coma or from intercurrent infection, such as pneumonia or tuberculosis.[8]

Not all practitioners felt helpless, though, when presented with a patient who was both pregnant and diabetic. Writing in 1915, Elliott Joslin admitted, "It is only fair to say that the general practitioner still has horror at the discovery of considerable quantities of sugar in the urine during pregnancy," recounting the case of a woman whose pregnancy, although "terminated" in the seventh month, nevertheless resulted in the death not only of the infant but also of the mother, with the bereaved husband subsequently committing suicide on the wife's grave. Such tragic cases notwithstanding, Joslin was characteristically more optimistic. He believed that "the secret of success in the treatment of pregnant women with sugar in the urine" consisted of having the "patients under constant supervision throughout the course of the pregnancy and for some months after confinement." The nature of treatment, he maintained, "should follow exactly the same methods which are employed in the treatment of the usual cases of diabetes," which to Joslin were the "rational" therapeutics pioneered in Europe by Bernard Naunyn and Carl von Noorden and, more recently in America, by Frederick M. Allen, consisting of carefully calibrated undernutrition diets.

To support his views, Joslin cited the observation, then being expressed by several physicians, that "the gloomy outlook for pregnant women showing large quantities of sugar" in their urine had been "modified when it was recognized that these cases could be divided into two groups, based on the appearance of sugar before or after the pregnancy began. If pregnancy occurred in diabetic patients the outlook was considered far more serious than when diabetes first appeared during pregnancy." Joslin then presented several cases, focusing especially on the experience of a thirty-one-year-old woman, "a physician's wife," who he first examined in December of 1914, in her sixth month of pregnancy. Despite the recent discovery of her urine containing 6.4 percent sugar, and her new symptoms of polydipsia and polyuria, Joslin felt that "the case appeared to me most favorable to attempt to carry through to term," due in part to the fact that "both she and her husband thoroughly appreciated the situation, each had a cheerful temperament and instantly showed that they would follow directions." A week later, she was admitted to the New England Deaconess Hospital, with the plan that she would "remain there until danger was over or until confinement [that is, birth of the baby] occurred." While Joslin thoughtfully regulated her diet, "she had the freedom of the hospital, took daily walks, and by her cheerful temperament contributed much to the happiness of other diabetic patients with whom she was associated." The "method of delivery was carefully considered," with Joslin and the obstetrician concluding that an elective cesarean section would be ideal, as it would minimize the physical exertion of the mother and the risks of delivery for the baby. Just as the pregnancy reached term, the cesarean section yielded an eight-pound baby, "normal in every way," and a healthy mother who made a complete recovery.

To this case of what might now be termed "gestational diabetes," Joslin added several others, many of which did not end nearly so happily, yet in these instances he cited errors in management of the diabetes, and not the diabetes per se, as the culprit. This type of error was rectifiable, in Joslin's view, and "the next few years may show that pregnancy can take place in diabetic patients far more readily than has ever been supposed." Joslin concluded his review prophetically, asserting, "It is certainly true that with the improvement in the treatment of diabetic patients [and therefore an unanticipated improvement in fertility], diabetic women will be less likely to avoid pregnancy."[9]

After 1922 and the profound transformation of the diabetic world wrought by insulin therapy, not only did the number of children living with diabetes increase, these youngsters began to mature into young adults. To handle the growing population of patients with juvenile-onset diabetes, the ever-forward-thinking Joslin hired a new staff member, Priscilla White, to assist him. Dr. White had still not completed her internship when she received the telephone call from Joslin offering her the position. Born in Boston in 1900, she had attended Radcliffe College and then Tufts University Medical College, graduating third in her class in 1923. Several months later, the twenty-four-year-old physician joined the Joslin Clinic, remaining on staff for the remainder of her long and remarkable career, in which she became an international expert both on childhood diabetes and on pregnancy occurring in the setting of diabetes. Half a century after her first day on the job, as part of a golden anniversary celebration, she recalled that "practically on my arrival Dr. Joslin assigned me to the study of diabetic children. As the youngest member of the team he thought that I would be close to them. This was true. A marvelous opportunity!"[10]

The children cared for at the Joslin Clinic during the 1920s, who were reared according to Joslin's doctrine of strict control, constituted the first long-lived cohort of juvenile patients. Soon, the young girls developed into women. In 1925, a teenage diabetic woman was reported to have resumed menstruation after starting insulin, and other accounts of diabetic children developing into fertile adults followed.[11] Many physicians worried that diabetic women, no longer protected by infertility, were now fully exposed to the frightful risks of maternal mortality that Duncan had described. Among sophisticated practitioners, however, insulin quickly changed the view that diabetes and pregnancy equaled a lethal coupling, with DeLee proclaiming in 1928, "The treatment of diabetes complicating pregnancy has undergone a complete revolution."[12]

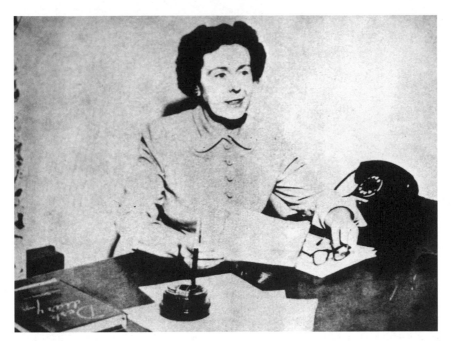

Priscilla White, M.D. Courtesy of the Joslin Diabetes Center Historical Archive.

White believed similarly that "the tragic end-results of diabetic preg-nancies are increasingly infrequent and with proper supervision and co-operation can be largely eliminated . . . our own case records show that diabetes is no longer a contraindication to pregnancy."[13]

Exactly what counted as "proper supervision and cooperation" was a moving target. For example, in 1932 White received a letter from a bereaved mother, whose daughter Janice had recently died late in her pregnancy. "She had been fine right along," the mother explained, "and she was down to see [her local doctor] a little over a week before she took sick and he said she was all right." A few days later Janice and her mother had gone "shopping and she walked a lot then came home and done some ironing, then after supper she started to vomit, and had a severe pain in the pit of her stomach." After a long night of relentless vomiting, the doctor was summoned and "when he came he ordered her to the hospital. He said she had albumin in the kidneys and toxemia poison, but oh what that poor thing suffered. If I could only get that out of my mind I could stand it." The next day, Janice's husband arrived back in town. "The poison killed the baby and it was born [that] night. A little girl, just what she wanted." The following morning, Janice "seemed better" but that evening "took convulsions" that recurred the following morning, "and after that they kept her full of morphine" until she died twenty-four hours later. The mother concluded with a lamentation: "I know we have to submit to God's will, but why one so good and patient as she always was should have to suffer so much I can't see. I don't know how to live without her. She was always so thoughtful and kind to me, and my only hope now is that I will meet her soon where parting cannot come."[14]

White subsequently wrote to the local doctor asking for detailed information, avoiding any hint of reprobation with her gently inquisitive tone. White then related her own experience. Although she claimed that the major problem was with the babies, she proceeded to recount the story of another patient who was married to the son of a gynecologist. This father-in-law physician had followed her pregnancy closely. One day in his office she had a convulsion and died soon thereafter. As a result of this tragedy, White noted, her group was "debating whether or not we should insist upon hospitalization of our young diabetics for a month prior to delivery, and Janice's case might influence us in doing this."[15]

In this decade following the discovery of insulin, the much-decreased incidence of maternal diabetic deaths stood in sharp contrast to the persistently high fetal and newborn mortality rates. As the focus of clinical concern shifted from mother to infant, the practical lessons that White and Joslin learned from an assortment of clinical tragedies was that good prenatal care was not good enough, close observation not close enough. Their mixture of mounting frustration and clinical perfectionism led to a new—and conspicuously aggressive—style of medical management.

MOUNTING INTENSITY OF CARE

The state-of-the-art approach that Joslin and White pioneered in the 1930s would prove to be prototypical of late-twentieth-century medical care in general: an intensive strategy of diabetes management, with weekly prenatal visits and an early and prolonged confinement, uniformly culminating with an elective cesarean section. In 1937, Raymond Titus—the obstetrician who collaborated with Joslin and White—described their approach after first observing, "Before 1920 diabetes and pregnancy made a discouraging association. The only encouraging part of this association was its actual infrequency." Titus wished, however, to recast the diabetic pregnancy more optimistically, emphasizing that "insulin has made medical history. Insulin is making obstetrical history." He noted, "Insulin is increasing every day the number of possible pregnancies in diabetics," and "insulin makes pregnancy safe for the mothers." While "present knowledge cannot guarantee living children," the Joslin group believed, "the baby is so very important in the severe diabetics and the 'insulin mothers' that, to avoid intrauterine death, the safest method is cesarean section when the baby seems quite big enough." The logic underlying this recommended mode of delivery appears to have been as much emotional as scientific, as Titus and his fellow clinicians "felt so badly about having lost a baby which died under our observation that the general rule was laid down to deliver all these insulin mothers and sick diabetics by cesarean section as soon as it was felt that the baby was viable."[16]

One woman who experienced the advent of this intensive management style was Susan Thompson. Fifteen years old when she first saw Joslin and White in 1928, Susan had begun to lose weight that spring, with polyuria commencing in September, urinary sugar detected in October, the initiation of insulin therapy in early November, and a trip from her home in Ohio to Boston by the end of November. Thereafter, she repeatedly drove the eight hundred miles by car to see her doctors. In the autumn of 1932, she sent the Joslin Clinic a card announcing her recent marriage. Several months later, an Ohio doctor wrote to Joslin about Susan. The nineteen-year-old woman had eloped and been married "a couple of months ago and now thinks she is pregnant—she did not consult anyone as to the danger of pregnancy in her condition." After noting that she had just had a twenty-four-hour urine sample free of any sugar and a fasting blood glucose level of 215 milligrams per deciliter (which Joslin would have considered slightly too elevated but most other physicians would have thought an acceptable level for a patient with diabetes), he asked Joslin, "What would be your advice about this case?" The doctor, alluding to Susan's previous impulsive actions, added, "The situation has sobered her and she insists she will be careful as to diet and hygiene."[17]

Joslin wrote back: "Despite all the sorrows with Susan there is something good in her I know and possibly it will now come out. We have quite a good many diabetic girls get pregnant and unanimously have reached the conclusion that the last three or four weeks of pregnancy must be spent in a hospital and, furthermore, that the patient must have a Cesarean section about two weeks before delivery." Joslin added, "We have gone through this on a good many cases and are simply sick at the thought of losing a nine pound baby which might be saved by a Cesarean."[18]

The Ohio doctor responded, thanking Joslin for his letter but asking whether he could have Joslin's "opinion of a therapeutic abortion in her case. She is only nineteen and quite irresponsible. Her parents feel she will not hold to her diet away from home and that a crisis might occur at any time." Expanding further on his rationale, the doctor continued, "If she were relieved of this pregnancy, . . . after she becomes more mature and acquires a greater sense of responsibility and has improved her habits, as she easily could, . . . a pregnancy could be carried thro' with more safety. . . . I shall be glad to have your opinion about Susan, having in mind her youth and irresponsibility."[19]

Joslin immediately shot back a reply, emphatically stating, "I could not approve of a therapeutic abortion in the case of Susan. I believe the girl is fundamentally a very nice girl and I believe her baby would pull her to her senses more quickly then anything else." He agreed that "it is quite a thing for a young diabetic girl to go through a pregnancy, but she can do it safely if she will only keep in touch with the doctor and I am sure she would do that." Joslin assured the physician, "I will do anything I can to be of assistance," noting not quite parenthetically that "only yesterday a woman came to the office and was grateful for her baby. She was older and, therefore, not as good a risk as Susan."[20] Despite Joslin's encouragement, though, the pregnancy was aborted.

Susan herself next wrote to Joslin in the spring of 1934. "I am going to have a baby in October," she declared, "and thought you might be interested. Is there any Doctor in Ohio you would recommend?"[21] Joslin responded by requesting more information while emphasizing, "I will do anything I can to aid you during your pregnancy but it must be done through your own local physician."[22] Following this advice, Susan apparently took matters into her own hands. Soon thereafter, Joslin received a letter from an Ohio obstetrician, telling him that "Mrs. Thompson appeared in my office this last week, requesting me to take care of her pregnancy. I am doing so with a good deal of trepidation, and am depending entirely on information which you may send me either by letter or through Mrs. Thompson, as to the procedure of prenatal care and of the delivery itself."[23]

Joslin replied, "The whole point is to have Mrs. Thompson keep in touch with your office so that you will know her diabetes is under reasonable control and that complications are being avoided." Joslin then recommended a precise regimen of diet and insulin and encouraged Susan's doctor to admit her to the hospital two weeks prior to delivery.[24]

After several more letters went back and forth, and after Susan went to visit the Joslin Clinic for a short while, Joslin wrote back to the obstetrician. While the best he could say about her laboratory studies were that they were "not dreadfully high," he nevertheless advised that "Thompson should go on with her pregnancy. She should be seen once a week. The last two weeks she should remain in the hospital. Presumably it will be safer for a Cesarean section to be performed a week or even more ahead of time and upon that occasion the question comes up about sterilization but one should be sure that all interested sign an agreement to it before carrying it out."[25]

After a healthy child was born by cesarean section in the late summer of 1934, the local doctor wrote to Joslin, sending him the details of Susan's somewhat complicated postoperative course (during which she developed an infection that lasted for several days), before concluding: "I want to thank you very much for your support and advice in this case. I have gained a lot of knowledge and information from this which I am sure will mean a great deal in my practice. Mrs. Thompson tells me to say 'Greetings' to you."[26] Several years later Susan wrote Joslin, telling him that she and her child were well and that "I have had no other pregnancies. One was plenty."[27]

Unlike Susan Thompson's experience, many pregnancies—despite intensive diabetic management—still ended with bitter disappointment. Writing in 1935, White observed that "stillbirths and the macerated fetus of the giant type are nearly as characteristic of diabetic pregnancies which are allowed to come to full term today as they were in the pre-insulin era."[28] Two years later, White again commented on this distressing clinical puzzle, noting, "Repeatedly it has been our experience, as well as that of others, that with a perfectly controlled case the fetus has died two, four or six weeks prior to term. Yet the opposite situation with acidosis and even coma has occurred in this same apparently critical period, and patients have later been delivered of normal living children."[29] So certain were White and her colleagues of their ability to control diabetes—or at least to determine when the disease was well controlled—that they were unable "to agree with the opinion that the accidents of diabetic pregnancies are caused by faulty management of the disease, diabetes, nor can we agree with the opinion that they can be prevented by adequate control of the diabetes."[30]

Such reasoning led the Joslin group to "search for some extra-diabetic factor common in diabetic pregnancies"—and by 1939 they pointed to "hormonal imbalance" as the much sought after cause.[31] Initially joining a research study of pre-eclampsia (the so-called toxemia of pregnancy that often lead to a stillbirth and could make the mother very ill) conducted at Harvard University by Drs. Olive Watkins Smith, a bio-chemist, and her physician-husband, George Van S. Smith, the doctors at the Joslin Clinic became convinced that not only could they predict threatening fetal demise by detecting a rise of a pregnancy hormone called chorionic gonadotropin, but they also could prevent stillbirths through "massive doses" of estrogen and progesterone. Whereas the pregnant diabetic had been "a nightmare to us, for we never knew by severity, duration, age or control of diabetes" how the pregnancy would fare, the authors concluded that hormonal testing "permits us to classify the patients according to hazard and to gauge the effect of therapy," which in their hands led more often to "the successful outcome of the pregnancy."[32]

The use of the potent hormone "diethylstilbestrol [DES] in the prevention and treatment of complications of pregnancy"[33] became a widespread practice for high-risk pregnancies until 1971, when exposure in utero to DES was linked to the subsequent development of adenocarcinoma of the vagina in young women.[34] While the carcinogenic effects of DES constitute a tragic legacy for the practice of hormone replacement, we can also see how fundamental aspects of this story continue to structure diabetic research and care, as clinical frustration spurs on the relentless pursuit of control, a motif that extends far beyond the management of just the diabetic pregnancy.

EXPANDING HORIZON OF MEDICAL MANAGEMENT

Seven-year-old Robin Jenner, a Connecticut schoolgirl who displayed her first diabetic symptoms in May of 1920, was diagnosed in September when sugar was found in her urine. A month later, her parents brought her to see Dr. Joslin.[35] Robin was one of the fortunate pre-insulin juvenile patients to survive long enough to benefit from the new discovery. Having started insulin therapy as a nine-year-old, she enjoyed good health throughout her adolescence. In 1929 Robin was enrolled by Joslin and White in a long-term follow-up study of juvenile-onset diabetics.[36] Ten years later, she replied to a questionnaire sent by Joslin informing him that she was "sorry to have to admit that I cannot really tell you anything definite about how I am getting along as since I went to work 2½ years ago, I have been careless in regard to properly caring for my health. I always have my Insulin twice a day, but I never get time, it seems, to make tests regularly or to even think of calories." Robin nevertheless expressed her gratitude for "your interest in me which has lasted thro' these seventeen years."[37]

In the summer of 1941 a formal note arrived at the clinic inviting Dr. White to Robin's upcoming wedding.[38] Four years later, after the cessation of the Second World War allowed wife and husband to be reunited, a few lines in the chart noted her admission to the hospital:

> *Old pt.* saw Dr. White at 81 By St. . . . Is *pregnant.* . . . Had *3 miscarriages* 1st @ 3 mos, 2nd @ 6 weeks, + 3rd @ 3 mos. gestation. Dr. White requested she come in for *Regulation + Observation.* Has been living in Georgia until 2 weeks ago. Has been taking *Belladonna + Phenobarbital* . . .— *no hormones.*[39]

Discharged a week later in the fourth month of her pregnancy, Robin was to receive daily intramuscular hormone injections of Proluton and Benzestrol and was scheduled "to see Dr. White 2 weeks hence in her office."[40] From December to February, Robin visited the Joslin Clinic eight times for close outpatient "regulation and observation," with the physicians noting briefly at each visit that she "looks wonderful" and the "baby active."[41] By mid-March, however, Robin's persistent elevation of blood pressure prompted another admission to the Faulkner Hospital, during which a cesarean section delivered an eight-and-a-half-pound girl who died shortly afterward.[42]

Robin and her husband soon thereafter adopted a child, who grew to be "just as precious as can be" in her adopted mother's eyes.[43] After this ill-fated pregnancy, though, Robin's medical problems quickly mounted. She already had been diagnosed as having "retinitis proliferans,"[44] and while the retinal eye disease seemed to remit during the mid-1940s, by the late 1940s Robin's vision began to fail. Whenever she visited Dr. White for a checkup, her blood pressure was usually markedly elevated and her urine contained significant amounts of protein.[45] And on top of these signs of physical deterioration, Robin continued to grieve the death of her infant, writing to White in 1949 how "it just seems as though I have really missed all the things that could have solved every problem, big and small, if only our own baby could have been saved. Death was not the end of that, but the very beginning of every unhappiness and longing, and we had to find substitutes."[46]

In the late spring of 1952, Robin's health suddenly deteriorated even further. In a follow-up note to a visit, White tried to offer reassurance. "Your diabetes was really under quite good control," she asserted, while going on to observe that "the blood sugar was 206 mg. With 0.2 per cent sugar and less albumin than previously in the urine. As I told you, the blood pressure was high, but you were extremely nervous during this examination."[47] That summer, Robin—already languishing in the uremia of chronic renal failure—suffered a stroke and was admitted to the Deaconess Hospital. After three days of diminishing consciousness, she finally succumbed to "acute heart failure." She was thirty-eight years old, having lived with her diabetes for nearly thirty-two years. White penned a letter of condolence to Robin's mother. "I cannot tell you how grieved we are over Robin's death though it was anticipated several months prior to the actual event." In particular, White regretted "so much that your last experience with the Deaconess was such an unfortunate and such an unhappy one. I wish we could have done more for Robin, but you must feel gratified that you kept her alive so many years. Her years of happiness and good health are largely due to the marvelous care you personally gave her."[48]

Cases such as Robin's led Dr. White and other physicians, by the 1950s, to elongate their time frame of clinical concern regarding diabetic pregnancies well beyond a nine-month boundary. In 1949 White had published her classification system for diabetic pregnancies, ranging from Class A (mild glucose intolerance) through F (mothers with already established kidney disease), a scheme that focused on the duration of diabetes prior to the pregnancy as a precursor state that posed a mounting hazard to mother and child.[49] Among "the objectives in the ideal management of the obstetrical diabetic patient" that White and her coauthors outlined in an article published in 1953, the first was "to insure maternal survival not only during pregnancy, but for a minimum of twenty additional years," specifically by protecting "the diabetic woman from the acceleration of malignant vascular disease to which she is liable."[50]

Accomplishing such a long-range objective—like many goals of managing the diabetic pregnancy—would require a team approach, as White had long suggested.[51] The rise of diabetes "experts" and the institution of such teams were but two of the several ways in which relationships between patients and their care providers, as well as their individual and shared responsibilities, would be reworked over time.

RECONFIGURING RELATIONSHIPS
AND RESPONSIBILITIES

Bernadette Dane was a junior in a Rhode Island high school in 1926 when her doctor found sugar in her urine after nearly a year of gradually worsening symptoms, including excessive appetite, thirst, and urination, and finally the cessation of her menstruation. Upon her diagnosis, she began receiving insulin immediately, meeting with Joslin for the first time six months later.

Joslin and White attended to every detail of her diet, exercise, and insulin. Since Bernadette was still growing into a young woman, the early years of her diabetic care were a balancing act, trying to provide enough calories and insulin to allow her to gain some weight and normal development while avoiding both low and high blood glucose levels. To this end, she would mail Joslin diet report cards, tallying her daily meals by food type, measured in grams. "I have added the two units of Insulin in the morning," she remarked in 1928, "but still the sugar seems to be most all in the morning test, even though I have a slight [hypoglycemic] reaction almost every day about one hour before dinner."[52]

In the late winter of 1936, Joslin sent notices to many patients regarding the new long-acting protamine insulin. "Thank you very much for your interest in me," Bernadette replied. "I have heard about the new insulin and have read an article about it. I hope to learn more about it and some day try it."[53] Joslin wrote back, enclosing a "reprint which tells something about the effects of the new insulin. As I do not have many copies of this article, will you kindly return it?"[54] Two months later, Bernadette wrote to say that she had made arrangements to spend a week at the hospital to be switched to the new insulin, adding that she also wanted "to know a little about the cost."[55] After an uneventful admission, Bernadette was admonished by Elliott Joslin's son, Dr. Allen Joslin, to "watch your specimens carefully during the next few days. . . . I hope that you will come up to see us in about a month's time so that we can be sure that you are doing satisfactorily with protamine insulin."[56]

Just what defined "satisfactory" was flexible. In public pronouncements, Joslin, White, and the clinic staff preached the gospel of strict glycemic control, attained through scrupulous adherence to dietary rules and the judicious use of insulin. In private, however, they were often considerably more accommodating. For instance, after a visit to the clinic in 1938, Bernadette was told in a follow-up note from Joslin that she "looked first rate" even though, he admitted, "it is true" that her urine samples contained more than 2 percent sugar and her blood glucose was markedly elevated (300 mg/dl) two and a half hours after lunch. "I understand," Joslin added in explanation, "that the second [urine] specimen [after rising in the morning] is sugar free and if that is the case, I would not suggest any more protamine insulin." He and his colleagues feared that patients like Bernadette, if given enough long-acting insulin to curb their blood glucose to acceptable levels during the day, would succumb to delayed-onset hypoglycemic shock in the predawn hours of the morning. Sugar-free urine in the morning was a sign that there was no more room to push the long-acting insulin without getting into trouble. But—as Joslin went on to say—if the second morning sample was not sugar free, Bernadette should add some regular insulin, six to eight units, with the morning protamine insulin.[57]

The mind-set of control extended beyond metabolic regulation to include—remarkably enough—marriage and reproduction. White and her colleagues believed that woman or men with juvenile-onset diabetes could pass the disease to their offspring as a Mendelian recessive trait. Therefore, marriage to a mate with the diabetic "taint" in the family was frowned upon.[58] "When I visited your office last June," Bernadette wrote, "I asked you about the possibility of my getting married. You seemed to have no objections providing the fellow is in good health, and you said that you would like to examine him. . . . He knows that I shall abide by your decision."[59] Apparently, the decision was favorable, and the couple was married in the fall. Half a year later she was pregnant.[60] And so began her quest for a live baby.

Having ceded control over many details of her life to White, Bernadette became anxious and annoyed whenever medical instructions were inconsistent or incomplete. She wrote after one of her first prenatal visits, "I received your report last week and started on my new schedule. However, I am a bit puzzled about testing and taking Insulin at noon and night. You said take 8-4-0 units, but I don't recall you telling me what color test to go by. I am doing my best, but wish you would let me know exactly what colors to go by."[61] White replied that she was "sorry I did not make the test clear. . . . Take 8 units if the test is red or orange and 4 units if yellow."[62]

Like many patients, Bernadette was not hesitant to express her frustration when she encountered difficulties and setbacks. As she put it in one note to "My dear Dr. White," "I certainly was disgusted, disappointed, and somewhat angry to arrive at your office last Saturday afternoon and find you not there. . . . Of all the hot days to take such a long ride for nothing. However, I suppose I must realize that you have many things to think of." Asking for another appointment, Bernadette added, "Please just don't lead me on another 'wild goose chase.'"[63]

Midway through the pregnancy, White placed Bernadette on DES and Proluton.[64] Marked swelling in her legs led to a hospital admission at the beginning of the seventh month. As she approached the anticipated date for the cesarean delivery, she was transferred to the Faulkner Hospital. There, the surgery delivered an eight-pound baby girl;[65] postoperative sterilization, which she and her husband desired and had consented to in writing, followed.[66]

A week or so later, the Joslin Clinic received a birth announcement: "There's Something New Under the Sun! . . . A Brand New Baby, Ester Nancy."[67] A month later, the "proud parents" received a letter from White, which enclosed "the bill which covers the entire cost of the Proluton." White wrote, "As you know, I only expect you to pay the amount which is correct for you. This does not have to be paid immediately. I would appreciate it if you would tell me the amount that you think is fair for you to pay and in what period of time. I do hope that everything is going along well with you and the baby."[68]

The strength and complexity of the ties between White and her patients are easily recognized. Bernadette once began a letter by inquiring about her insulin but then moved onto what appears to have been her main agenda: "Now I must tell you about Ester. She is just fine and adorable, of course. . . . I still can't believe that she is really mine, and how thankful I am to you and Dr. Titus for bringing us both through so well. . . . Sometimes I feel that I am alone a great deal, especially this wintry weather when Ester and I can't go out much; but then I thank God that I have Ester to keep me occupied and give me company."[69]

Bernadette was not the only woman who strove to maintain the intense ties that had developed between patients during their pregnancies and this particular doctor. White lavished her patients with "charismatic attention,"[70] and some patients appear to have become thoroughly enmeshed with their physician, desiring to extend the realm of intimacy beyond the hospital and examination room, into their homes and domestic lives. Bernadette confided to White, "We often speak of you and wonder how you are. I suppose you are as busy as can be."[71] In another letter from the autumn of 1943, she told White that "we are still hoping you can get to visit us, but suppose that can't be until this war-torn world gets back to normal."[72] White reciprocated these sentiments, responding, "I too am hoping that I can visit you sometime. It looks as if the war is not going to last too long now."[73] And, as she often did in closing a letter, signifying the emotional dimensions of the relationship, she added: "Give my love to the baby."[74]

LIFE AFTER PREGNANCY

The relational bonds forged between patient and physician during gestation were reconfigured yet again when the interlude of the pregnancy ended. For many women, the medical challenges posed by their diabetes in the context of pregnancy faded considerably into the background of their lives as they assumed the chores of motherhood or struggled with the loss of the baby. For some mothers, though—and for most, eventually—the problems of living with diabetes continued to dominate their lives.

Within a few weeks of giving birth to Ester, Bernadette reported anxiously in the autumn of 1941, "These past three or four days my feet and ankles have taken to swelling again, and I am beginning to worry about it. Does that mean that the edema is coming back?"[75] Although White encouraged Bernadette to "not be discouraged about the swelling," as it was "possibly in relation to an attempt to menstruate again,"[76] this accumulation of fluid in her legs and other tissues of her body would become a recurrent problem for Bernadette, probably due to abnormal cardiac valves (perhaps damaged from rheumatic fever) and the consequent strain this placed on her heart. Several office visits over the ensuing years also revealed erratic blood glucose control at best, with as many measurements above 250 mg/dl as below; the physicians, though, were gentle and reassuring, with White even commenting that she was "pleased with your report."[77]

In the winter of 1947, Bernadette suffered a severe setback, with "pronounced and progressive edema" leading to a month-long admission at the New England Deaconess Hospital. She eventually was diagnosed with endocarditis (an infection of the heart valves) caused by the bacteria *staphylococcus albus*. Massive doses of the still-novel drug penicillin cleared the infection over the course of eight weeks, which included four weeks of home-administered antibiotics.[78] Upon discharge, White's instructions were typical of how "heart patients" were treated at midcentury: "You are to continue with complete bed rest for a period of two weeks. At the end of two weeks you may get up to the bathroom once a day. At the end of three weeks you may get up to the bathroom whenever necessary and at the end of four weeks you may sit up for one-half hour a day adding one-half an hour with moderate activity until you are up twelve hours out of the twenty-four. I would like you to have help in your house for six months."[79] A fortnight after going home, Bernadette wrote to White, "Everyone says that I look so much better. They all say that I should be up. However, I know they are just kidding, and I am following your instructions." Her husband was doing "very well giving the penicillin morning and night, and the district nurse comes in the afternoon." She concluded by asking "one favor," namely would White "please write down the name of the 'germ' that I had. I can't remember it, and the folks think I'm 'stupid' when I say I don't know."[80] White promptly replied, spelling out *staphylococcus albus* and commenting, "I am pleased that you are much better."[81]

The remaining five years of Bernadette's life were marked by recurrent exacerbations of her congestive heart failure. Her body flooded with accumulated fluid, she would feel profoundly fatigued and struggle to breathe, especially at night. Even the strongest diuretics eventually failed to ameliorate her symptoms. In response to White's request for an update on her health in the late summer of 1953, Bernadette wrote, "Sorry to have to report that I am not pleased with the way I feel. I am O.K. if I can stay in bed as I did in the hospital [during a recent admission], but I do not like to become a complete invalid. As soon as I am up doing things I get edema and shortness of breath and feel so weary." Despite this grim synopsis, she saw "no immediate need of traveling to Boston, because I imagine you could only advise more rest and that I know is up to me, so I'll keep trying."[82] The theme of personal effort and responsibility was struck up again six months later when, after yet another hospitalization, she assured White, "I finally have a girl to come in and work 3 out of 7 days each week; and am trying harder to be more inactive. . . . I realize it is all up to me to behave. . . . I'll try hard to follow orders. I know you have done all you can."[83]

Throughout these years of travail, Bernadette worried not only about herself but her daughter as well. As far back as Ester's second birthday, the mother had sent White a photograph of the child and wished aloud that "my only hope is that Ester will never have [diabetes]."[84] Despite White's reassurance that "I think Ester will escape,"[85] Bernadette remained worried, and her medical record reveals that she had her daughter's blood and urine tested for sugar on several occasions.[86] (Diabetics' concerns about their offspring developing diabetes were reflected in several of the archived medical records. As another mother explained in response to an inquiry from Dr. White regarding her health in 1937, "I am keeping a close watch on my [three-year-old] son for any signs of 'trouble,' but so far he is perfectly healthy. I can only hope and pray that he will always be that way."[87])

When Bernadette died in the mid-1950s, her husband sent White a clipping of the obituary from the local newspaper along with several lines of further explanation. After months of struggling with her congestive heart failure, he wrote, Bernadette actually had had a remarkably lively day until "in the evening, we sat chatting, when in the middle of a sentence she just slumped down in her chair and passed on seemingly without pain for which we are all very thankful. May I thank you for all you have done to ease her suffering these many years."[88] A letter of condolence soon followed from White, thanking Bernadette's husband for writing. "We are sorry that she had so much suffering during the past few years," White lamented, "and wish that we could have done more for her."[89]

CULTURAL LOGIC, SOCIAL CONSTRAINTS,
AND MEDICAL INNOVATION

The twentieth-century history of pregnancy for women with diabetes mellitus is both the sum of myriad individual stories and the product of deeper emotional, social, and cultural forces that tie many of the idiosyncratic stories together with common themes. I have sought to illustrate this perspective by situating the stories of Janice, Susan Thompson, Robin Jenner, and Bernadette Dane within the framework of four enduring themes: a migrating focus of clinical concern, a steadily mounting intensity of care, a gradually expanding horizon of medical management, and a constant reconfiguring of relationships and responsibilities between patients and providers. While each woman's story differed, due to factors that ranged from physiology to personality to personal circumstances, their stories were also shaped by larger aspects of the system of health care and how it changed over time.

One such larger aspect was technological innovation, which yielded what can only be thought of as "miraculous" success in improving the health outcomes for mothers and their babies.[90] The questions posed by Priscilla White on behalf of young adult women living with diabetes in 1948[91]—will I be able to conceive, survive my pregnancy, and deliver a healthy child who will be unlikely to develop diabetes?—had grown relatively outdated by the 1990s. While concerns for fetal and maternal well-being continue to guide the medical management of diabetic pregnancies, these worries largely have been supplanted by newer concerns regarding the impact of pregnancy on the mother's health in the years and decades following parturition, as well as long-term outcomes for the growth and development of children born from a diabetic pregnancy.

This shift in concern over time speaks to a culturally specific logic of innovation, which constitutes the second embracing attribute of the system of health care that has influenced the experience of would-be mothers with diabetes. For patients and physicians operating within the American health care system, this logic has consisted of certain basic rules, such as "do not be satisfied with less than perfect health outcomes" and "if problems do not yield to hard work, work harder," which in turn have been underwritten by fundamental values esteemed in American culture. The logic has also consisted of social constraints, especially the limits that patients, providers, and health care payers have placed on the financing of care and the workload imposed by care regimens. Furthermore, societal tolerance of variable access to and quality of care has meant that the successful fruits of technological innovation have not been enjoyed by all. In our account, we have mapped out the operation of this logic through a description of the four motifs, each of which represent a way in which the pursuit of control was manifested in the concrete terms of clinical actions and redesigned procedures or systems of care. These motifs are emblematic of how modern medical care has developed over the past fifty years—a direction of development likely to continue into the twenty-first century. If the patterns established during the past century persist, then we should anticipate that diabetes care in the future will be more intense and have a wider purview, focused less on immediate or short-term problems and more on primary prevention and the long-term enhancement of quality of life for people with diabetes. And as far into the future as we can see, concerns regarding payment and burden of work will likely continue to keep in check certain innovative possibilities regarding care and how it is delivered.

We have seen how a diabetic woman's experience of pursuing motherhood has been drastically reshaped by what may be thought of as external forces: technological medical innovation and an operating logic specified by cultural values and social constraints. Yet we also have ample evidence that the women who constitute this history each had an interior driving force motivating her pursuit. In the stories recounted above, we caught glimmers of longing. While the letters did not contain enough detail for us to fully comprehend the nature and source of these feelings, we would be foolish to ignore their significance. If we are to truly understand how the experience of living with diabetes was transformed during the twentieth century—to deepen our sense of the ecology of chronic disease—we need to examine the realm of desire and identity, to appreciate the structure of human motivations and the intimate workings of the maintenance of hope. To this more subtle realm of history we turn next.

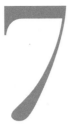

PREDICAMENTS OF
DANGEROUS SAFETY:
IDENTITY, RESPONSIBILITY,
AND LIFE WITH A CHRONIC
ILLNESS

*Remedies are not useless because they fall short of
their full scope. It is better to keep a man on the edge
of a precipice, if you cannot pluck him away from it,
than to let him fall over. And many diabetic patients
are kept in this predicament of dangerous safety.*
—Thomas Watson, 1836–37

Throughout the twentieth and early twenty-first centuries, to live with diabetes has meant living with duties and chores that burden the present and difficulties and uncertainty that loom in the future. Certain experiences of people inhabiting the diabetic world have been quite concrete, such as how they manage the daily work of diabetic self-care, or how they have sought, in their own fashion, to control the effect of the disease upon their lives. But patients with diabetes have also encountered a less tangible level of experience, pervasive and influential yet elusive, as they have grappled with the question of responsibility.

This question of responsibility—which was a core issue for most people who lived with diabetes in twentieth-century America—is highlighted through the following diabetic stories of three patients, one of whom died before 1922, the other two of whom were born after the discovery of insulin. Their experiences (which include one patient's attempts at motherhood, here set into a more complete life history) will broaden our notion of the question, refine our sense of how it played in their lives, and enhance our appreciation of the ironies—some dignified, others disturbing—found within the answers that they or their physicians devised.

THE ARRANGEMENT OF RESPONSIBILITY
BEFORE INSULIN

In November of 1915, Elliott Joslin received a telegram from a Seattle physician, Dr. Peabody, regarding a boy named Sander Flowers. The doctor informed Joslin of the pertinent details:

> PATIENT EIGHT YEARS | DIABETES THREE WEEKS | SEVENTY SIX OUNCES [OF URINE] | SIX PERCENT SUGAR | AFTER FOLLOWING YOUR PAPER [IN] MEDICAL SCIENCES STARVATION CARBOHYDRATE FREE DIET SUGAR DISAPPEARED | LATER ONE PERCENT AND LESS DUE [TO] LACK [OF] MY EXPERIENCE | CAN YOU GIVE FAVORABLE PROGNOSIS | PATIENT CAN START AT ONCE FOR BOSTON | ANSWER QUICK[1]

Joslin must have dashed off a "favorable" response, for the next day a second telegram from Peabody arrived:

> YOUR TELEGRAM RECEIVED | YOU[R] REPUTATION EXPLAINED TO PATIENT | I ADVISED PLACING THEIR SON IN YOUR CARE UNTIL YOU ARE SATISFIED WE CAN GET ALONG HERE BY CORRESPONDING WITH YOU | AS YOU WOULD BE BETTER PREPARED TO INTELLIGENTLY ADVISE US MRS FLOWERS AND SON LEAVE HERE NOV[EMBER] FOURTEENTH FOR BOSTON[2]

Sanders and his mother traveled to Boston over the course of a week. During that interval, Joslin received a long letter from Peabody. "These people," the doctor explained to Joslin, "are not only patients of mine but very intimate friends of my family, and I believe I would be derelict in my duty if I did not recommend they consult you and especially knowing as I do about the original work you have done along these lines."

Peabody let Joslin know that "Mr. Flowers is well able from a financial standpoint to have the best Medical authorities in this or any other country, and should I fail to make such recommendations, they and their friends would forever censure me." The Seattle physician further assured his Boston colleague that he would "find Mrs. Flowers an exceptionally intelligent woman, eager and anxious to follow all your instructions in every instance regardless of her own convictions and the protests from the patient." Sander was an only child, "and both Mr. and Mrs. Flowers are exceedingly anxious for his recovery and will spare nothing to accomplish this if such a thing is possible."

Peabody confided to Joslin, "As a matter of fact[,] this is the first child to come under my care suffering from this disease, and I feel my short-comings in comparison to the enormous experience you have had, and if these people are able to profit by anything you may offer why should they not have it?"

"Keep them in Boston under your care," Peabody continued with more than a trace of anxiety, "just as long as you deem it advisable and whenever you consider that I can continue treatment under your advice by letter or telegram, then it will be soon enough for them to return home."[3]

When the patient in question finally arrived in Boston, Joslin observed that Sander was "cachectic, frail, pale" with a trace of sugar and diacetic acid in his urine.[4] Joslin made plans to admit the boy to the hospital but received yet another telegram from Peabody, who evidently had been contacted by the boy's mother. Peabody asked:

> CAN YOU MAKE IT POSSIBLE FOR MRS FLOWERS TO STAY AT HOSPITAL WITH PATIENT UNTIL HE GOES TO SLEEP | OR MAYBE A SPECIAL NURSE WILL SOLVE THE PROBLEM | I AM VERY ANXIOUS TO KEEP HIM UNDER YOUR CARE FOR A WHILE

On the bottom of the telegram, Joslin jotted a brief note: "Told Mrs. Flowers yesterday she could stay at hospital from 6 A.M. to 10 P.M."[5]

Once Sander was tucked into his hospital room, Joslin fasted him and then advanced the child's diet ever so slowly, according to the Allen treatment scheme.[6] Joslin also had another Boston physician come by and recommend some exercises appropriate for an eight-year-old child.[7] By the time Sander left for home in mid-December of 1915, his blood sugar was down to 0.14 percent, a nearly normal value that was well out of the immediate danger zone.[8]

A year passed before Joslin made another entry into Sander's medical chart. During that period, Joslin's relationships with Sander, the Flowers, and Dr. Peabody evolved from "acute" interactions into a "chronic" arrangement. Unlike the weeks that Sander spent hospitalized, when Joslin and his staff assumed most of the responsibility of providing care, the time after the boy returned home blurred the lines of responsibility that connected the specialist to his far-removed patient, family, and local physician, and the ever-present disease. Joslin had already done most of what he could to aid this child; thereafter, as a Hippocratic writer had asserted more than 2,000 years earlier, in the struggle with disease, "it is not enough for the physician to do what is necessary," since the path back to health required the patient and family members to "do their part as well, and the circumstances must be favorable."[9]

In January of 1917, Joslin sent a note to the family in Seattle. Someone returned the note to Boston with a little message scribbled on the back, informing Joslin, "At this time Sander Flowers is taking per twenty four hours Fats 73 grams, Protein 71 grams, and Carbohydrate 33 grams. His weight is 38 pounds." As Joslin could have calculated, this diet provided the boy with 1,073 calories a day—not nearly enough for a boy to grow normally but evidently just sufficient to keep him alive.[10]

Three months later, however, Peabody wrote Joslin "to report to you of the death of Sander Flowers which occurred on March 6th about three o'clock in the afternoon." The boy "had been in his usual condition up to Sunday March 4th, when his Mother noticed that he was more languid than ordinarily, but she gave it little thought because it was his starvation day and for this reason contributed to his condition because he always had more or less of a dread of that particular day." Instead, though, Sander was lapsing into diabetic coma.

> In the evening he began to vomit and complained of intense thirst and dyspnoea [frequent deep breathing] was marked. He was restless all night but toward morning he went into a deep sleep lasting until the middle of Monday forenoon, and during the day he was conscious at times and semi-conscious at others, this condition lasted until about ten-thirty P.M. when we noticed that he was in a deep comatose state which terminated in his death on Tuesday afternoon.[11]

The story of Sander Flower suggests that the manner in which parents and physicians handled a case of juvenile diabetes in the time before insulin reflected their circumstances and beliefs. When Sander took ill, the Flowers and Dr. Peabody had to contend with a disease that was lethal—and often swiftly so. Peabody, knowing the family as "very intimate friends" and fearing that he would not be able to keep the boy alive, believed that Joslin—as the expert doing the most "original work" in diabetic therapeutics—would provide the best care. The Flowers had the money to seek this care for their son, and Mrs. Flowers was sufficiently "eager and anxious" to make the cross-country journey. The Flowers and Peabody were quite willing to defer to the famous Boston specialist, and Joslin agreed to serve as a long-distance consultant, proffering his advice to the anxious Dr. Peabody by telegram or mail. The family may well have followed Joslin's "instructions in every instance" when the boy returned home, keeping him on a curtailed diet with Sunday fasts. Sander—still a child when he died—had little to say, as his "protests" and "dread" of fast days were to be disregarded.

Such were the relationships among an inexperienced doctor, a wealthy family, a distant expert, and a youngster suffering from a deadly disease. These were the ways they sought to manage this disease, thinking that the best hope was offered by strict dietary treatment that required "enormous experience" on the part of the supervising clinician. And these were their means of dividing responsibility, demonstrating not only the serious nature of juvenile diabetes and the limited therapeutic repertoire but also their trust in medical expertise, their desire to seek "recovery," and their willingness and financial ability to "spare nothing to accomplish this." In sum, the Flowers, Peabody, and Joslin arranged responsibility in a manner that expressed their economic capabilities, social values, and cultural beliefs.[12]

Their relationships and handling of responsibility also reflected a specific period in the life course of patient and physician. Sander lived and died as a youngster; his relationship with those caring for him never had the chance to mature. His interactions certainly would have changed had he been able to grow old with his disease, passing from childhood into adulthood, perhaps marrying, raising a family, and eventually retiring. Equally, the inexperienced Dr. Peabody probably altered his manner of relating to his patients, their parents, and other physicians as he grayed. Had Sander lived and remained in Peabody's care, the balance of responsibility and authority between the two would likely have shifted back and forth, in keeping with the maturing capabilities and experience of patient and doctor.

Sander did not live, nor did most other youngsters who became diabetic before insulin arrived. From 1922 forward, though, children did grow into adulthood. Insulin stretched the arrangement of responsibility beyond the acute period, even beyond the chronic childhood phase, and extended it into an unprecedented realm: the chronic relationships between physicians and patients who have lived with juvenile diabetes for decades. And it was here, in this uncharted territory, that they confronted the long-term sequelae of a miraculously "successful" medical intervention.[13]

The management of responsibility in this time after insulin had implications that were both traditionally medical and deeply personal. In the following stories of Tracy Pike Villars and John Hansen, the question of responsibility took on compelling importance as these two patients grew older. Tracy and John each had to confront, in different ways, therapeutic "failure," arguing with their doctors whether this "failure" was in any way their or their physicians' "fault"—or whether circumstances were simply and inscrutably unfavorable. These arguments, viewed at the end of these patients' life courses with illness, allow the question of responsibility to be exposed and dissected, revealing at its core the interplay of uncertainty, authority, and morality.

THE ARRANGEMENT OF RESPONSIBILITY
AFTER INSULIN

When insulin arrived in 1922, it vitalized not only the patients of Dr. Joslin but their venerable physician as well. Already fifty-three years of age, Joslin subsequently redoubled his efforts to attain diabetic control both for his own patients and for diabetic individuals across the nation. During the remaining four decades of his life, Joslin persistently reminded his fellow doctors and diabetic patients that diabetes was still a lethal disease. He believed adamantly that the lessons and practices of the pre-insulin era, although set in a more optimistic setting, were now even more important. Insulin—a mighty but imperfect gift—should not be squandered in a profligate manner.

Joslin began this campaign for conscientious diabetic control as early as 1923, when he cautioned the readers of the *Journal of the American Medical Association* that, while "there has never been anything discovered as valuable for the diabetic as insulin," both patient and physician had to realize that "diabetes, although subdued, is not yet conquered."[14] Similarly, in the 1923 edition of his textbook he warned that the diabetic was still prone to complications of coma, pneumonia, tuberculosis, arteriosclerosis, heart disease, neuritis, Bright's disease, and gangrene. Patients still needed to adhere to a strict regimen of diet and exercise.[15]

And so insulin joined forces with the other, older means of obtaining diabetic control. As we have seen, the idea of control served as a composite motif, one that mixed together notions of biological relations, social order, and personal character. Insulin was simply another tool—albeit a potent one—to achieve control. As Joslin himself metaphorically put it, "I look upon the diabetic as a charioteer and his chariot as drawn by three steeds named (1) Diet, (2) Insulin and (3) Exercise." With skill acquired through practice and instruction, the diabetic pa-

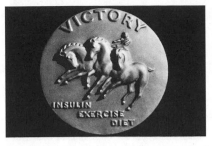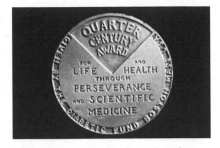

The Victory Medal (front view, left; back view, right). Photograph taken by author of medals from the archival collection of the Countway Library Rare Book Department, Harvard Medical School, Boston.

tient could drive his or her disease away from morbidity and toward victory.

This idea of directing the course of one's disease toward "success" through the exercise of self-discipline and adherence to regimen led Joslin to create the Victory Medal. Beginning in 1947, Joslin would give a Victory Medal to any patients who had had diabetes for twenty-five years or longer and were found—after a thorough physical and oph-thalmologic examination, an X-ray study of the major arteries, and an analysis of the urine—to be in perfect health. Embossed on one side of the medal was the three-steed chariot, while on the other was en-graved the phrase "For Life and Health through Perseverance and Sci-entific Medicine." Several years later, Joslin introduced a second medal for those patients who had outlived their normal life expectancy. He justified both awards by equating a patient's willpower with "successful" long-term results. In Joslin's view, a diabetic patient who achieved last-ing health had (as the Life Span medal pronounced) earned "A Scien-tific and Moral Victory."[16]

These medals embodied the apotheosis of Joslin's moral conception of the fight against diabetes. Other members of the diabetic world, how-ever, chose not to subscribe to Joslin's puritanical approach to diabetic salvation. To these individuals, the medals came to symbolize an un-compassionate, even arrogant, example of medical authority. For the implicit logic of Joslin's creed led to a disturbing conclusion: tight con-trol would prevent complications; patients could control their disease if they followed the rules set down by doctors; completing the syllogism, patients were responsible for their health, good or bad. Since both the minor and major premises were unproven—and since the conclusion

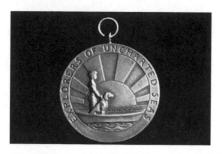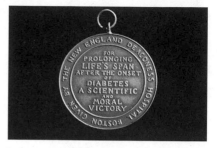

The Life Expectancy Medal (front view, left; back view, right). Photograph taken by author of medals from the archival collection of the Countway Library Rare Book Department, Harvard Medical School, Boston.

was, prima facie, emotionally unacceptable—many patients and physicians rejected the contentious notion that patients were to blame for the long-term complications of diabetes.

Joslin heard his critics—just as he had heard them when he used the Allen diet to treat diabetic children prior to 1922—and he sought to answer them. "The idea has been raised," he lectured to an audience in 1958, "that a diabetic should not feel he has done wrong if he has a poor Benedict test. I disagree." Joslin felt that he had both a duty to warn and an obligation to praise: "When I see a red test, I know, if uncorrected, that patient is headed for destruction. I believe he should be happy when he knows his faithful following of the rules ends with a blue victory."[17]

These were the words of an aged physician, late in his eighth decade of life, who had been fighting diabetes for sixty years. They were the expression not only of his vast clinical experience but also of what he felt to be his role as the elder statesman of diabetic care in a world where laxity was a perpetual temptation. Joslin spoke like a preacher to shore up the will of his flock. His words and their underlying therapeutic view, however, played quite another role in the lives of young diabetic patients who were only just learning about the pursuit of blue victories.

ESTABLISHING ONE'S SELF IN A DIABETIC WORLD

How children or teenagers entered the diabetic world and "became" diabetics affected, in a subtle but lingering fashion, how they lived with diabetes for the remainder of their lives. When youngsters first came to the Joslin Clinic, they had yet to establish a firm sense of who they were. Growing into adulthood, they then had occasion to build large parts of their personal identity around their diabetes and to carry with them lessons and values they had learned as juveniles. Whether these once-young patients went on to embrace or defy medical authority, their subsequent mature views and behaviors hearkened back to their early experiences in the diabetic world and their initial encounters with physicians.

Tracy Pike Villars

Fifteen-year-old Tracy Pike became diabetic in December of 1923 but did not travel from her home on Cape Cod to see Joslin until March of 1925. Although her medical record does not specify what exactly prompted this journey, when Tracy arrived in Boston she probably felt sick, as she had "+++" diacetic acid in her urine. She spent twelve days in the Deaconess Hospital while her diet was advanced from an initial fast to 1,461 calories. The physicians gave Tracy only three units of insulin on the first day, eventually supplying her with ten units twice daily. This restrained course of therapy did not render her urine sugar free until the ninth day. But by the time she was discharged, Tracy had a blood sugar of 0.14 percent (which was a good level)—and no doubt had received twelve days of thorough diabetic education.[18]

Three years passed before the next entry was made in Tracy Pike's medical record. During the interval, she had married, and when she wrote to Joslin as a nineteen-year-old woman in August of 1928, she had a question to ask. "Is it safe," she wondered, "for a diabetic to have babies[?] I had a little girl two months ago and it was dead, due I believe to riding [an automobile] too much, rode 200 miles the week before it was born a premature birth." Tracy added that the child was not only "dead but also deformed. Its body was perfect but its head was deformed. Mother claims that it was marked by some dead puppies. My dog had pups when I was first sickly and four were dead. I brought them into the house in my hands and was very excited for I love dogs and I buried the dead pups myself." She concluded the letter on a plaintive note, telling Joslin, "I love children and so does my husband. Do you think we would have better luck next time?"[19]

Like so many other patients, Tracy wanted to find meaning in this sad and worrisome event. Similar to the experience of women who confronted misfortune in the previous chapter on pregnancy and diabetes, her search for meaning became a search for the cause, attempting to divine who or what was to blame. And when patients in these circumstances turned to their physicians, the explanations offered by each individual doctor—perhaps unavoidably, given their specific needs, values, and experiences—often sounded quite different.

In this instance, Joslin responded reassuringly yet firmly. He told her that he thought she "probably would get on better the next time if pregnant, provided you are sugar free generally." After suggesting that she see him in Boston for an examination, he mentioned that he took "no stock at all in the dog story and the best thing for you is to forget it. If you keep talking about it with your family it would simply get on your nerves and annoy you. If there was any truth in any such statement there would practically never be a decent baby born."[20]

Two years later, in 1930, Tracy wrote to Joslin again, telling him that she had been "confined Sat 15, Sick nine hours. A girl was born weighing over 11 lbs, In perfectly normal shape and healthy looking, but she was stillborn." While "the Dr. did not have an idea of cause of death," Tracy continued to seek an explanation for the mishap. She told Joslin that she had "raked up the yard a week before it was born, would that have killed it? I shall keep on trying until I have a live baby. . . . Am sorry I did not see you this time."[21] Joslin replied that he was "ever so sorry that you had the misfortune with the baby." He reassured her that "the fact that she was a well developed baby and of full weight makes me feel quite confident that you would be able to have a living child." Due to the big babies that diabetics were prone to have, however, he suggested that "in order to save these babies if they are the first or even if the second pregnancy it would be safer to resort to a Caesarian section."[22] A few days later Joslin reiterated his views. "The babies of diabetic patients," he observed, "are often quite large and very well developed and that is one difficulty there is in the birth." He also let Tracy know that he was "wondering if I ought not to make a rule to advise diabetic patients to have their babies in hospitals where it would give the obstetricians a better chance. I should be glad to know what your doctor would think of such a plan."[23]

As these letters attest, in 1930 even a renowned diabetes specialist still might "wonder" whether his high-risk patients should go to the hospital for their births; not until 1938 did hospital births outnumber home deliveries. Joslin, always careful to defer to the local physician, had to negotiate for what he felt was the best means of care. As discussed in Chapter 6, while Joslin and Priscilla White's emerging intensivist strategy of managing diabetic pregnancies (with weekly prenatal visits and then prolonged confinements ending in cesarean delivery) was strikingly modern, it was built upon a therapeutic reliance on expertise—an expertise that was just being established as legitimate in the "woman's sphere" of birthing.[24] Joslin's willingness to share management decisions and responsibilities with patients and their local doctors gave these relationships a quality of reciprocity that may seem to be separated from modern therapeutic relationships by much more than the intervening seventy years. Joslin's judgments of therapeutic failure, however, based as they were on the ideals of tight control and close management (both born from his pre-insulin experience), were not so flexible.

John Hansen

In the winter of 1940, John Hansen, a fifteen-year-old Scandinavian boy living on the outskirts of Boston, began to lose weight and feel poorly. His regular doctor quickly recognized the classic diagnostic triad of polyuria, polyphagia, and polydipsia and confirmed his suspicion of diabetes by finding sugar in the young man's urine. The physician immediately referred John to Joslin, who saw the patient the very next day at 81 Bay State Road. After reaffirming the diagnosis, Joslin sent the boy across town to the Deaconess Hospital, where a social worker arranged for John's mother to pay only the room charge of four dollars a day, with all other services covered by a charity fund, and all professional fees waived.[25]

The subsequent week-long stay in the hospital, when John learned about his new illness and how to adjust his diet and administer his insulin, marked the beginning of his career as a diabetic. Here his doctors—especially Priscilla White—inculcated a set of defining values into John's life. Two weeks after he was discharged, his mother wrote to White that her son "feels splendidly and relishes his food so much, downing every morsel with much satisfaction!" According to the mother, John's "attitude remains excellent, with a continued desire to follow his diet rigidly. . . . We are not discouraged because we realize that there is much to be Thankful for, especially since we have you to guide us in the right direction."[26] White replied with thanks for the note, commenting, "It is fine that your attitude and John's toward diabetes is so good. John was most cooperative, learned a great deal about the care of diabetes and should do very well."[27]

Here, as elsewhere, White emphasized attitude, cooperation, and knowledge. These might very well have been the three steeds of the chariot that Joslin spoke of: they were seen as the virtues that one needed in the mortal and moral confrontation with diabetes. They also were key terms in the implicit contract between doctor and patient that governed the proper conduct of their relationship: the doctor was responsible for educating the patient and providing the optimal regimen, but it was the patient's attitude and cooperation that ultimately determined the outcome. John "should do very well" because he was cooperative and learned a great deal, not because of some internal, biological predisposition to do well.

During the next two relatively uneventful years, whenever John would see White she would examine him and conduct a few tests, such as blood sugar measurements or an annual chest X ray, which took several hours to complete. White would then notify John and his mother of the results by mail a day or two after their visit, usually also including a few supportive comments. According to White, John's tests were "perfect" and he remained "really in fine condition." In one follow-up note, she even continued their conversation from the office visit, as she offered her final words of counsel on choosing a college.[28]

The interpersonal politics of praise, however, implied the possibility of failure and censure. When John was eighteen years old, two and a half years after he became diabetic, he failed to live up to the strict standard. As White stated in a curt note to John, his test three days previous was "not as good a test as you should have and I don't think you have been trying quite as hard as you should." White may have based her suspicion on things John had told her during the office visit, and they may have already discussed redoubling his self-care efforts. In her note, White instructed him simply to increase his insulin dose and, perhaps trying to firm up John's resolve, added, "I shall want to see you in a month and with better tests."[29]

Notably, within a month John had written White two letters that essentially reestablished his credentials as a "good patient." In the first letter, he told her that he had recently declared his diabetes on a draft questionnaire and that he needed a letter from her attesting to his diagnosis.[30] A week later, John wrote to White that "due to the current food shortages, my Mother has had difficulty in obtaining meat and butter as required on my diet." He asked her to suggest substitute foods or some way that his mother could "buy the required weight of meat and butter so I can continue on my regular diet." He added, plaintively, "As it is now I cannot eat the type of menue [*sic*] prepared for the rest of the family without violating my diet. . . . I would appreciate a letter telling me what to do in a situation of this kind."[31]

In response to these requests for White to use her authority and knowledge, she sent two letters. The first came with a note that she had written for the draft board, which provided details of his case; she reassured John that, when he showed the note to the draft board, "I am sure they will send you home at once."[32] Several days later she dictated a full typed page of instructions to guide John in substituting cheese for eggs and bacon, bread for cereal, margarine for butter, cod liver oil for cream, and fish, liver, heart, sweetbreads, or nuts for meat. She entrusted him to figure out the vegetables and fruits exchanges according to the rules that he had been taught.[33]

Although outwardly both letters are simply informative, they suggest a subtext of reconciliation after John's poor November test results: through them, White provided evidence that she still cared. Collectively, the correspondence also indicates how much John depended on this relationship. Two months after the exchange of letters, John told White that he had applied to a local college for the approaching fall term; he also had told the college that he was diabetic and took the "liberty" of putting her down as a reference. As he explained, he felt "that through our relationship as doctor and patient you must have formed a personal opinion of me. I realize how very busy you are, but hope you will be able to find time to fill out the enclosed blank."[34] John's feeling that she "must" have formed a personal opinion hints at his uncertainty regarding the nature of their relationship (was he really important enough to warrant a personal opinion?) and indicates that, in his mind, she had authority that entitled her to an opinion that a college would value.

A year later, now attending his college of choice, John visited White, which prompted a follow-up note several days later. Addressing him as "Mr. Hansen" (a change from previous letters, when he was "John"), White told him, "You are doing splendidly." She closed with the comment: "Take no chances with yourself but keep on as you are doing. I do think it advisable for you to be checked up at least every three to four months. It does not take very long. You can bring a book with you if you need to wait."[35]

Americans who have made the typical transition from adolescence to adulthood during the twentieth and early twenty-first centuries usually have assumed new roles that carry more autonomy and responsibility. For people with diabetes, this transition led not only to additional family and occupational commitments but also to further responsibilities in living with their disease. As they aged, patients came to shoulder more of the burdens—financial, social, personal—of being chronically diabetic.

Tracy

After Tracy had lived through the two stillbirths, she entrusted herself to Joslin and his collaborating obstetrician, Raymond Titus, when she next became pregnant in the fall of 1930. She visited Boston for a day in January of 1931, when four months pregnant, and was examined by Titus and Joslin. Titus informed Joslin that he thought "with any degree of luck we ought to be able to guarantee her a baby."[36] Joslin then wrote Tracy, outlining his proposed plan of care. "Within four weeks and preferably within three weeks," he stated, "I would like to see you. I think in the meantime your physician at home must know that you are coming to see me and that you intend, eventually, to be confined here in Boston under the care of Dr. Titus." Joslin emphasized optimistically, "We must all do the best we can for you and then good results will accrue." He even told Tracy that he thought she was "so important a case that I would be willing to let one of the diabetic nurses go down and stay two or three days at your house to help find out about your diet and dosage of insulin and how to arrange the same." Joslin also let Tracy know that he "could not do this, however, unless your doctor said he will welcome such a nurse and would chaperon her medically while she was there."[37]

A week later, Joslin wrote again, presumably in response to a telephone call or an unfiled note from Tracy. "You ask me about what charge I should make," he began. "Gladly will I say that your total charges to me and my group, as shown on the heading of this letter, until you go home after your confinement will not exceed $50. If this is more than you ought to pay please let me know."[38] Apparently, Tracy felt that this was a suitable arrangement, for she came to Boston and saw Titus ten days later.[39] Then, a month later, Tracy spent a few days at the Deaconess Hospital—her boarding costs cut in half by the Joslin group—and was made sugar free on 48 units of insulin a day. She was sent home after being told that the next months were critical to delivering a healthy baby.[40]

That delivery occurred after eleven days of confinement. Tracy spent nearly all of that time at the Deaconess Hospital (with blood sugars measured only every two or three days), until the final stage, when she was transported to the nearby Faulkner Hospital, where all the diabetic deliveries took place. Finally, an induced labor gave Tracy her first live baby, weighing just over nine pounds, in May of 1931.[41]

The legacy of this medically managed pregnancy was not only the healthy child it produced. It also put Tracy in debt, thus linking her diabetic experience with that of many other American patients. As was mentioned in Chapter 3, health insurance was largely unavailable prior to the 1940s; not until the 1960s did private and public insurance expenditures approach the amount paid by patients out of pocket.[42] For uninsured and underinsured patients throughout the twentieth century, the costs of medical care have often been a major concern. Finances have had a direct bearing on what therapeutic courses patients pursued, and presumably on the nature of the relationship that they had with their doctors. The Great Depression accentuated the impact of financial constraints on health care.[43] The Depression evidently restrained diabetic patients who otherwise might have traveled to the Joslin Clinic, as the yearly enrollment of new patients into the clinic (a figure that had grown substantially after the First World War) dipped when the Depression commenced in 1929 and did not regain its previous growth rate until nearly a decade later.[44] Perhaps even more powerfully, though, the influence of medical costs on strained budgets can be seen in the choices made by individual patients such as Tracy.

Three years after her delivery at the Faulkner Hospital, Tracy wrote Joslin in August of 1934, telling him that she was six months pregnant and that she "would like very much to be under your care and for Dr. Titus to take care of the confinement. However I am afraid Dr. Titus will not take my case. You see we are still in debt to him for that other confinement." She mentioned that she had "had one baby stillborn since Dr. Titus had my case and have had so much expense that we have been unable to pay him." Hoping that her circumstances would mitigate his judgment regarding the debt, she reassured Joslin that if he "would ask [Dr. Titus] the price and if he will take my case this time I will try to raise enough money by the time he is ready to perform the operation to pay him."[45]

When Joslin received this letter, he outlined the situation to Titus and remarked, "Just how one can handle a case of this sort is a question. I shall be guided by your advice." Titus replied, "The [Villars] are still in arrears to the tune of $195.00, having paid $5.00 on their previous statement. However, I shall be very glad to take care of her again."[46]

Apparently, though Joslin and White both wrote to Tracy, she did not learn of their willingness to treat her gratis until it was too late. Tracy told White, "Your letter arrived too late for me to come up to the Deaconess. I was already in this hospital. I waited to hear from my last letter to Dr. Joslin to know about money arrangements but did not hear until you wrote." Nevertheless, Tracy wanted to let White "know about how things have turned out thus far." The baby had been "taken" by cesarean section. Tracy's local doctor had "got me sugar free and acid free before the operation and without any breakfast took me to [the] operating room. There with a small hypo.[dermic injection] I had something to quiet me, then they injected spinal injections which deadened me from chest down. I was conscious all through the operation, and was given orange juice and water." Although she was "a little sick" to her stomach after the operation, "since then I have been O.K. and getting along very very well. Doctors were very pleased. The baby was taken to Boston Thursday night for X Ray treatment and given a blood transfusion Friday. He was a 8 mo[nth] 4 day baby [who weighed 7¼ pounds]. Is getting along well now." Tracy signed off: "Thanking you for your letter and all you have done for me."[47]

John

In the summer of 1945, John married. Two years later he wrote to White of his plans to pursue a Ph.D. in chemistry once he graduated from college that spring. In his letter, after asking White for the name of a good doctor near his Midwestern university, he proceeded with a series of harrowingly blunt questions. First, he observed that he would be twenty-seven years old when he completed the Ph.D., then asked whether his "normal life-expectancy is long enough to warr[a]nt my spending another four years in school. For instance, if my life-expectancy were only 35 years, it would seem wiser for me to accept a position now, and thus be able to provide my wife with a home and family for a maximum length of time." He then wondered if White would "advise my having children. That is, what is the probability of a child of mine being diabetic (there is no record of diabetes in my wife's family)." Finally, he requested that White recommend some accessible medical writing on diabetes since his current knowledge was "limited to what I've gained from Dr. Joslin's 'Diabetic Manual.'" He was particularly keen "to gain a more technical knowledge, especially concerning what parts of my body will be most likely to fail in later life, and the detrimental (if any) effects of prolonged use of insulin." He also wanted "to follow current developments in diabetic research work."[48]

While John's questions and subsequent decisions about marriage and continued education imply that he did not truly believe his life would end prematurely at thirty-five years, he was clearly aware of the possibility of complications and early death. Additionally, his emphasis on knowledge and research, fitting for a chemist, signaled a redistribution of authority and responsibility in his relations with White and Joslin. As his rephrased remarks (from solicitations of advice to requests for factual information) suggest, he seemed to have matured as a patient to an interim stage, no longer a completely dependent child but still not a fully emancipated adult in the doctor-patient relationship.

White responded to John's letter, first reassuring him that "your life expectancy is certainly long enough to warrant your spending another four years in school." She stated that the life span of a diabetic is three-fourths the normal length, "and of course treatment will be improving during the next few years." She also offered reassurance that "there is no probability of diabetes in your children providing your wife's family history is absolutely correct [that is, 'untainted by diabetes']." She recommended the most recent textbook that Joslin, White, and others had written on diabetes, and several doctors whom he could contact near his university.[49]

In the summer between his first and second years of graduate school, John took a temporary job at a manufacturing plant in a southern state to learn firsthand how his research was applied in industry. On arrival, he was required to take a physical exam. "A doctor (of questionable mentality)," he told White, "placed a stethoscope in the center of my chest for fully three seconds, and then after checking me for hernia was about to pronounce me a perfect physical specimen until I was naive enough to tell him I was diabetic. Visibly shaken, the doctor made several hurried phone calls while watching me to see when I would fall into coma." John then was told that it was company policy not to hire diabetics. After some hasty negotiation, he was retained because he had already been hired; but instead of working throughout the plant, he "would be confined within the safe walls of the laboratory."[50]

John fumed. He exclaimed to White that he was "not ashamed to be a diabetic, and until now I have never hesitated to admit it. . . . My health is perfect, I feel fine. . . . Yet, because some moron employed by the mill has gone into coma several times, they believe that all diabetics will do likewise." He then asked White, "a recognized authority," to send the company doctor a letter to clear up his misconceptions and thus "make it possible for capable and intelligent diabetics to secure jobs in the future—jobs that they have no right to be denied." Mentioning a newspaper article he had recently read that advocated prohibiting diabetics from obtaining a driver's license, he summed up his feelings: "This type of hog-wash makes my blood boil! I see no reason for the thousands of sensible diabetics to be looked upon as 'industrial hazards' merely because of the mistakes of a few, too idiotic to care properly for themselves."[51]

White replied with an even-handed explanation of why such discrimination existed, and why it was no longer appropriate. Previously, she maintained, companies feared that a diabetic who sustained a slight cut or other injury on the job might become deathly ill due to their well-known susceptibility to bacterial infections. With the advent of antibiotics in the late 1930s and 1940s, however, "this danger has been completely wiped out but industry in general doesn't appreciate that this has altered the diabetic's position." The second fear was that the diabetic would suffer a sudden hypoglycemic reaction, lose consciousness, and injure himself or his coworkers. This remained a problem, although the most recent insulin, NPH 50, with a slower onset and more sustained effect, might eradicate such reactions. White also enclosed a letter to the company doctor, telling him that chemotherapeutic treatment of infection in diabetics was very effective, "so that no longer do we fear infection as we did formerly." Furthermore, White testified that John "is an extremely intelligent and cooperative patient, recognizes his insulin reactions and I think the hazards from this point of view [are] also very slight."[52]

This exchange of letters and views bespoke a deeper mutual understanding—dating back to John's first hospitalization—of the key principles of diabetic management as preached by Joslin and White, and believed adamantly by John: knowledge, attitude, and adherence. John had built his diabetic identity around being an intelligent and conscientious patient; White corroborated and even nurtured this view. Knowledge was John's talisman, attitude his defensive weapon, and adherence to regimen his protective armor. Little did he realize how heavy this manner of combating diabetes would become.

COPING WITH THERAPEUTIC "FAILURE"

To say that juvenile diabetic patients, diagnosed as youngsters and kept alive through medical intervention, could experience therapeutic failure—decades after they otherwise would have died—is to speak right to the heart of the frustrating reality of modern diabetic history. For their dramatically prolonged lives represent a stunning therapeutic success, as insulin restored a semblance of balance to their metabolism and enabled many of these boys and girls to grow into reasonably healthy adults.

And yet this delicately maintained equilibrium of well-being could not endure indefinitely. For these two diabetic patients, like so many others, the final stages of their lives were fraught with difficulty. Their cases become studies of stress and coping, as they attempted to maintain hope, come to grips with frightful disappointment, and apportion responsibility between themselves and their doctors for the long-term effects that living with diabetes had wreaked upon their bodies.

In some of the medical records that I examined, diabetic patients did not express their thoughts and feelings on these final matters to Joslin or his staff, even though for decades they had articulated a wide range of their experiences. For these men and women, such as Sally Kramer from Chapter 3, the muted end of their stories exemplify a pattern whereby disease—or, more exactly, the collective response on the part of the patient, family, and physicians to the patient's mounting disability—rewound the life-cycle clock from independent adulthood back toward dependent childhood. As I described previously, for most children with diabetes (but not all) the mother was the principal manager of relationships with Joslin and his staff, shepherding the child to office visits or through hospitalizations, negotiating medical bills, and handling correspondence. The task of patient-physician relationship management was assumed by the patient when she or he reached late adolescence or young adulthood, and that became the status quo—unless the illness intensified with a succession of late-onset sequelae, in which case the mother or the patient's spouse became the chief liaison between patient and physicians. The patient, from the vantage of the medical record, fell silent.

Other diabetic individuals, however, spoke quite forthrightly about the problems and disappointments they encountered near the ends of their lives. Tracy and John were two such patients, and their views emphasize that living with diabetes involved far more than coping with the physical manifestations of this disease.

Tracy

Reading the letters that Tracy sent to the Joslin Clinic, one sees a woman maturing, almost using her diabetes as a source of psychological empowerment: having dealt with the disease continuously, she seems to have viewed her achievements in life as particularly significant. Soon after the medal was established, Tracy wrote Joslin telling him, "I am very interested in the Victory medal. As your record shows I have had diabetes 27 years. At this time I am sound and healthy." She pointed out, with pride, that she was "bringing up a fine daughter and son, alone. This in itself is a job these days. Of course my two a[re] the best ever." Then, as a reminder of their decades-long relationship, Tracy jotted beneath her signature, "one of your diabetic children."[53]

Joslin replied pleasantly that he was "ever so glad to get that nice letter from you. . . . It is splendid that you have done so well and have accomplished so much." Mindful that every patient of his who earned a medal was yet more anecdotal proof that his emphasis on diabetic control was efficacious, he was quick to suggest that if she was "ever in this vicinity come in and we would love to check you over and see whether you would fit in to the Victory Medal Group."[54]

There the issue lay until four years later, when Tracy again broached the subject with Joslin. At the end of a letter in which she mentioned her recent hospitalization for recurrent, painful bladder infections, the upcoming marriage of her daughter to a man who she did not respect, her own second marriage, and other sources of "nervous strain," she moved on to tell him of a recent eye exam that documented twenty-twenty vision and then proclaimed, "Please Don't Disappoint me. Can I *have* the medal *now.*" She argued, "As far as diabetes and control of same doesn't this letter speak for itself and my record. I could go on page after page as to my activity in the 30 years I have had diabetes, but enough of your valuable time. Please let me know. Can I have the medal now."[55]

Joslin knew that Tracy had only minor signs of retinopathy; nevertheless, if his medal winners were to provide the irrefutable evidence that diabetic control mattered, then he needed to adhere to strict standards. He denied Tracy's request, which only fanned her desire for the medal, and her frustration at not receiving it. She sent a letter to White, telling her,

> Doc Joslin said I could not get Victory medal on account of my eyes, and yet I have 20.20 sight, and am a thirty year diabetic. As this medal is for 25 year diabetics under control, *Why* can't I get it? My eyes are remarkable as I have been told several times by your eye doctors. [Doc Joslin] said I would have to live a few more years for the life medal. Well if I live a few more years I guess Doc Joslin will be dead by the time I get either medal. I am disappointed and Doc Joslin who has been so wonderful in everything. What has got into him that he won't give me this medal. Has anyone lived 30 years and is perfectly healthy with diabetes, if so I'd like to see them. Please speak in my behalf and let me know what happens.[56]

White wrote explaining that although Tracy was in "wonderful condition," she had small retinal hemorrhages that disqualified her for the medal. White added, however, that the clinic "should have a blue ribbon for those who *almost* get the medal and you would certainly win this award."[57]

Despite this strain on Tracy's relationship with her physicians, she still expressed genuinely warm and grateful feelings toward White and Joslin. Over the next few years, she sent White two announcements regarding the birth of grandchildren.[58] She also wrote Joslin (after watching him on television lay the cornerstone of the new Joslin Clinic building) a letter of thanks, telling him, "If it had not been for my early training as a diabetic I would not have lived through to the age of 47 next month. Doc. Pris White has been my good Samaritan and advisor, as well as yourself and others on your staff."[59]

But the medal was still on Tracy's mind. Two years later, in 1957, she received a standard note from the clinic inquiring after her health, and asking whether there was anything they could do for her. Tracy did not hesitate. "Yes! *Give me a medal for living so long* and *still having good dia-*

betic control." As she noted, she was "STILL ALIVE," and although she had what appeared to be anginal chest pain, Tracy considered herself to be a "35 year diabetic under good control. (God's been good)."[60] Joslin, when he wrote back a few days later, assured her that "you certainly deserve credit for having had diabetes for more than 33 years, raising up two children and keeping your diabetes so well controlled. In fact, it is because of that [that] you have done so well." Always the teacher, Joslin added that he wished "you were here so that I could show you off to the patients in class because it would encourage them so."[61] Tracy died less than a year later of a heart attack.

Tracy's story highlights the dissension that often occurred when patients and doctors tried to assign responsibility for the damage caused by diabetes. In part, such disputes arose from deep-seated philosophical differences regarding what constituted therapeutic "success." Tracy judged success as an enduring act of will, striving for control, and as the sum total of her personal accomplishments, diabetic and otherwise. The physicians, in contrast, steadfastly measured patients' achievements against a benchmark of no physical complications whatsoever. This high and narrow standard of "success" and its underlying moral premises about salvation through self-control—the basis of the Victory Medal award—consigned certain patients not only to ill health but also to moral failure.

While the end of Tracy's life story was shaped by this contentious debate of what amounted to therapeutic success, John's experience had far more to do with the ravaging effects of the disease itself—and how he fought back.

John

After leaving the manufacturing plant and returning to graduate school, John enjoyed robust health for nearly a decade, as his occasional visits and letters to Boston document.[62] In 1959, however, John's fortunes took a turn for the worse—drastically so. He wrote Joslin, "requesting information concerning my diabetic condition and to obtain any possible advice or help from your clinic which may help prevent my becoming blind." He had suffered a "massive hemorrhage" in one eye, followed shortly thereafter by a hemorrhage in the other. He told Joslin that he "would greatly appreciate your advice or comments as to anything I can possibly do to save what sight I have left. I understand

Dr. Root [one of Joslin's associates] has been conducting research in this area."

Drawing his letter to a close, John wanted "to add some personal comments." As a chemical engineering professor at a major university, he assured Joslin that he could "appreciate the tremendous research problem involved in this blood vessel damage." What shocked John, however, was his "own naiv[ete] about this problem. From the meager statistics I now can find, I should have expected this development." Then, pointing a recriminating finger, he asserted, "I do not fear the truth, but I do fear ignorance, and therefore I resent very deeply not being informed truthfully." Feeling that Joslin had not been forthright with him about this well-known diabetic complication, John contemplated "the personal hell I have gone through trying to rationalize my coming blindness. I am horrified to think of all the others having to face the same problem with no warning. Yet, I hasten to add, I have been grateful for every day of life I have had since first becoming diabetic. I've always regarded each day as a sort of bonus."[63]

The danger that diabetes posed to eyesight long had been a major concern for doctors. Joslin responded to John's letter that "although what I write will not restore your eyesight, I think you will be thankful to learn what is going on." He informed John that "it is a fact that we have 90 patients who have been awarded our Quarter Century Victory Medal because their eyes were certified perfect by [an] expert ophthalmologist" and that the Joslin Diabetes Center had recently "spent over $200,000 on research for a single year . . . and I imagine this year we will do the same and even more." Near the end of the letter, Joslin reiterated his opening caveat: "What I write does not bring back your eyesight but it shows we are not idle and I feel reassured that our patients are living three times as long as formerly and the children with onset in the first decade who have died, have lived some 24 years compared with 1 year at the beginning of the century." He closed by offering his advice to John's doctors regarding how best to manage his diabetes and eye disease.[64]

Whenever a complication such as blindness arose, both patient and physician had to cope, but the tasks they faced and resources at their disposal differed. John suddenly had to confront his own mortality and his feelings of anger, fear, and grief. His protests that he had been left uninformed, although perhaps true in an explicit sense, defy his earlier references about diabetic manuals and textbooks, all of which discussed the complications at length, and his previously blunt understanding about a possible early diabetic death. Just as he had as a younger man, nurturing his prolonged education and high aspirations, John continued to look to his physicians for guidance and hope. Most poignantly, as he tried in the final sentences of his letter to strike a balance between outrage and gratitude, John showed how deeply committed he was to this ambivalent relationship.

Joslin's response, on the other hand, was typical for him: he took the long view. Emphasizing the progress of diabetics as a group, and steadfastly looking forward to yet more research and more progress, Joslin elevated himself above the misfortunes of a given patient (as a doctor who had cared for thousands of fatal cases over decades could do—and perhaps would have to do). In the end, physician and patient each tackled the emotional work of coping in ways consistent with his own personal history.[65]

Three years later, John elected to try and save his vision through an experimental operation that removed part of his pituitary gland. Subsequently, his eye disease seemed to have ameliorated, probably more by chance than by the dubious efficacy of this surgical intervention. John's overall condition, however, continued to deteriorate. And when he died a few years later—still in his early forties—among the several factors that led to John's death was the diabetes insipidus that the surgical removal of the pituitary stalk had itself caused.[66]

RESPONSIBILITY AND THE SEQUELA OF "SUCCESS"

Stories about patients, doctors, and their relationships with each other are tales of cooperation and resistance, indoctrination and resilience. Through them, we gain a better appreciation of the past experiences of patients and practitioners, and how their choices and constraints, their disappointments and hopes were rooted in history—medical, social, and cultural. New therapies have transmuted juvenile diabetes, providing young patients with the chance to grow old. Beyond medical interventions, factors such as family support, financial circumstances, and other aspects of patients' social environment have affected their experience of illness. Cultural beliefs have also modified this illness experience, as the values of self-discipline and the moral battle against disease have directed the pursuit of diabetic control. These general patterns, however, have little meaning unless they are situated in individuals' personal histories. Through the accounts of people who have lived with a transformed illness, these patterns come alive, complete with their attendant uncertainty, contradictions, and trade-offs that have long made living with a chronic illness inherently difficult. While the incredible impact of insulin on the diabetic metabolism has long cast this entire history as a "success" story, focusing on the lives of patients as well as their physicians clarifies how long-term success has meant not only the marked extension of life span, but also—and fundamentally—the successful navigation around the predicaments of dangerous safety over the course of a lifetime.

Elliott P. Joslin, M.D.

Joslin had an eminently successful career. By the end of his tenure in medicine, he had grown old in a manner that cannot be gauged by simply counting the number of years. A pious doctor of the nineteenth century, one well acquainted with suffering and faith, Joslin was still practicing medicine in the middle of the twentieth century. During his ninety-two years of life, he had seen the landscape of American medicine and its institutions change in a manner comparable to that of a quiet neighborly town developing into a large bustling city—change that engendered, for many Americans, ambivalent feelings of awe and nostalgia, excitement and unease. Working within this larger domain, Doctor Joslin and his diabetic patients had refashioned many aspects of the diabetic world. As therapeutic innovations repeatedly revised the medical road map of disease problems and treatment options, they also worked at a private level, navigating new courses along this ever-changing route of health, illness, and medical care.

Although Joslin died in 1962, his influence endures through certain indelible features of the modern diabetic world. The clinic that Joslin built in Boston has remained vibrant and central. The Joslin Diabetes Center continues to expand its facilities, renovating clinical areas while adding new laboratory space. There, the legatees of Joslin's entrepreneurial vision—clinicians and scientists—still care for and study diabetic patients under one roof. In addition, Joslin's publications continue to appear in revised editions. His textbook, *The Treatment of Diabetes Mellitus,* now in its fourteenth edition, provides one of the most complete discussions of diabetes available. Successive editions of the *Diabetic Manual,* as well as the countless other manuals that other physicians have written for diabetic patients, attest to the lay public's sustained interest in this genre of diabetic guidebooks that Joslin pioneered.

These books have carried forward Joslin's ideals that diabetic care should provide the patient with a "liberal diabetic education" and that physicians should guide patients in a practical manner to live with this disease for a lifetime.

Other aspects of Joslin's career, however, seemed curiously dated even before he died. In 1959, for instance, the *New England Journal of Medicine* dedicated an issue to diabetes in honor of Joslin's ninetieth birthday. Looking back over his seventy years of clinical practice, many notables of diabetes research contributed their reminiscences of the "*doyen* of physicians interested in diabetes," the "High Priest of the treatment of diabetes," "a physician devoted to his profession as a sacerdocy," a "BELOVED PHYSICIAN."[67] Yet amidst such words of adoration, Joslin himself occupied an increasingly awkward place in mid-century American medical research. The articles in this Festschrift addressed only the most current laboratory understanding of diabetes and its basic biomedical defects; unwittingly, these papers indicated how peripheral Joslin's brand of clinical tabulation and investigation had become, and how his meticulous attention to details of home care could no longer readily find its way onto the pages of medical journals. By the late 1950s, academic medicine had largely marginalized Joslin's prescient concern for the public health dimensions of diabetes along with his belief in epidemiological reasoning in the clinic and across the nation. Joslin had become an anachronism—revered but seemingly irrelevant.

Of late, Joslin's vision of the comprehensive management of patients and their problems has acquired newfound appeal in this era of cost containment and competition between hospitals. Specialty clinics for diabetic patients have been joined by self-styled "comprehensive care centers" for cancer. Meanwhile, Joslin's interests in clinic-based and populationwide epidemiology have enjoyed an intellectual resurgence, spurred on as the field of health services research and the discipline of general internal medicine began to blossom in the 1980s.

Such recent reincarnations of Joslin-style medical practice, however, are distinguished from their earlier versions by more than just new therapeutic technologies, research techniques, and financial incentives. For better and worse, they lack Joslin's animating moral vision. Three distinctive attributes of his style of medical practice—his self-consciously paternalistic manner with patients, his ready professions of Christian belief, and his morally charged rhetoric of diabetic control—no longer have a comfortable place in American medicine. While current ethical sensibilities might feel no pangs of loss at the departure of these attributes from medical care, something quite important and worthy of reflection might also be jeopardized by the fading of such sentiments. For out of this unique mix of motivation and behavior emerged a patient-centered orientation that, for seventy years of practice, made Joslin an outstanding clinician for the thousands of patients that he treated. Was he perfect?—no, of course not. Was he deeply dedicated?—yes, and the roots of that dedication warrant attention and the fruits of his labors command respect.

Each Day as a Sort of Bonus

What has "success" meant to diabetic patients who lived with a disease that once was swiftly lethal? As the experiences of diabetic patients conveyed on these pages suggests, it meant many—sadly divergent—things. These people have seen both the best and the worst that medicine offers, and many have viewed "each day as a sort of bonus" while lamenting the devastation that the disease wreaked upon their lives. This divergence of meaning has created its own sort of problem, one that has caught patients in a bind of conflicting emotions and contrasting interpretations. People with diabetes, since 1922, have lived with the ironic dilemma of therapeutic success: how should we think or feel about a remarkable medical achievement that gives with one hand and, years later, takes away with the other? How can one be ungrateful for a miracle, one that extends life and hope?

This dilemma can turn into a trap for people with disease and those who care for them. As medical science achieves greater "success" at treating diseases, transmuting their courses onto more chronic paths, we must as individuals and as a society beware of being caught in this dilemma of success, pulled along by what seem to be therapeutic imperatives. The experience with juvenile diabetes and insulin—one of the most spectacular successes of modern medicine—suggests that the dilemma will always look less problematic and more appealing at the outset, only to grow more complex and somber as time passes.

Perhaps these stories of people who have lived with diabetes—viewed across the course of their lives—will temper some of the allure that medical innovations command in our imagination. Perhaps they will help us to understand the long-term emotional sequelae of therapeutic success that ends not in victory but in disappointment. Perhaps they will give us pause when we discuss individual accountability for the effects of chronic disease upon the body.

All these points converge on a perspective that does not refute modern medical achievements or personal responsibility but rather places them in a wider, more complicated context so that we can see them afresh. To avoid the emotional and moral traps of success too narrowly conceived, or responsibility too severely defined, we must constantly strive for the broader and longer view. This exhortation is not specific to medicine and disease. The experiences of illness speak about the world of the healthy as well as the world of the sick; success has its ironic consequences in many areas of life. Both privately and publicly, we must live with this inescapable fact responsibly.

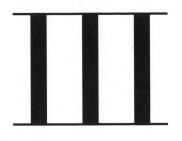

III

Illness and People Care Tomorrow

Before this strange disease

of modern life,

With its sick hurry, its

divided aims.

Matthew Arnold,

The Scholar Gipsy, 1853

8

MEDICINE AND THE MARSHALING OF HOPE: CONFRONTING THE INCREASINGLY COMPLICATED CHOICES OF INCOMPLETE CONTROL

Perfection of means and confusion of goals seem—
in my opinion—to characterize our age.
—Albert Einstein, *Out of My Later Years,* 1950

The best practice of medicine, observed the Renaissance physician Paracelsus, combines science and art. Five hundred years later, this dual nature of health care is evident to me, as a pediatrician, every day. Tending to sick or injured children, I have learned that most patients and their families want not only to acquire information regarding their diseases and treatment options but also to be understood by those caring for them, to have their social circumstances recognized, their cultural values respected, their fears and anxieties, aspirations and dreams acknowledged. Through a fusion of clinical information and mutual understanding, they strive to develop a helpful—even healthful—perspective on their medical conditions, on the predicaments these conditions create, on the meaning of their lives now altered, perhaps permanently, by illness. They seek, in other words, the best that scientific medicine can offer in terms of knowledge and therapeutic interventions, set into a humanistic context of understanding, discernment, and empathy.[1]

Serving the science and the art of medicine requires health care providers to attend to both aspects. Those physicians, nurses, and other healers who enable the science of medicine to flourish in their practice do so through their commitment to lifelong learning, keeping abreast of medical progress, searching for the most recent and rigorous studies, conversing with their colleagues, and scrutinizing the results of their own clinical care. For health care providers to also nurture the art of medicine necessitates a different kind of continuing education, one focused on the humanity of health and illness.

One of the fundamental goals of this book has been to contribute to this continuing education in the art of medicine. To this end, recounting the history of diabetes in twentieth-century America, in and of itself, has been a worthy undertaking. Why? Because the saga of diabetes so clearly demonstrates the human consequences—good and bad—of medical progress, tracing how patients and doctors have fared in an era of vaunting technological expectations. But beyond the particular context of diabetes or the specific chain of events set in motion by insulin and other medical interventions, the chapters of this book have also brought to the fore general concepts of disease transmutation and illness transformation, and far-reaching themes of management, control, and responsibility. These concepts and themes contribute not only to our knowledge about diabetic history but also to our understanding of medical technology and how it impacts our lives.

The wise use of this technology is a central challenge for the artful practice of medicine. I am not alone in my belief that our ever-expanding ability to *do* is overwhelming our capacity to *choose*. In order to address the emerging predicaments presented by our remarkable health care system and its formidable technology, we need a framework both subtle and imaginative, one that can assist us in contemplating the dilemmas posed by imperfect miracles and incomplete control, one that can frame our efforts to grapple with the fundamental human experiences of hope and sorrow. If this book culminates by helping us to better apprehend these issues, and hence confront them in our lives with greater awareness, then I believe it will have achieved its goal of advancing the art of medicine.

RECKONING WITH IMPERFECT MIRACLES

What did insulin mean to doctors and patients in those years shortly after its discovery? Clearly, the drug had profound meaning for physicians such as Joslin. Having introduced insulin into his clinical practice in August 1922, the fifty-four-year-old Joslin challenged the reader of his 1923 textbook to "imagine the feelings of a doctor with a background of 1000 fatal cases, who has lived to see what the ages have longed for come true with the discovery of insulin. . . . Who wants a vacation when he can watch mere ghosts of children start to grow, play and make noise and see their mothers smile again."[2]

Teddy Ryder was one patient who traversed the precarious bridge

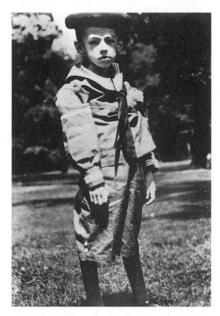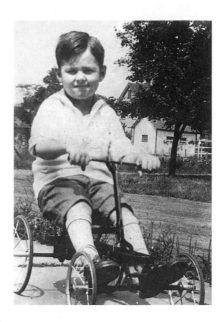

Teddy Ryder just before starting insulin therapy (left) and one year after.
Courtesy of the Thomas Fisher Rare Book Library, University of Toronto.

spanning the pre- and post-insulin eras. A five-year-old with diabetes from New Jersey, Teddy had been kept alive through the Allen starvation diet treatment until he received his first injection of insulin on the tenth of July, 1922, in Toronto General Hospital. Dr. Banting directly supervised Teddy's care for three months until the boy had regained enough vitality to return home. On the anniversary of that initial dose of insulin, the now-robust child had his photograph taken; comparing this image to his frail shadow of a year previous, he seemed indeed to have gained entrance to the Promised Land, where he resided for the ensuing—remarkable—seventy years.

The pictures of Teddy and other patients, beyond any scientific merits, convey deeper sentiments, as though bearing witness to a pilgrimage from suffering to salvation: from bodies emaciated by disease and barely sustained by a disciplined faith, to bodies restored by a wonder drug that raised them from the near dead. In such a reading, the photographs have become symbols of a common "story" that we Americans told ourselves throughout the twentieth century, in which technological progress has solved—or is on the verge of solving—a vast array of problems that trouble our lives. This broad belief in the beneficent powers of technology has especially framed the way that we have come to think about living with disease and struggling against death.

Joslin, illustrating poignantly how faith in technology can create meaning surrounding the death of these children, believed that "insulin redeemed diabetics."[3] Implying that the drug had formidable—almost magical—powers, Joslin had written a letter in 1926 to the brother of a long-deceased patient. "You will remember that in July 1915 I took care of your sister, and she had diabetes at the Deaconess Hospital." As Joslin went on to explain, he thought about her "a great deal because if I had seen her a year later it is just possible I could have kept her alive by fasting and under-nutrition for a good many more years until 1922 when the insulin redeemed diabetics."[4]

Yet in what sense did insulin redeem diabetics? Certainly, children and adults who once would have died now live, sustained by this extraordinary substance. In 1922, just prior to insulin's arrival, children who developed what we now think of as Type 1 diabetes had subsequent life spans measured in days, months, or, at most, a few years. By the year 2000, most young patients newly diagnosed could anticipate living for three decades or longer with the aid of insulin and other health care interventions, reasonably expecting further improvements in future generations.[5] This life-extending capability of insulin might incline many Americans to believe that the drug has been redemptive in the sense of buying back lives that otherwise would have been lost to suffering and death.

Despite this virtually miraculous power, however, insulin has not proved to be an immaculate blessing for those who live with the disease. Rather, children who develop diabetes still face a two- or threefold greater risk of dying than their nondiabetic peers, and they continue to be threatened by the short-term specter of diabetic ketoacidosis and the debilitating long-term diabetic sequelae of kidney failure, nerve damage, impotence, atherosclerosis of the arteries of the heart and limbs, leading to heart attacks and amputations, and injury to the retina of the eye, leading to blindness. Furthermore, insulin treatment itself poses the hazards of insulin-induced hypoglycemic episodes, which can lead to loss of consciousness, seizures, and even (rarely) death.[6] These health problems, coupled with the daily drudge of diabetic self-care, all argue that insulin has not been a panacea. Many of the chores and dilemmas that patients, parents, and physicians had encountered prior to

1921 merely became protracted after insulin's discovery, stretching over decades, and the suffering and death was significantly forestalled but not prevented. From this point of view, the twentieth-century transformation of diabetic experience after insulin is fundamentally connected to the pre-insulin history of how diabetic children, their parents, and physicians had dealt with the disease, their private dramas of sorrow and hope.

Call insulin, then, a precious but flawed miracle. Herein lies a central paradox of assessing remarkable health care interventions: in proportion to which they offer incredible benefits in certain regards, medical technologies often make life more onerous or complicated in other regards. We typically purchase enhanced control in one realm at the expense of diminished control in another. Examples of this phenomenon of "problem exchange" abound in technologically sophisticated hospitals, including the children's hospital in which I work. For instance, children with malignancies have a much greater chance, compared to pediatric cancer patients twenty or thirty years ago, of having their cancers put into remission through extremely intense chemotherapy or bone marrow transplantation; but now they confront the problems of therapeutically induced injury to the brain, heart, endocrine glands, or reproductive organs, and of new tumors arising due to the very therapy that beat back the original cancer. Other children who have had one of their major organs fail—including the kidneys, liver, heart, lungs, or parts of their bowels—can undergo transplantation of these solid organs, but they typically have to receive immunosuppression for the remainder of their lives in order to prevent their bodies from rejecting the transplant, and this immunosuppression can weaken their bones, cause them to gain weight, predispose them to certain forms of cancer, and make them more vulnerable to infections. Finally, perhaps the most dramatic—and eerie—intervention occurs when an infant or child whose lungs or heart have failed is placed onto what is called ECMO (for extracorporal membranous oxygenation), a type of heart-lung machine that takes blood out of the body, fills it with oxygen, and then pumps it back in through the major vessels of the neck. Although ECMO's ability to rescue a child from certain death in many cases is astonishing, survivors often have substantial cognitive deficits, and for those patients who do die despite ECMO, the technology ensnares them in a macabre web of tubing and wires, isolating them from their family members during what too often is a prolonged and utterly dehumanized dying process.

Whenever therapeutic trade-offs prove to be inevitable—and I maintain that such trade-offs occur more often than not—the choices that they pose are usually not straightforward. The noted essayist and cancer researcher Lewis Thomas, after surveying American health care in the 1970s, pointed to a variety of medical treatments that palliated but did not cure disease, coining the phrase "half-way technologies" to describe these sources of therapeutic disappointment. Thomas's perceptive analysis, however, proceeded only halfway itself toward the broader and more difficult truth.[7] Years earlier, René Dubos—a microbiologist who was also an ecologist and historian—composed a remarkable book, *The Mirage of Health*, that came much closer to grasping the essential quandary of therapeutic advances: cures are inherently elusive and transitory, while patients and physicians chronically overestimate the ability of human intervention to alter lives for only the better and not the worse.[8] The reality is that our medical care is encumbered not only by halfway technologies but also by excessive expectations of what drugs and devices can do to promote our well-being. In the end, if redemption is to be found in the history of living with diabetes, the technological redemption offered by insulin has been etched as much by irony as gilded by grace.

A LIFE OF MANAGED HOPE AND SORROW

As the stories of patients told across the preceding pages have illustrated, the broader saga—the compelling yet often contradictory contour of the transformation of diabetes during the past century—defies any concise synopsis or list of simple lessons. A more nuanced understanding is required. To that end, narrative accounts of patients' experiences, if told with enough detail and attention to the interplay of personality, circumstances, and the operation of chance, reveal important contradictions in our struggles with illness, contradictions of thoughts and emotions, of goals and actions, contradictions that our society has grown so accustomed to that they are no longer seen. Through individual cases, compiled and juxtaposed, we have come to a particularly realistic view of not only what this history has been but also—by revealing our contradictory tendencies to ourselves—what this history can mean to us.

Joslin himself made liberal use of case histories, one of which is particularly fitting as we consider the implications of this history of transformed disease. In 1922, delivering his Shattuck Lecture regarding the treatment of diabetes before the Massachusetts Medical Society, Joslin had spoken with unbridled enthusiasm of the discovery of insulin in Toronto. "Now there is no longer need to say '*Hope long deferred maketh the heart sick,*'" for with insulin to fortify the treatment of diabetes, "the promised land is plain in view."[9]

When uttering those words, Joslin had Maria Hanka in mind. Eight years earlier, Maria had been a cheerful toddler, "extraordinarily" healthy and happy, when she became irritable and developed polyuria in January of 1914. Her diabetes presented so gradually that diagnosis was delayed until January of 1915; she was then treated for six months with "codeia and bromid" until she visited Joslin in July of 1915. From that summer until the spring of 1922, she saw Joslin intermittently.[10]

Maria appears to have been either a very mild diabetic or under immaculate control. About once each year, she would visit the Deaconess Hospital and stay for a spell. When entering the hospital these times, at most she would have in her urine a small amount of sugar (which would clear by the second day) and no diacetic acid until her 1920 admission. Over these years, the diets prescribed upon her discharge shifted away from fat and toward more carbohydrates; the caloric content ranged from 500 to 1,000 calories per day.[11]

Through these visits, Maria and her parents grew quite attached to Joslin and his wife, Elizabeth Denny Joslin, and the feelings might easily have been reciprocated. Prior to one trip to Boston in 1920, eight-year-old Maria wrote (in her own well-schooled handwriting) to "My Dear Doctor Joslin: Mother and I are coming up with pleasure next Friday. And will be delighted to spend the night with Mrs. Joslin." The precocious patient let her physician know that "last night I didn't sleep a wink, at least I had my eyes shut but I wasn't asleep[,] I was twisting and turning all night long. First I was too hot, then I was too cold, then I wanted a drink of water, and so on and so forth." Maria also kept him abreast of her social life. "My two dolls," she noted earnestly, "are kicking up their heels, especially Polly the oldest one, who can't even walk yet, though she is thirteen." Quite dramatically she then noted that, "as I am sitting up in bed I hear the wind howling outside," before she signed off with "Love."[12]

Maria's parents watched their daughter carefully. Throughout 1916, they frequently sent Joslin the typed results of urinalysis—comprising more than two hundred daily entries—all of which were "negative for sugar and albumin." Like other children, however, as Maria grew older she also grew more difficult to control, both physiologically and behaviorally. Occasionally, the family turned to Joslin for help or support. In 1920, while the Hankas were busy moving house, the father explained to Joslin how "a week ago someone gave [Maria] some candy, and then when she was all right again, or nearly so, she did some foraging on her own account, getting some cold sausage and some potted meat." Maria had spent two days in bed recovering. Given these episodes and the tumultuous nature of packing and moving, "Mrs. Hanka does not feel that she can properly look out for her for a few days while getting settled in the house we have taken. . . . Hence the request to take her in at the Deaconess Hospital and that you have arranged it makes everything simpler. Thank you very much indeed."[13]

Two years later, Maria's mother, Amelia Hanka, lamented, "It is difficult for me to be accurate about her diet—for I am not always with her + she has been seen with an ice cream cone—and once with a bar of chocolate." Mrs. Hanka told Joslin that "at home we keep her on as light a diet as possible to compensate for these lapses" and assured him that Maria "is looking extremely well + in high spirits." Still, Mrs. Hanka knew that Joslin would "understand the sorrow it is to me to be unable to control what she eats and you would hardly believe the numbers of people who give her things thinking 'it won't hurt her'—."[14]

Hope and sorrow, huddled close together, were the weight and counterweight of Maria's life with diabetes—as they were, and have continued to be, for countless other patients. Joslin, as an expert on a uniformly deadly disease, tried to balance the one against the other, helping patients and parents and practitioners manage the emotional battles of living with diabetes. In his eyes, Maria was an inspirational patient, so much so that in his Shattuck Lecture, he highlighted her case for his audience. Joslin was discussing the "prognosis in diabetic children." He observed that "tender-hearted parents sometimes ask, and sympathetic friends nearly always ask: 'Since diabetes is always fatal in children, why prolong the agony? Why not let the poor child eat and be happy while life lasts?'" In reply, Joslin offered three reasons to persist, even though, after learning the diagnosis, a family's "hope often falls to nearly nil." For one, "the mother must not be forgotten, [and] we cannot do her the injury of killing hope, of admitting, 'Yes, popular belief is true: your child can never grow up." For another, "courage has lengthened the lives of many diabetic children, and no man knows but that the cure may be at hand within the year—even the month." Finally, "many of these children get a lot of fun out of life. Who but a moron will maintain that cripples are not often both more cheerful and braver than many of our intellectual, social, political leaders!"[15]

And then Joslin offered up the "exceptionally happy" example of Maria. "*After eight years and four months of diabetes she is now 9 years and 9 months old.*" He rattled off her diabetic facts and figures, focusing on the intermittent appearance of sugar in her urine, her mildly elevated blood sugars, and her weight of "47.4 pounds naked" and height of "45.5 inches tall, without shoes." He also mentioned that in 1918 she had sold "Liberty bonds, and a year ago was kind enough to sing for the New England Pediatric Society, to show that a diabetic child was happy." Aside from these details, Joslin did not dwell upon the difficulties that the mother confronted when managing the child's diet and regimen, or the sorrow she felt over her daughter's situation; he was content to pose "this bright, attractive and plump little creature" as an example of hope well managed.[16]

Shortly after the lecture, as Joslin had predicted, the dream of "cure" arrived in Boston. On the seventh of August 1922 (as described in Chapter 4), Joslin's colleague Howard Root injected the first dose of insulin into forty-two-year-old Elizabeth Mudge.[17] After this successful initiation of insulin therapy, Joslin set about informing all of his severely ill patients and their parents about the new drug and its availability.

"You have probably seen more or less about the pancreatic extract in the papers," Joslin wrote to Mrs. Hanka in September of 1922. "I have had it for some weeks, and it really works quite well. It is possible that it would help Maria a good deal." Joslin recommended that, if Maria was "as comfortable as she was," they should delay giving her insulin "until possibly the first of October. All of us will be more experienced with it then. On the other hand, if Maria is in a critical state, of course, I should want to give it to her at once." Joslin also let Amelia Hanka know that he had written to her "confidentially, because it is not generally known that I was given this extract, and it would embarrass me should it come to light, because of the number of people who would want it."[18]

Mrs. Hanka replied immediately. "Dear Dr. Joslin—I was perfectly delighted to get your note today + feel that there is a new chance for Maria—Her general health is splendid, her step light, and color + spirits good—so that there is no urgency." Indeed, Maria had "just had a part in the Art Association Pageant + won much approval," according to Mrs. Hanka. How the once constricted and gloomy future must have suddenly changed shape and color in her mind as she signed off: "With many thanks—and love to Mrs. Joslin—I am always—Faithfully Yours, Amelia Hanka—."[19]

Inscrutable fate interceded, however, before the promise of this brighter future could be realized. Although no letters provide details, the medical record of Maria Hanka ends with a simple entry, noting that she died in coma at the end of 1922. The case file does not indicate whether she received insulin during the fall or early winter. She probably did, yet fell ill with a cold or infection and lapsed into coma despite the insulin. During the early years of insulin, such events were not uncommon. Whatever the circumstances of her death, Maria's life of managed hope and sorrow had ended, leaving a saddened physician and grieving parents behind, encircled by the cold fire of loss. Thinking back over the case of Maria, and all the children who died before insulin could save them, perhaps Joslin reflected—as was his style—upon this verse from Ecclesiastes: "I returned, and saw under the sun that the race is not to the swift, nor the battle to the strong."[20]

HISTORY, MEDICINE, AND FORMS OF IMAGINATION

Maria Hanka's case strikes some of the most resonant chords in the experience of diabetes during the twentieth century: uncertainty, sadness, and hope reverberated throughout this child's life, as they have for so many other patients living with diabetes. These quintessentially human qualities appeared almost sacrosanct to me, when I first read through the notes and letters contained in Maria's record, and the records of others, a decade ago. My regard for the intimate aspects of chronic illness was then amplified by the intervening years of medical training and practice, and has spurred my attempts to envision the day-to-day realities, emotional as well as physical, of living with this disease, both as a historian and a physician.

Hewing close to the experiences of the people recounted in this book has deepened—and perhaps darkened—my historical account, as I have grappled vicariously with the intractable realities of illness and the inherent limits of medical technology. My perspective on the history of diabetes in modern America, emphasizing less the technological wonder and more these intractable realities and inherent limits, runs counter to the technological enthusiasm of our times. Occasionally, I have wondered whether my interpretation reflects a poverty of imagination, whether in this era of multi-organ transplants and bold plans for gene therapy I have failed to exercise sufficient imagination regarding what the future might bring. One could argue that too much skepticism and not enough commitment to explore the unknown would slow medical progress, preventing us from seeing how a series of innovations might someday help people who suffer and die. And I would, in a limited sense, agree: optimism is essential for technological imagination, which flourishes best in an atmosphere of can-do bravado.

Yet the untrammeled pursuit of cure also suffers from an impoverished imagination, one lacking a dedicated and constant awareness of the person who is the patient. The history of insulin and diabetes provides ample evidence for this countervailing viewpoint, contrasting with the technological ethos and its vision of health care, emphasizing the need for a different kind of imagination. As I have learned while writing this history and practicing medicine, too little skepticism toward health care and too much commitment to technology can lead to individual tragedies: patients who live with the isolation that too often accompanies chronic illness and who die in the embrace of machines rather than family and friends. These lives and deaths argue, paradoxically but compellingly, that without what we might call a humanistic, empathic, or moral imagination, our society and its astonishingly sophisticated medical system—overly committed, as it is, to the radical cure of disease— can never care properly for people who live with chronic illness or those who approach death.

THE CONSTANT PRESENCE OF THE PAST

In the stories that compose this book, both forms of imagination—the technological and the humanistic—have been at work to reconstitute the substance of these people's lives. While the protagonists of the preceding pages are all now long dead, the concepts and themes identified in their lives persist, shaping the types of medical care that patients receive and the nature of their experiences. In the world of people living with transformed illnesses, the past, in a remarkably tangible sense, is constantly present.[21]

Consider, first, the continued trends of disease transmutation and mounting intensity of care. Since Joslin's death in 1962, a host of new medical interventions have continued to modify the physiological trajectory of juvenile diabetes. Vascular surgery, renal dialysis, and kidney transplantation had appeared on the therapeutic scene in the 1950s, but their impact on the lives of diabetics escalated sharply from the late 1960s onward. Newer versions of drugs to treat high blood pressure and weakened hearts likewise became much more effective after Joslin's time. In addition to these improvements, innovative diagnostic and therapeutic techniques further altered the biological course of events. Home blood glucose monitors, which are portable and relatively inexpensive machines that determine the sugar level from a single drop of blood, have been the most pervasive. In the medical office, the monitoring of hemoglobin A1c (a protein in the blood that will have more sugar attached to it if the blood sugar level has been consistently elevated) and the review of blood glucose measurements from home (recorded electronically so that the data can be analyzed on a computer) have provided new information for the continuing pursuit of diabetic control. And then there have been diabetic individuals who have been treated with what once were experimental therapies, such as retinal photocoagulation (which uses tiny laser burns to arrest diabetic eye disease), or the use of small insulin infusion pumps (attached to the body via fine tubing and needle inserted just under the skin, supplying a steady infusion of insulin along with easy-to-administer additional doses whenever the blood sugar rises), or most recently the transplantation of pancreatic tissue (so as to replace the insulin-making β cells that were destroyed).

Second, people with diabetes live in the context of a ceaselessly transforming illness experience, one that underscores the fundamental role of human choice in the technological victories and tragedies of medical care. While the evolving form of the disease has been altered by innovative medical treatments, this alteration has not been dictated by technology but rather by individual decisions, social circumstances, and uncertain consequences, and each of these have an influential history. In other words, insulin and other interventions are potent tools that have developed in response to the concerns of patients, physicians, and researchers. These interventions in turn have been deployed as medical therapies in a series of individual decisions and behaviors, guided by specific values and beliefs, and played out in the setting of particular constraints, all of which change over time, the past influencing the present and thus shaping the future. For instance, patients who ascribed to the goal of attaining stringent diabetic control, and possessed the financial means to pursue this objective, were able to utilize insulin and monitoring technologies in a way that physically inscribed the history of these beliefs and choices on their bodies. Exactly what course this history would ultimately take—whether triumphant longevity or complicated tragedy—has and continues to be determined by processes that lie just outside the reach of human manipulation, amenable to influence but still prone to the capriciousness of fate that brought Maria Hanka's life to an end. Such is the reality of living with a disease in motion, confounding simple dichotomies between natural physiology and unnatural intervention, between value-neutral technologies and the value-laden choices that determine how they are used, between events we can manage and events beyond our control.

Third, the ramifications of the biological transmutation and the social transformation of diabetes have been wide-ranging, carving themselves into the broader history of our nation. The disease has gone from an ailment that was spoken of in hushed terms, if at all, to a condition that has fully entered the national stage. "National Diabetes Week," first sponsored by the American Diabetes Association (ADA) in 1948 and now expanded to a month, has led to the testing of countless adults for diabetes and enhanced public awareness of the disease. A more recent screening program, which tests all pregnant women who receive prenatal care for gestational diabetes, has changed the experience of pregnancy for many women. The 1972 enactment of Public Law 92-603 provided end-stage renal disease patients with funds through Medicaid for chronic renal dialysis and, in a more limited manner, for kidney transplantation. During the same period, the Juvenile Diabetes Foundation was established in 1970 by parents of diabetic children. These parents, angered that a definitive cure for juvenile diabetes still was not in hand—and that the ADA seemed complacent—created an organization that has since generated substantial public interest and research funds for finding a cure.[22]

Finally, at an intimate level, the three transformational themes that we have tracked over time—the daily realities of management, the ceaseless pursuit of control, and the problematic repercussions of responsibility for patient, family, and doctor—still permeate the diabetic world. Every day throughout the past century, people living with juvenile diabetes have performed the work of illness self-care. The managerial work of strict dieting may have been replaced by the work of insulin injections, and urine testing may have been supplanted by blood sugar monitoring, but the fact is that managerial work remains. Patients still have to find ways to manage their disease and its medical treatment along with conducting the rest of their lives. Patients and physicians still debate the place of tight diabetic control in treating this disease—and thus in shaping patients' lives. And these men and women still wrestle with the contentious issue of responsibility, regarding both the daily management of diabetic care and the personal accountability for diabetes-induced disability and death. Insulin may have alleviated the threats of coma and other acute medical problems from the lives of young patients—but insulin did not, and could not, remove all the burdens of living with chronic illness.

INEXTINGUISHABLE TENSIONS

Although the implications of disease transformation are profound, they have not yet been fully appreciated. Too many doctors still believe too readily that medical orders should dictate the order of a patient's life. For example, consider the Diabetes Control and Complications Trial (DCCT), which was conducted under the aegis of the National Institutes of Health between 1983 and 1993 at many clinical sites across America. The DCCT demonstrated that strict diabetic control—testing blood sugar four to ten times a day, injecting insulin several times if indicated by the tests—reduces the risk of blindness, kidney damage, and blood vessel disease (yet raised the risk of hypoglycemic spells). The leaders of this study had thought that diabetic patients would flock to the offices of their doctors, seeking to be put on the more rigorous regimen. Many patients, however, realize that their lives consist of far more than their chronic disease, that they have more to do than simply manage their diabetes. And so, while some people with diabetes expressed enthusiasm regarding the DCCT findings, far fewer patients than the researchers had imagined came to their physicians asking to tighten their control through more intensive therapy.[23]

This mixed reception to the results of the DCCT was, given the history of diabetes that we have covered, rather predictable. The behavior of diabetic patients reflects a set of tensions that have been at work throughout the twentieth and early twenty-first centuries, tensions evident in the chronically ill patient's archetypal dilemma: how to reconcile the pursuit of control over a disease with the pursuit of living well with that disease. Differences in how these two pursuits frame the problems presented by chronic illness are crucial. Viewing illness through the reductive focus of cure or treatment simplifies therapeutic decision-making by limiting the range of considerations factored into decisions of how to proceed. The more holistic perspective of how an individual can best live with the ailment and its treatment, on the other hand, considers a broader range of issues that are important to people living with a disease yet makes decisions more complicated, as patients must balance the demands of their illness against the demands of managing families, jobs, social activities, and personal identities.

The juxtaposition of reductive and holistic thinking is linked, in our current American health care system, to a group of other dichotomous concepts or approaches to the pursuit of well-being:

Reductive	Holistic
Disease-specific care	Patient-centered care
Emphasis on cure or outcome	Emphasis on caring or process
Intervention key activity	Interpretation key activity
Technology oriented	Relationship oriented
Activism against disease and death	Acceptance of mortality and its limits
Quantity of life	Quality of life

While these opposing viewpoints do not line up as precisely as this listing might suggest, overall they represent ends of a spectrum of alternative perspectives on the goals, and thus the tasks, of medicine. Reconciling these perspectives is no mean feat, and yet this is precisely what has to happen, explicitly or implicitly, every time a patient and doctor interact. To a degree, our culture provides some biases in favor of one perspective over another, preferring for example to "wage war" against various diseases, seeking the total victory of cure rather than the negotiated agreement of life with a chronic or life-threatening ailment, or preferring high-technology over low-technology solutions to a wide range of problems. But these biases, although influential, have never determined the course of therapeutic events. Whenever patients have opted—either on their own or jointly with their physicians—to strive for increasingly stringent diabetic control, or to tend to other areas of their lives, their decisions have represented individualized resolutions to the tensions between these opposing points of view.[24]

These tensions are inextinguishable: they will never go away. No care pathway or disease management system can forge a lasting resolution. Nor would we want them to; for any one-size-fits-all, permanent resolution would need to be forced upon people whose values differ from the values that guided the formulation of these protocols. While pathways and protocols can assist us greatly in improving the quality of specific services, they cannot decide what services a particular patient wants to receive. Such a decision requires, now and always, an individualized resolution.[25]

CONFRONTING THE CHOICES
OF INCOMPLETE CONTROL

Complicated choices arise wherever medical technology has transmuted a disease into a chronic condition, as has been the case for premature birth, some congenital defects, many cancers, most heart diseases, certain neurological ailments, and countless other conditions. Questions regarding management, control, and responsibility suffuse every medical encounter and all acts of self-care. As patient and physician work to manage a disease, they seek that ideal yet elusive resolution of those inextinguishable tensions, striking a balance between striving for greater control versus making the most of the status quo, between assuming responsibility for what happens versus acknowledging that the outcomes of events often fall beyond the ambit of human control.

All too often, however, this balancing act is performed implicitly and quite imperfectly, resulting in frustration and disappointment, anger and guilt. Furthermore, advances in medical technology likely will create increasingly complicated choices in the years to come, making the achievement of balance far more difficult. These problems affect all areas of medical practice. A conspicuous example in the realm of care for adults involves the determination of risk for diseases such as breast cancer through genetic testing. What is a woman to do, if presented with test results that indicate she has an elevated risk of developing breast and ovarian cancer compared to most other women? Undergo prophylactic bilateral mastectomy and oophorectomy, as some choose?

These kinds of complicated choices, with perhaps less draconian yet still arduous options, are on the horizon for a host of other diseases, from Alzheimer's to arthritis, with some degree of genetic influence. Within the field of pediatrics, prenatal diagnosis by genetic testing or ultrasound presents similar dilemmas (especially since termination of pregnancy is not a therapy but rather only an extremely unhappy solution, and fetal surgery, despite the hoopla surrounding it, is still an impressively unusual and unproven intervention). Since the 1950s, neonatologists have dramatically lowered the gestational age at which point infants who are born prematurely have a fighting chance to live, yet in so doing they have fostered a whole area of bioethics that hotly debates when these tour de force efforts have gone too far, creating unacceptable suffering or disability for the children, generating crushing financial and social burdens on their families, or consuming inordinate amounts of health care resources. Even the treatment of far less dangerous or far more common problems, such as attention deficit and hyperactivity disorder with the stimulant methylphenidate (Ritalin), or therapy for asthma with inhaled steroid medications, or the prevention of infectious illnesses with immunizations, presents trade-offs that must be sorted through in order for us to make good decisions.

What can be done to improve our efforts to make better choices in an increasingly complicated health care world? Since the 1960s, American society has embraced the concept of informed consent as a method to assist patients in making difficult choices (as well as a means to safeguard their rights).[26] Accurate information alone, though, is not sufficient to make good decisions. Rather, this information must be brought into a solid decision-making process, which interprets this information in the context of values and deeply considered objectives.[27]

One hundred years ago, Joslin reflected on how a patient and a doctor should interact: "Between the two a partnership must be formed."[28] While Joslin did not always himself succeed in forging ideal partnerships, he was well ahead of his time with this invaluable insight. An essential task for the patient-doctor partnership is to pilot a course of action based not only on the interpretation of clinical information but also on the contemplation of what issues matter most to the patient. Both patient and physician need to contribute substantially to this process. Often, complicated medical decisions arise when we want to accomplish several objectives (for example, to have both a longer life and a life of higher quality) that are not fully compatible with each other and create tremendous confusion and strife when they are left vague or ill-defined. Just as the notion of therapeutic "success" cannot be defined without regard for people's underlying preferences and ambitions, deciding what therapeutic course to pursue requires consideration of these same values and goals. When we have thoughtfully asked what, over the span of our lives, would really constitute "success," we begin to escape the seductive entrapments of wondrous technology, with its monomaniacal focus on the prolongation of life, and start the process of answering how to steer our course through the myriad options that medical care poses.

The straightforward act of specifying the problems that we want our medical care to address can have substantial implications, even for decisions that seem to have an "obvious" preferred course of action. For example, what person with Type 1 diabetes would, if asked, choose not to take insulin? Is there really a choice here? Yet choice is still fundamental, perhaps not so much regarding whether to take the drug but how to: Should we inject once or twice a day in the privacy of home, or maybe settle into a more open approach injecting with every meal or using the infusion pump? Do we adopt a more intensive regimen of monitoring and insulin dosing in order to prevent high blood glucose levels, knowing that we will then experience more episodes of hypoglycemia? This constellation of problems and trade-offs, in my experience, is appreciated better when framed in the broader context of how to live life, not just how to treat the diabetes or some other medical condition. This broader perspective can be helpful throughout the course of therapy but is especially valuable when major decisions need to be made, in response to new information or therapeutic options, or because the original treatment plan is not working, moving further away from the desired objectives, and not closer. Without a broader perspective, perceiving when medical therapy has strayed from the desired path is nearly impossible, and care, as a consequence, suffers.

In my own practice of medicine, I have found that examining the hopes and therapeutic aspirations of patients and families, with empathy yet quite forthrightly, can be of inestimable value. For gravely ill infants or children in the hospital, when the hope of curing the condition or extending the patient's life span substantially has dwindled, this examination can enable other hopes to surface, perhaps of minimizing suffering while maximizing comfort, or of striving to return home or accomplish a dearly wished-for activity, or of gathering family members for religious ceremonies or other mutually supportive activities. For chronically ill patients, reconsidering what hopes, beliefs, and values underwrite the goals of care—and then reconsidering these goals themselves—can lead to breakthroughs in realizing that certain medical tests or treatments make no sense (because they would yield information that would not change the treatment plan, or cause too much discomfort, or make care much more burdensome for the family), while other treatment options may be crucial in order to accomplish the clarified goals of, say, enhanced quality of life. Even for children with conditions like attention-deficit and hyperactivity disorder, clarifying the goals of therapy with the family—centering on issues such as buoying the child's sense of self-esteem, building skills of self-management, and bolstering the ability to attend and hence learn—can put this aspect of the child's life into a much more salubrious perspective.

What does such a process of medical decision-making look like? Several central features are illustrated in Table 8.1, which depicts a scenario in which a patient is facing a life-threatening condition. Discussion with the patient (or parent, if the patient is a child) about important goals results in a list of six major objectives, including maximizing the chance for a cure, minimizing the risk of future disability, and maximizing the patient's connectedness to family. These objectives represent, in a concrete sense, what this patient is hoping for. While the physician should facilitate this process, the patient, and only the patient, can define and prioritize this list of objectives. The medical condition is usually treated one of three ways, ranging from the most intensive therapy A (focused on cure), to treatment option B (focused on aggressive long-term management), to treatment option C (focused on palliation). The physician must then inform the patient how these treatment options differ in terms of how likely they are to accomplish the patient's listed objectives. Treatment A is clearly the best if the pursuit of cure is the only objective. But if the chance of cure is, at best, remote, and other objectives are added to the decision, the best choice becomes less clear-cut. Indeed, after examining how treatment options B and C each offer real advantages to accomplishing some, but not all, of the goals, the patient and physician could conceive of combining those two approaches, creating a nonstandard therapeutic course that is tailored to the specific situation and goals of this particular patient. As clinical events then unfold—such as the disease relapsing, disability sequelae arising, or pain increasing—the patient and doctor can return to this framework and reconsider what to do next.[29]

If such a scheme for framing our struggles with disease would improve the medical decisions that we make (a conjecture that still needs to be proven), we should investigate how to best help individuals consider their values and goals, identifying what they are hoping to accom-

TABLE 8.1. Framework for Considering the Impact of Treatment Options on Treatment Goals

| | TREATMENT OPTIONS | | | |
| | Most Intensively Focused on Cure | Spectrum of Treatment Focus | | Most Intensively Focused on Palliation |
Important Goals or Objectives	Option A	Option B	Combination of Options B & C	Option C
Maximize chance for cure	Best			
Minimize risk of death in short term		← Best ? →		
Minimize risk of future disability		← Best ? →		
Minimize pain and suffering				← Best ? →
Maximize enjoyment of activities			← Best ? →	
Maximize connectedness to family				← Best ? →

plish. We also need to develop techniques to assist people in weighing the trade-offs between alternative courses of action, to help them grapple with the uncertainty that surrounds all efforts to predict the future, and to confront the specific emotional challenges posed by medical prognostication.[30] Last but not least, we need to acknowledge and work within constraints, imposed not so much by the costs of health care (although such monetary issues can be extremely confining) but by our mortality. One of the insights I gained from this historical study—which may seem obvious—is that, eventually, everyone dies. Of course, at some level I have long known that we all die. Yet as I followed each of the cases from the time of diagnosis until, sooner or later, the time of death, I felt at times overwhelmed, surrounded by all this death, in each instance unprepared emotionally for its arrival. I came to realize that, like our culture generally, I was far from fully acclimated to the inevitability of death; it still felt like cold brutal winter to me, and I would shiver and turn away. Now, as a physician, I see quite clearly that I must constantly work to become more comfortable with death if I am to really help those who are dying. And so must anyone else who cares about taking care of mortal beings. Until we can confront death without turning away, planning how to make the most of the life we are granted, right to the very end, is likely to never receive the attention it warrants.

We also need, at the level of national policy, to come to grips with the implications of transformed diseases and their associated complicated medical decisions. When we interrogate aspects of our health care system (In what direction should we steer our complex system of health care? How should we train our young physicians? What research should we fund?), our answers must be built on the reality that disease will always be with us. Control over human health and disease, as I have stressed repeatedly, is an alluring yet elusive goal. Our approach needs to be balanced. On the one hand, I encourage ambitious medical investigators to dream of eradicating ill health, one disease at a time, through the power of genetic medicine, or of compressing the period of disability or suffering that so often accompanies the end of our lives down to a fleeting minimum. Yet—and this is a crucial point—I also encourage these or other equally ambitious and talented investigators to consider how the processes of disease substitution and transmutation will continue to create health problems with which we shall have to live. For while we should continue efforts to reduce disease and disability, we need a matching commitment to improve the experience of living with disease—and to do this we must realize that such a transformation of experience will be accomplished not so much with wonder drugs that cure but with people who provide attentive and compassionate care and policies that support these people and the provision of care. We need to expand our thinking, in other words, beyond the confines of a health care system that treats patients, to envision a people care system that takes care of people.

MARSHALING HOPE

Ultimately, as one of the humanities, historical study ought to augment our humanity. I cannot rightly say whether this book, tracing a remarkable transformation of human illness, has accomplished this goal. At least I cannot say so for others, who read only what I have written. What I can attest to is that the process of researching and writing this book has been a remarkable personal experience, one that has affected me as a physician and a person. In attempting to tell the stories of people who have lived with diabetes, I confronted the challenge alluded to in one of the epigrams that opened this work. Laboring to understand the people described upon these pages—who became characters in my own emotional and moral life—I tried not to turn from their suffering and instead sought to follow compassion wherever it led. Through this effort, I came to regard the changes wrought by medical interventions as powerful but limited, to respect more deeply the capacity of people to live with disease, and to appreciate more fully the fundamental, and precarious, role that hope plays in our lives.

Hope: that feeling that defines a perspective that becomes a motive force in our lives when control over events eludes us. Surprisingly, we know so little about hope, as though the topic is too maudlin or effusive. Yet few aspects of our private or public lives are more powerful. My own education in this subject has been conducted, for the most part, through observations made in my clinical practice and the research and writing of this book. For I believe that this complicated and ironic saga of a dreaded disease and a miraculous drug is, at core, a history of hope. For although hope is so intimate, what we hope for simultaneously reflects our society and the opportunities it affords, our culture and the values it promotes. Weaving together our individual lives and collective experiences, hope is a verb, active and powerful, capable of learning and adapting, moving us forward. Physicians and other providers who ply the art of medicine, in their roles as mediators and purveyors of hope, need to understand and mobilize this force better. Such an ac-complishment would not result in lives lived without illness but rather a different prospect: of lives still often beset by illness but lived better nevertheless because proper attention is paid to making choices conso-nant with our deepest values and marshaling our hope with a clearer vision and sense of purpose.

NOTES

Preface

1. Best to Hugh Lyle Stalker, 17 March 1965, H MS c 3.2, in the Charles Herbert Best Papers, Fisher Rare Book Library, University of Toronto, Canada.

2. Readers who are interested in pursuing the medical aspects of diabetes further might turn first to those books written with the lay reader in mind, such as the most recent version of *Joslin Diabetes Manual*. Alternatively, they could peruse one of the magazines dedicated to diabetic patients; for example, *Diabetes Self-Management* (for information and subscriptions, write P.O. Box 52890, Boulder, CO, 80322, or at <www.diabetes-self-mgmt.com> [accessed 1 August 2002]). For more extensive scientific discussions, I would begin with a general textbook on diabetes or on medicine, such as *Joslin's Diabetes Mellitus* or *Harrison's Principles of Internal Medicine*.

3. I hope that what these pages sacrifice in terms of thoroughness or accuracy is compensated, at least in part, by their being brief and readable. I am indebted to the many fine teachers at the University of Pennsylvania School of Medicine, and in particular, Dr. Francis H. Sterling, for their diligence in helping me to understand endocrinology.

Chapter One

1. The estimated annual incidence of Type 1 diabetes mellitus in the United States is between 12 and 18 new cases per year, per 100,000 children zero to six-

teen years of age. Given an estimated 66 million children in this age bracket in 1997, approximately 22 to 32 new cases should be diagnosed each day of the year, with more cases presented in the late fall and winter than in the spring or summer. On incidence and prevalence, see LaPorte et al., "Pittsburgh Insulin-Dependent Diabetes Mellitus (IDDM) Registry," and Kurtz, Peckham, and Ades, "Changing Prevalence of Juvenile-Onset Diabetes Mellitus." The estimate of one million Americans with Type 1 diabetes is based on the estimated total prevalence of diabetes cases in the United States and the 5 to 10 percent estimated proportion of these cases as being due to Type 1 diabetes; see the fact sheet published by the Center for Disease Control and Prevention, which can be found at the following internet address: <http://www.cdc.gov/diabetes/pubs/factsheet.htm> (accessed July 2002).

2. For a discussion of the *Papyrus Ebers,* see Sigerist, *Primitive and Archaic Medicine,* 310–15. On diabetes in non-Western medical writings, see Frank, "Diabetes Mellitus in the Texts of Old Hindu Medicine."

3. Aretaeus (ca. 81–138 A.D.), "On Diabetes," and "Cure of Diabetes." I have revised the translation of the opening phrase slightly, rendering it as "mysterious illness" instead of "wonderful affection."

4. Willis, "Section IV, Chapter III" and "Chapter IV."

5. Willis, *Pharmaceutic Rationalis,* 79. I have modernized spelling to make the passage clearer.

6. Dobson, "Experiments and Observations on the Urine of a Diabetic."

7. Rollo, *Account of Two Cases of the Diabetes Mellitus.* The "animal diet" is fully described by Rollo in the case of Captain Meredith, appearing on pages v–xiii and 1–69. A year after the first edition was published, Rollo issued a second edition, which included additional correspondence that he had received from other physicians regarding diabetes and its treatment, but he otherwise left the two case reports unaltered; see ibid.

8. Joslin et al., *Treatment of Diabetes Mellitus,* 8th ed., 318.

9. Major, "Treatment of Diabetes Mellitus with Insulin," 1597–1600.

10. For examples, see Bliss, *Discovery of Insulin,* and the American Diabetes Association, *Journey and the Dream.*

11. Collins, "Diabetes, Dread Disease."

12. "Ex-Secretary Lansing, Ill from Diabetes."

13. Frederick Allen, "Methods and Results of Diabetic Treatment."

14. Wrenshall, Hetenyi, and Feasby, *Story of Insulin,* 21.

15. Howell, *Technology in the Hospital,* discusses a similar set of values and beliefs that I am here labeling as a "technology ethos" as he describes the adoption of new technologies into the world of hospitals during the early part of the twentieth century.

16. Estimating the prevalence of diabetes in America is difficult because so many adult diabetics with an indolent form of the disease are never diagnosed. Nevertheless, the evidence of the burden that diabetes imposes upon patients is incontrovertible. See U.S. Preventive Services Task Force, *Guide to Clinical Preven-*

tive Services, 193–94; "Incidence of Treatment for End-Stage Renal Disease"; and Geiss et al., "Surveillance for Diabetes Mellitus."

17. Bliss, *Discovery of Insulin.* Bliss continues his account of the credit dispute in "Rewriting Medical History."

18. Holt, *Elliot Proctor Joslin;* Tompkins, *Continuing Quest.*

19. American Diabetes Association, *Journey and the Dream;* Walker, *Chronicle of a Diabetic Service.*

20. Barach, "Historical Facts in Diabetes"; Harris, *Banting's Miracle;* Nothman, "History of the Discovery of Pancreatic Diabetes"; Wrenshall, Hetenyi, and Feasby, *Story of Insulin;* Papaspyros, *History of Diabetes Mellitus;* Hall, *Invisible Frontiers;* von Engelhardt, *Diabetes.* My research was furthered by Presley's "History of Diabetes Mellitus," a dissertation principally concerned with the causes of the persistently high diabetic death rate and the relative neglect of dietary therapy.

21. Ackerknecht, *Malaria in the Upper Mississippi Valley;* Dubos and Dubos, *White Plague;* Rosenberg, *Cholera Years;* McKeown, *Role of Medicine;* Ettling, *Germ of Laziness;* Brandt, *No Magic Bullet;* Harden, *Rocky Mountain Spotted Fever;* Temkin, *Falling Sickness;* Grob, *From Asylum to Community;* Patterson, *Dread Disease;* Haber, *Beyond Sixty-Five.*

22. Joslin, "Metabolism in Diabetic Coma." Joslin refers to the patient with the initials "A. W." in the text of the article, but "Alvin Wilson" is a pseudonym based on these initials that I conceived.

23. Joslin, "Metabolism in Diabetic Coma," 306–7.

24. Rich sources are necessary to produce "thick description" of patient experience. While the historian's ability to create a thick description is often constrained by limited sources of information, I use the phrase to indicate my regard of enthnography as a means to understand how people deal with problems. See Geertz, *Interpretation of Cultures* and *Local Knowledge,* and the collection of essays edited by Alexander and Seidman, *Culture and Society.* Van Maanen, *Tales of the Field,* clarified issues regarding style of thought and writing.

25. The historical collections that I consulted are listed in the bibliography.

26. I am indebted to the center's Committee on Human Studies for granting access to their records.

27. American Association for the History of Medicine, "Report on the Committee on Ethical Codes."

28. White, "Natural Course."

29. The caveat to this claim is extremely important, since we have no data regarding the proportion of children who died of their diabetes prior to being correctly diagnosed or shortly thereafter. Quite possibly, Joslin's panel of young patients reflect a kind of selection bias called "length bias," whereby those patients who survived long enough to be seen by Joslin (or any other diabetes "expert" physician) had a disease process less fulminant than other children. If this was the case, the longer length or duration of their clinical course explains how they survived long enough to become one of Joslin's patients but also distorts our sense of what was occurring for the other children. The more certain claim I am making,

though, is that the astonishingly emaciated children seen in some of the photographs surely do not represent the common experience of that era.

30. Joslin, "Changing Diabetic Clientele," 304.

31. To examine the change in the duration of illness over time, epidemiologists would now use methods of life table analysis or survival analysis, methods that were not available to Joslin. Joslin's method most likely underestimates the true life expectancy, as it considers only the cases of diabetes that have died, failing to account for those cases with long duration illness still alive.

32. Joslin, "Changing Diabetic Clientele," 305.

33. Moderation of the birthrate has also contributed to the demographic redistribution of age groups.

34. The quotation is from Joslin, "Changing Diabetic Clientele," 305. My notion of "supplantation of disease" is drawn from the ideas presented by McKeown, whose work culminated in *Origins of Human Disease;* Omran, "Epidemiologic Transition"; Peery, "New and Old Diseases"; and Weindling, "From Infectious to Chronic Diseases." The field of evolutionary medicine—which seeks to explain individual- and population-level disease phenomena in terms of genotype, phenotypic expression, Darwinian fitness, and related concepts—has developed similar thoughts; for examples, see Gerber and Crews, "Evolutionary Perspectives on Chronic Degenerative Diseases," and Smith et al., "Evolution of Non-Infectious and Degenerative Disease."

35. Crosby, *Colombian Exchange;* McNeill, *Plagues and Peoples.*

36. Burnhan, *Bad Habits;* Bartecchi, MacKenzie, and Schrier, "Human Costs of Tobacco Use."

37. Lederberg, Shope, and Oaks, *Emerging Infections;* Berkelman, "Emerging Infectious Diseases in the United States, 1993."

38. Kunin, "Resistance to Antimicrobial Drugs"; Iseman, "Evolution of Drug Resistant Tuberculosis"; Poit and Islam, "Sexually Transmitted Diseases in the 1990s"; Brandt, *No Magic Bullet.*

39. A thought-provoking history of a disease transformed by medical intervention is Peitzman, "From Dropsy to Bright's Disease." For a sociological perspective of this phenomenon, see Strauss et al., *Social Organization of Medical Work.* For epidemiological discussions of the changing morbidity profile of diabetes, see Davidson, "Continually Changing 'Natural History'"; Krolewski et al., "Changing Natural History"; and Krolewski et al., "Evolving Natural History."

40. Dutton examines the last three of these examples in *Worse than the Disease.* For a sobering assessment of the artificial heart and transplantation, see Fox and Swazey, *Spare Parts.*

41. Wiener et al., "Trajectories, Biographies, and the Evolving Medical Scene"; Jain and Vidyasagar, "Iatrogenic Disorders"; McCormick, "Survival of Very Tiny Babies."

42. Hammond, "Late Adverse Effects of Treatment."

43. Peitzman, "From Dropsy To Bright's Disease."

44. Ackerknecht, "Plea for a 'Behaviorist' Approach"; Reverby and Rosner, "Beyond 'the Great Doctors'"; Grob, "Social History of Medicine"; and Porter,

"Patient's View." I was first introduced to the perspective on the history of medicine through the encouragement of Charles E. Rosenberg and his work, typified by the essays collected in his *Explaining Epidemics and Other Studies*. Keith Wailoo put many of these and other ideas to exemplary use in *Dying in the City of Blues*. Among other chronic diseases, tuberculosis has received perhaps the most historical attention. In my own research and writing I have been influenced by the following historians, both in conversations with them and through their works: Barbara Bates, *Bargaining for Life;* Rothman, *Living in the Shadow of Death;* and Lerner, *Contagion and Confinement*.

45. See Engel, "Need for a New Medical Model"; Kleinman, *Illness Narratives;* and Eisenberg, "Science in Medicine."

46. For an overview of these aspects of diabetic history, which figure only in passing in this book, see the American Diabetes Association, *Journey and the Dream,* 35–57.

47. Indeed, a sense of frustration permeates many areas of medical "progress." This was nicely captured in Knowles, *Doing Better and Feeling Worse.*

48. Blotner, "Coronary Disease in Diabetes Mellitus"; Root and Rogers, "Diabetic Neuritis with Paralysis"; White and Hunt, "Cholesterol of the Blood of Diabetic Children."

49. Kimmelstein and Wilson, "Intercapillary Lesions."

50. The sociological framework employed by Becker in *Art Worlds* has proved extremely useful, as the art world and the diabetic world share striking similarities in the ordering of life and coordinating of collective activity. Many of the ideas that Becker presented in *Art Worlds* have been elaborated further by him and others; for an overview, see Becker and McCall, *Symbolic Interaction and Cultural Studies.*

51. My concern for the inner workings of character, motivation, and personal relationships was initially fortified by a conversation I had with Bob Coles, after I had read his book *Call of Stories.* In recent years, concern for these aspects of the patient and physician experience has burgeoned into a new model of medical practice; for an overview, see Charon, "Narrative Medicine."

52. A few such works are Spence, *Death of Woman Wang;* Davis, *Return of Martin Guerre;* and Darnton, *Great Cat Massacre;* and in the history of medicine, Ulrich, *Midwife's Tale,* and Rosenberg, *Trial of the Assassin Guiteau.*

53. For a theoretical examination of the "social microscope," "microhistory," "polyphonic" history, and "braided" narratives, see Burke, *History and Social Theory,* 38–43, 126–29, 163.

Chapter Two

1. A photograph of Joslin's office is reproduced in the *Pulse,* 3. Donald M. Barnett, M.D., helped me to identify Baker. The weather was described in the *New York Times,* 22 December 1961, 44.

2. Joslin, "Pathology of Diabetes Mellitus"; *Treatment of Diabetes Mellitus,* 1st ed.; and *Diabetic Manual,* 1st ed. The textbook is currently in its 14th edition, published in 2003, and the manual is in its 12th edition, appearing in 1989.

3. As mentioned in Chapter 1, for an intimate and sympathetic biography of

Joslin, providing details about his childhood and early education, see Holt, *Elliott Proctor Joslin*.

4. Quotations, respectively, from Priscilla White's recollection in the booklet Barnett and Younger, *In Celebration of the Golden Anniversary*, 8, and in Holt, *Elliott Proctor Joslin*, 43.

5. Estimate of 1,900 new patients in 1961 is from the "Black Book" entries of new patients that Joslin kept for that year. The lifetime estimate of 50,000 patients is from Holt, *Elliott Proctor Joslin*, 63, and the substantial obituaries, "Elliott Proctor Joslin, M.D.," appearing in the *New England Journal of Medicine*, and "Elliott P. Joslin, M.D. Sc.D.," in the *British Medical Journal*.

6. I owe the story of watching low-orbiting satellites and their remnants flying overhead to my friend Jim Warram, who remembers seeing the bright reflective signs of change from the perches of the rooftops in Boston.

7. EPJ memorandum to "Members of the Joslin Clinic," 21 December 1961, JDCA. In the Bible, the beginning of the passage actually reads: ". . . and, behold, *they were* very many in the open valley; and, lo, *they were* very dry." In Joslin's quotation, I have inserted preceding verses and italicized the biblical text for clarity. Just after Joslin's death, his colleague of forty-odd years, Howard F. Root, recalled that Joslin had often quoted this passage; see his "Dr. Elliot P. Joslin," 2. Indeed, in a dedication speech at the opening of the Lilly Research Laboratories in 1934, Joslin cited this verse; see Bliss, *Discovery of Insulin*, 164–65.

8. Root, "Dr. Elliott P. Joslin"; Meek, "Eulogy for Dr. Elliott P. Joslin"; Holt, *Elliot Proctor Joslin*, 66–67.

9. Geiss, "Surveillance for Diabetes Mellitus."

10. Joslin himself identified several "eras" and tagged each with the name of a famous diabetologist: Naunyn (1897–1914), Allen (1914–22), Banting (1922–36), Hagedorn (1937–43), and Best (1944–50). See Joslin, "Half-Century's Experience in Diabetes Mellitus."

11. White, "Natural Course."

12. Davidson, "Continually Changing 'Natural History'"; Krolewski et al., "Changing Natural History" and "Evolving Natural History."

13. Knowles, *Doing Better and Feeling Worse*.

14. Holt, *Elliot Proctor Joslin*, 19–23, 30, 33. I learned about Joslin's two-year stint at the Boston Dispensary, from 1898 to 1900, from a letter he sent to a patient: EPJ to patient, 5 February 1947, JDCA. For a history of dispensaries, see Rosenberg, "Social Class and Medical Care." For more on the role that hospitals played in the careers of ambitious physicians, see Rosenberg, *Care of Strangers*.

15. Joslin's lecture to the Boyleston Medical Society of the Harvard Medical School appeared as Joslin, "Pathology of Diabetes Mellitus." In this publication and others, Joslin refers to Mary Higgens by name. Joslin later recalled that his fascination with diabetes became so well known that his "classmate, Harvey Cushing [soon to become a pioneer in neurosurgery]—always up to jokes—in an after-dinner speech presented me with a bouquet of sweet peas!" This reminiscence introduced the Ninth Banting Memorial Lecture of the British Diabetic Association, 1955, published as Joslin, "Diabetes for the Diabetics."

16. All quotations of Joslin's remarks regarding Mary Higgens are from this typed report, which is filed in the JDCA.

17. For a detailed account of the constitutional treatments for tuberculosis during the late nineteenth and early twentieth centuries, see Barbara Bates, *Bargaining for Life.* As Joslin was considering the constitutional aspects of Mary's treatment, this framework for thinking was about to be marginalized in mainstream American medicine; for its subsequent fate, see Tracy, "George Draper and American Constitutional Medicine."

18. On use of opiates at the Massachusetts General Hospital during the nineteenth century, see Warner, *Therapeutic Perspective.*

19. Case record, JDCA.

20. Ibid.

21. Ibid.

22. For an examination of the origins of the acid intoxication metabolic theories, see the four lectures given by Holmes, collected in *Between Biology and Medicine.*

23. Frederick Allen (1879–1964) produced two extensive treatises based on his work during this period: Allen, *Studies Concerning Glycosuria and Diabetes,* and Allen, Stillman, and Fitz, *Total Dietary Regulation.* For an overview of Allen's career, see Henderson, "Frederick M. Allen, M.D."

24. Private correspondence and papers from James D. Havens's daughter to Chris Feudtner, July 1995; and intake sheet, JDCA.

25. Private correspondence and papers from James D. Havens's daughter to Chris Feudtner, July 1995.

26. LMD to EPJ, 17 April 1918, medical record of JDH, JDCA.

27. LMD to EPJ, 24 October 1921, JDCA. "Water vegetables" would have meant items such as lettuce, celery, spinach, and other leafy greens.

28. EPJ to LMD, 26 October 1921, JDCA.

29. Bliss, *Discovery of Insulin.* Bliss subsequently examined Banting's life in greater detail in *Banting.* These two books inspired the public television miniseries "Glory Enough for All."

30. Rollo, *Account of Two Cases of the Diabetes Mellitus.* On Bernard, see Young, "Claude Bernard."

31. Von Mering and Minkowski, "Diabetes Mellitus nach Pankreas Extirpation." For the story in context, see Houssay, "Discovery of Pancreatic Diabetes."

32. Opie, "Relationship of Diabetes Mellitus." See also Giacometti and Barss, "Paul Langerhans."

33. Medvei, *History of Clinical Endocrinology,* 160–62.

34. On these early attempts to isolate the internal secretion of the pancreas, see Bliss, *Discovery of Insulin,* 25–42.

35. Ibid. For reports from the first clinicians to use insulin, see Allen, *Journal of Metabolic Research;* while this book is listed as appearing in 1922, it was actually published in May of 1923. Nonetheless, one can now hardly imagine any drug moving from newly discovered to widely marketed so quickly.

36. J. Williams, "Clinical Study."

37. Bliss, *Discovery of Insulin.*

38. JDH's father to friend, 12 August 1922, JDCA. I do not know how this letter found its way into the medical record; I suspect that, realizing the historical significance of this early use of insulin, either the friend sent it to Joslin or Jim or his father retrieved the letter and gave it to Joslin. Details have also been supplied from correspondence from JDH's daughter, July 1995, and from Bliss, *Discovery of Insulin.*

39. J. Williams, "Clinical Study."

40. Bliss, *Discover of Insulin,* 172–73. I also uncovered, scattered across the records of many patients, numerous references to these obstacles that thwarted the early use of insulin.

41. Peterson, "Social Aspects of Diabetes." Peterson had performed her study at the Mayo Clinic, where Russell M. Wilder and Frank A. Allan ran a renowned diabetes clinic.

42. On the standardization of insulin, see Sinding, "Making the Unit of Insulin"; Lacey, "Unit of Insulin"; Murnaghan and Talalay, "H. H. Dale's Account" and "John Jacob Abel"; and Krall, Levine, and Barnett, "History of Diabetes," 5.

For some perspective on how clinician-researchers handled the transition between one form of insulin and another (in this case, from regular to protamine insulin), see Hagedorn et al., "Protamine Insulinate"; Root et al., "Clinical Experience with Protamine Insulinate"; and Joslin et al., "Protamine Insulin."

43. JDH to EPJ, 3 November 1927, JDCA.

44. Ibid., 20 January 1930.

45. Ibid., 22 March 1938.

46. Ibid., 25 March 1939.

47. Ibid., 31 January 1944.

48. Ibid., 19 January 1956.

49. Ibid., 3 November 1927.

50. Table 1.8 in Pasko and Seidman, *Physician Characteristics.* The precise figures for the United States are: 412 physicians identified themselves as diabetologists, 4,073 as endocrinologists, and 633 as pediatric endocrinologists.

51. JDH to EPJ, 29 June 1933, JDCA.

52. EPJ to JDH, 30 June 1933, JDCA. It appears that this proposed meeting never took place.

53. JDH to EPJ, 31 January 1944, JDCA.

54. All quoted passages are from EJP to patient, 30 November 1953, JDCA. Other details are found in Holt, *Elliot Proctor Joslin,* 42–43.

Chapter Three

1. One of the best overviews of the 1920s remains Leuchtenburg's *Perils of Prosperity.*

2. Intake sheet note, 19 August 1922, JDCA. The local doctor had graduated from Middlesex College of Medicine and Surgery in 1918, according to the *American Medical Directory.*

3. Anselm Strauss and his collaborators have examined the experience of sick-

ness through an analysis of the work it entails; for example, see Corbin and Strauss, "Managing Chronic Illness at Home." This approach was elaborated at greater length in their earlier study by Strauss et al., *Social Organization of Medical Work*.

Three additional articles helped me to focus on the tasks that patients and family members perform: Beneliol, "Childhood Diabetes"; Grey and Thurber, "Adaptation to Chronic Illness in Childhood"; and Gerhardt and Brieskorn-Zinke, "Normalization of Hemodialysis at Home."

4. This situation parallels the irony of housewives overburdened by the assistance of domestic technology such as washing machines, an irony explored in Cowan, *More Work for Mother*.

5. See Chapter 5 for more on the debates over diabetic control.

6. For sociological studies of responsibility and its manifestations, see Bluebond-Langner, *In the Shadow of Illness*, which examines the phenomenon in families of children with chronic illness; and Heimer and Staffen, *For the Sake of the Children*, which focuses on how issues of responsibility are handled surrounding the care of premature infants.

7. The classic definition of the social norm for the "sick role" appeared in the work of Talcott Parsons, whose initial formulation appeared in "Illness and the Role of the Physician." Parsons then expanded and refined his ideas in chapter 10 of *The Social System*. Although Parsons, even in this early work, had pointed out that the rules varied according to the type of illness and whether the patient resided in a medical or home setting, the four aspects of the sick role that he delineated were more apropos to the situation of acutely ill patients. Near the end of his career, Parsons formulated a final overview of his views and the criticism of them; see "Sick Role and the Role of the Physician Reconsidered."

8. Two historical studies of tubercular patients that demonstrate this point with detail and poignancy are Barbara Bates, *Bargaining for Life*, and Rothman, *Living in the Shadow of Death*.

9. While thinking about how the issue of responsibility factored into the relationship between patient and physicians, and how this drama is correlated to broader social values, I have been particularly influenced by Renée C. Fox and her book *Experiment Perilous*. Although Fox conducted her fieldwork in an acute-care setting, her account overlaps with mine geographically (Boston's Peter Bent Brigham Hospital is three blocks from the Joslin Clinic) and temporally (she studied Ward F-Second during the early 1950s), and I have learned much from her thematic and morally resonant "participant-observer" approach.

10. The literature on human development is legion. For a brief introduction to the psychoanalytic perspective, one might look to Erikson, *Life Cycle Completed;* for sociological views, see Rose, *Socialization and the Life Cycle;* and for historical analyses, Graff, *Growing up in America;* Haber, *Beyond Sixty-Five;* and Clarke, "Women's Health."

11. See Charmaz, *Good Days, Bad Days*.

12. My interest in the diabetic-life-history aspect of the chronic illness experience was piqued by Erving Goffman's seminal study of illness as a career, "The

Moral Career of the Mental Patient," in *Asylums*. An analogous train of thought on life history and illness (focusing on "mini-ethnographies") is developed by Kleinman in *Illness Narratives*.

Strauss and colleagues use the metaphor of "illness trajectory" to capture the sentiment that I am trying to express in "diabetic life history." I choose not to use "trajectory" for several reasons. First, it carries the unwanted connotations of momentum and an almost ballistic course that is determined initially and then unaltered. Second, objects typically have trajectories, not people, and the term thus sounds somewhat inhuman. Finally, the term "trajectory" takes on its full significance (as rendered by Strauss) only as these authors affix more meanings onto it, none of which are intuitive connotations of the term itself.

13. Sally's mother to EPJ, 28 May 1924.

14. Past medical history included on Joslin Clinic intake sheet, 19 August 1922, JDCA.

15. EPJ to LMD, 12 March 1924, JDCA.

16. "Surgery and Diabetes." The author drew upon the surgical experience in the New England Deaconess Hospital, as presented in Jones, McKittrick, and Sisco, "Surgical Treatment of Gallbladder Disease in Diabetics," and Jones, McKittrick, and Root, "Abdominal Surgery in Diabetes." These early post-insulin papers led eventually to the book by McKittrick and Root, *Diabetic Surgery*.

17. LMD to EPJ, 16 September 1924, JDCA.

18. EPJ to LMD, 18 September 1924, JDCA.

19. EPJ to Sally's mother, 15 October 1928, JDCA.

20. See Rosenberg, "Social Class and Medical Care."

21. *Medical Care for the American People*, 5–9.

22. On the history of health insurance, see Hoffman, *Wages of Sickness*, and Numbers, *Almost Persuaded;* and for a brief synopsis, see Numbers, "Third Party," where the quotation regarding compulsory insurance is cited on page 181. Health insurance is set within the context of hospital development by Stevens, *In Sickness and in Wealth*. One of the best examinations of the business of medical practice appears in the posthumously published work of Rosen, *Structure of American Medical Practice;* see especially pages 32–36 (on "dispensary abuse"), 49–53 (on "hospital clinic abuse"), and 108–15 (on the insurance debate of 1912–20).

23. LMD to EPJ, 17 November 1929, JDCA. The textbook that Dr. Jones referred to was DeLee, *Principles and Practice of Obstetrics*, 4th ed.

24. Stemming from now-classic studies on the adoption of new drugs, the study of regional variation of medical knowledge and practices has become a fast-growing field for health services researchers. For an overview, see John Eisenberg, *Doctors' Decisions*, and Dartmouth Medical School, *Dartmouth Atlas*.

25. Details about Dr. Jones's practice were gleaned from the *American Medical Directory*.

26. EPJ to LMD, 22 November 1929, JDCA.

27. Ibid., 26 November 1929.

28. Ibid.; Titus to EPJ, 10 December 1929, JDCA.

29. SMK to EPJ, 5 February 1932, JDCA.

30. LMD to EPJ, 22 July 1932, JDCA.

31. PW to LMD, 9 August 1932, JDCA.

32. Marble to LMD, 9 August and 8 September 1932, JDCA.

33. PW to LMD, 2 November 1932, JDCA. "Macerated" indicates that the child's skin was swollen with fluid and beginning to slough.

34. LMD to PW, 4 November 1932, JDCA.

35. LMD to EPJ, 6 March 1933, JDCA. The penultimate section in Ladd-Taylor's *Raising a Baby the Government Way,* titled "I have children so fast it is wrecking my life," discusses the problems that women of this era had in obtaining birth control and limiting their pregnancies.

36. PW to SMK, 16 March 1933, JDCA.

37. For more on the history of the diabetic pregnancy, see Chapter 6 and Feudtner and Gabbe, "Diabetes and Pregnancy."

38. For a widely influential counterexample of military history written from the soldier's perspective, see Keegan, *Face of Battle.* For criticism of medical history dedicated to notable physicians, see Reverby and Rosner, "Beyond 'the Great Doctors.'"

39. For a useful overview, see Foner, *New American History.*

40. As an introduction, see Hunt, *New Cultural History.*

41. SMK to EPJ, 23 September 1936, JDCA.

42. SMK to PW, 4 April 1939, JDCA.

43. Ibid., on back of follow-up letter from clinic staff, 15 July 1941.

44. On well-baby visits and the growth of pediatrics as a specialty, see Stern and Markel, *Formative Years;* Halpern, *American Pediatrics;* Meckel, *Save the Babies;* and Brosco, "Sin or Folly."

45. Root, "Association of Diabetes and Tuberculosis," 203 and 205. This dream of early treatment leading to better "cures" was widely shared; see Dubos and Dubos, *White Plague,* 154–72, and Barbara Bates, *Bargaining for Life.*

46. SMK to HFR, 10 May 1937, JDCA.

47. HFR to SMK, 19 June 1937, JDCA.

48. LMD to HFR, 27 July 1937, JDCA.

49. SMK to EPJ, 4 March 1942, JDCA.

50. On "take up thy bed" attitudes, see Fox, *Experiment Perilous,* 143–47. The quest for "normalcy" by chronically ill patients is an important issue and one that I feel is part of a wider cultural phenomenon. For some works that touch on this theme, see Marchland, *Advertising the American Dream,* and Riesman, *Lonely Crowd.* For the effects of the Second World War on American views of "normal" behavior, see Fussell, *Wartime.*

51. SMK to EPJ, 29 February 1948, JDCA.

52. EPJ to LMD, 20 March 1948, JDCA.

53. William P. Beetham to EPJ, 4 August 1950, and unsigned letter to LMD, summarizing four-day admission at the New England Deaconess Hospital, 21 August 1950, JDCA.

54. Sally's mother to RFB, 7 February 1951, JDCA.

55. Robert F. Bradley (RFB) to Sally's mother, 9 February 1951, JDCA.

56. Sally's mother to RFB, 13 February 1951, JDCA. Bradley's response was not enclosed in the chart.

57. RFB to LMD, 30 March 1951, JDCA.

58. Sally's mother to RFB, 3 May 1951.

59. Sally's mother to EPJ, 28 January 1953.

60. The few historical works that have used patient records and other historical materials to construct patient-oriented accounts provide some guidance. The late Roy Porter has been one of the most prominent advocates of patient-oriented history; see his works cited in the previous chapters and the bibliography. Some of the most useful examples of how to write patient-oriented narrative have been MacDonald, *Mystical Bedlam;* Lane, "'Doctor Scolds Me'"; Barbara Bates, *Bargaining for Life;* Ladd-Taylor, *Raising a Baby the Government Way;* Rothman, *Living in the Shadow of Death;* Leavitt, *Typhoid Mary;* and Leopold, *Darker Ribbon.*

61. Charmaz, *Good Days, Bad Days.*

62. On the significance of patient accounts and interpretations of their illness, see Kleinman, *Illness Narratives,* and Feudtner, "Patients' Stories and Clinical Care."

Chapter Four

1. EPJ to patient, 17 November 1955, JDCA.

2. I use Elizabeth Mudge's real name, since it is cited in numerous published sources and she was proud of her place in diabetes history. My account is, for the most part, gathered from her medical file, which is kept in the JDCA. That Mudge had become a shut-in prior to receiving insulin comes from the report issued by Joslin, Gray, and Root, "Insulin in Hospital and Home," which was actually published in 1923 and summarized the Joslin experience with insulin from August 1922 until the end of January 1923.

3. Bliss, *Discovery of Insulin,* 74–78, 120–21, 149–50. The group of American diabetes specialists consisted of Frederick Allen, Henry Geyelin, Elliott Joslin, Russell Wilder, John Williams, and Rollin Woodyatt; see the unnumbered preface to *Journal of Metabolic Research* 2 (1922).

4. Mudge's treatment was recorded on treatment flowsheets in JDCA; her February status is from Joslin, Gray, and Root, "Insulin in Hospital and Home," 651.

5. Mudge's death due to myocardial infarction was determined by autopsy, 28 May 1947, JDCA.

6. Joslin, Gray, and Root, "Insulin in Hospital and Home," 662–63; the enclosed quotations are presumably from reports given by either Dorothy's parents or a local physician.

7. For analyses of the experience of sickness in terms of the work entailed, see Corbin and Strauss, "Managing Chronic Illness at Home"; Beneliol, "Childhood Diabetes"; and Charmaz, *Good Days, Bad Days.*

8. In my description of 81 Bay State Road, I lean heavily upon the details provided by Holt, *Elliott Proctor Joslin,* 24–25. A photograph of the building, circa 1912, appears on page 15 of Barnett, *Elliott P. Joslin, M.D.* I also draw upon my own visit to the building, which now seems to house graduate students at Boston University.

The estimate of fifty thousand patients is based on the fact that, between the end of 1905 and the end of 1956, the Joslin Clinic added 48,628 new medical record numbers to its rolls.

9. The "instructions" to bring a urine sample are from the chapter on "Efficiency in Visits to a Doctor" that appeared in the first ten editions of Joslin, *Diabetic Manual.* This chapter will refer to this and earlier versions of the *Manual* often. For clarity, I will refer to specific editions by year of publication, which were 1918, 1919, 1924, 1929, 1934, 1937, 1941, 1948, and 1953; newer editions continued to appear after Joslin's death in 1962.

10. Joslin, *Diabetic Manual* (1919), 45. The same wording is used in the *Diabetic Manual* (1959), 75.

11. The wording is from *Diabetic Manual* (1919), 44. The same passage in *Diabetic Manual* (1959), 72, differs chiefly in that it specifies that thirty minutes are "allowed for the length of a return visit."

12. Guy Rainsford's cartoons are kept in the JDCA; details about his medical history are from the intake sheet that Joslin completed.

13. Benedict, "Detection and Estimation of Glucose in the Urine."

14. Joslin, "Diabetes for the Diabetics," 143.

15. Sigerist, *Primitive and Archaic Medicine* and *Early Greek, Hindu, and Persian Medicine;* Rosenberg, "Therapeutic Revolution."

16. For a more thorough discussion regarding this managerial style of Joslin's medical practice—which I view as the prototype of modern systems of disease management and care pathways—see Feudtner, "Pathway to Health." For Joslin's seminal article, see Joslin and Goodall, "Diabetic Chart."

17. Joslin, *Diabetic Manual* (1919).

18. American Diabetes Association, *Journey and the Dream,* 49–50.

19. Joslin, Gray, and Root, "Insulin in Hospital and Home," 695.

20. Blotner, "Use of Insulin in an Out-Patient Department." For more on the safety of home insulin use, see Joslin, "Routine Treatment of Diabetes with Insulin."

21. See Joslin, *Diabetic Manual* (1937), from which I draw the following illustration.

22. Ritholz and Jacobson, "Living with Hypoglycemia."

23. Joslin, "Insulin in the Routine Treatment of Diabetes."

24. Research Laboratories of Eli Lilly and Company, *Treatment of Diabetes Mellitus,* 24–25.

25. American Diabetes Association, *Journey and the Dream,* 121.

26. Joslin, *Diabetic Manual* (1937), 120.

27. This wording was used in ibid., 117.

28. Retinal eye disease secondary to diabetes was described in 1921 by Wagener and Wilder, "Retinitis of Diabetes Mellitus." Yet at the end of the 1920s, concerns regarding diabetes-related eye damage focused chiefly on cataracts, which were not common among patients with juvenile-onset diabetes; see Joslin and White, "Diabetic Children." By 1934, however, the importance of retinal disease to patients with diabetes was fully recognized with the publication of a much more

extensive report from the Mayo Clinic by Wagener, Dry, and Wilder, "Retinitis in Diabetes."

29. One of the first historians to attend to this aspect of the patient-doctor relationship was Rosen in *Fees and Fee Bills.*

30. Joslin, *Diabetic Manual* (1919), 32.

Chapter Five

1. Intake sheet, 22 March 1927; and, on back of intake sheet, past medical history in Priscilla White's handwriting; both in JDCA.

2. EPJ to LMD, 29 March 1927, JDCA.

3. Ibid., 14 April 1927.

4. Hudson, in *Disease and Its Control,* has examined past attempts to control disease as mediated (in the broadest sense) by understanding disease either ontologically or physiologically. This chapter operates within a different analytic framework, as it tries to understand more explicitly the connections among ideas of disease, therapeutic ideals, and actual patient care. Two major studies of therapeutics that have considered aspects of these relationships are Ackerknecht, *Therapeutics,* and Warner, *Therapeutic Perspective.*

5. A similar tale has been told of renal dialysis and organ transplantation by Fox and Swazey, *Courage to Fail.*

6. For a thoughtful discussion on the historical use of medical records, see Risse and Warner, "Reconstructing Clinical Activities." Two examples of medical records used in a manner that has influenced my approach are Dwyer, *Homes for the Mad,* and Barbara Bates, *Bargaining for Life.*

7. The comments by Dr. Liebmann appeared in the report from the Clinical Section of the Suffolk District Medical Society, "Treatment of Diabetes."

8. Private-duty nurse to EPJ, 6 November 1916; and patient's father to EPJ, 17 November 1916, JDCA.

9. Private-duty nurse to EPJ, 26 December 1916, JDCA.

10. Ibid.

11. Patient's father to EPJ, 30 April 1917, JDCA.

12. Ibid., 31 December 1917.

13. Patient to EPJ, 11 November 1917, JDCA.

14. Ibid., 27 December 1917.

15. B. H. Ragle to EPJ, 26 February 1920, JDCA.

16. The most outspoken advocate of telling patients the truth was Richard C. Cabot; see his "Use of Truth and Falsehood in Medicine" and "Doctor and the Community."

17. EPJ to B. H. Ragle, 2 March 1920, JDCA.

18. B. H. Ragle to EPJ, 18 October 1920, JDCA.

19. B. H. Ragle to patient's mother, 18 October 1920, JDCA.

20. Ibid.

21. B. H. Ragle to EPJ, 8 September 1921, JDCA.

22. Joslin, "Shattuck Lecture," 833, 835, 836, and 852, respectively.

23. Bliss, *Discovery of Insulin;* Barach, "Historical Facts in Diabetes"; Nothman,

"History of the Discovery of Pancreatic Diabetes." This genealogy of the theory was put forward by just about every contemporary physician that commented on the discovery of insulin, including Joslin.

24. Joslin, "Changing Diabetic Clientele," 304. Only Banting and Macleod were awarded the prize, which served to further inflame the credit dispute within the group (Bliss, *Discovery of Insulin*). Michael Bliss ("Rewriting Medical History") has recently reevaluated Best's role in the discovery and development of insulin.

25. Joslin continued his line of thinking further in his article "Routine Treatment of Diabetes with Insulin": "Insulin does not allow a diabetic to eat anything he desires. . . . It is true that heretofore there has never been anything discovered as valuable for the diabetic as insulin; but diabetes, though subdued, is not yet conquered" (1581).

26. The sense in which insulin "conquered" diabetes—and how clinicians thought about the impact of this dramatic but noncurative treatment—is strikingly analogous to the "conquest" of pernicious anemia through the use of the liver extract therapy developed by Minot and Murphy; see Wailoo, *Drawing Blood*. Analogous thoughts and behaviors can also be found regarding not just other potent biological compounds but also remarkable technological innovation such as renal dialysis and organ transplant; see Fox and Swazey, *Courage to Fail*.

27. Priscilla White (1900–1989) will figure prominently in Chapter 6, where I will introduce her in greater detail. My understanding of Dr. White was deepened by her colleague, M. Donna Younger; the quotation regarding ice cream is from an interview that I conducted with Dr. Younger on 1 July 1992 at the Joslin Diabetes Center. I have also been guided by White's personal papers, which contain many heartfelt letters from patients; these are housed in the Schlesinger Library on the History of Women in America, Radcliffe College, Cambridge, Mass. For a glimpse at White's extensive work on diabetic pregnancy, see White, "Diabetes Mellitus in Pregnancy."

28. EPJ to EB, 17 April 1928, JDCA.

29. EB to EPJ, 22 November 1930, JDCA.

30. EPJ to EB, 24 November 1930, JDCA.

31. In 1934, a social worker estimated that the weekly cost of insulin and other routine materials was $1.75 (Peterson, "Social Aspects of Diabetes"). In 1947, Joslin reported that the average diabetic hospitalization cost totaled $269; see "Cost of Hospital Care."

32. EB to EPJ, 8 February 1929, JDCA.

33. Ibid., 9 February 1932.

34. Outpatient chart, 30 March 1933, JDCA.

35. EB to EPJ, 12 April 1933, JDCA.

36. Joslin, "Cost of Hospital Care"; numerous letters to patients and doctors contained in other medical records document his waiving of fees.

37. Joslin, "Abolishing Diabetic Coma" and "Diabetic Coma," 1007.

38. One record from the JDCA indicates that a young man had first come to Joslin in 1926, having "two days ago omitted insulin because he was out of insulin and alcohol. . . . Does not know how to test urine." Later, he died after lapsing into

coma in his hometown hospital, where (according to the LMD) "insolin [sic] and glucose injections were of no avail." Reports of such events were not uncommon in the charts I have examined.

39. Inpatient medical chart, 7 July 1934, JDCA. Arnold was admitted in coma, with a blood sugar of 0.68 percent (that is, 680 milligrams/deciliter [mg/dl] of blood) and blood carbon dioxide of 11 volumes percent. He was treated with 750 cc of intravenous normal saline, a 1,500 cc clysis, and insulin, as follows: 20 units every half hour from 6:40 P.M. until 9:10 P.M., then 40 units at 9:25 P.M. and 9:50 P.M. His blood sugar at 10 P.M. was 0.19 percent; at 5 A.M., 0.04; he was given 5 grams of glucose intravenously for a reaction at 6:30 A.M.; he then stabilized.

40. PW to EB, 16 July 1934, JDCA.

41. Although this fact is beyond the scope of this chapter, I should note that, from the particular crisis of coma, Joslin and his colleague extended the operational paradigm of intensive control to other diabetic problems, such as pregnancy (which we will consider further in Chapter 6), then to the treatment of infections (especially after the advent of antibiotics), and more broadly to the daily management of a patient's regimen of diet, exercise, and insulin.

42. R. T. Woodyatt to Elmer L. Sevringhaus, 26 December 1929, Sevringhaus Papers, American Philosophical Society Library, Philadelphia, Pa.

43. For a summary of these diets, which, along with those of Newburgh and Marsh, permitted much more fat than had become customary, see Woodyatt, "Objects and Method of Diet Adjustment in Diabetes."

44. R. T. Woodyatt to Elmer L. Sevringhaus, 26 December 1929, Sevringhaus Papers, American Philosophical Society Library, Philadelphia, Pa. The portrait of Rollin Turner Woodyatt (1878–1953) is based upon materials in the Woodyatt obituary file (including a typescript copy of the 21 December 1953 eulogy delivered by Arthur R. Colwell), which is held in the Faculty Members Biographical Files, 1837–1942, at the Rush-Presbyterian–St. Luke's Medical Center Archives, Chicago, Ill.

45. The position outlined by Woodyatt, in both its scientific reasoning and its assessment of "the good life," was held by many physicians. The controversy over the need for "tight" control raged from the 1940s onward, with Edward Tolstoi often championing a de-emphasis of glycosuria; see Tolstoi, "Treatment of Diabetes Mellitus."

46. This point, in a different context, is made by Warner, *Therapeutic Perspective*.

47. EB to PW, 5 May 1938, JDCA.

48. PW to EB, 9 May 1938, JDCA.

49. EB to PW, 27 May 1938, JDCA. These hypoglycemic reactions were precisely what Woodyatt, in his therapeutic strategy outlined above, wanted to avoid.

50. This vigorous image of success was literally the "portrait" presented in the frontispiece of Joslin's 1928 textbook (which displayed a photograph of a twenty-year-old woman, ten years after her diagnosis of diabetes, grasping a tennis racquet). Joslin continued to project similar images of vitality throughout his publications, culminating in the numerous photographs contained in his 1956 manual. In a similar vein, but without the visual rhetoric, Priscilla White presented statis-

tical data regarding various measures of "achievement" of her juvenile patients; see White, "Natural Course."

51. "Of What Shall Diabetics Die?"

52. Kimmelstiel and Wilson, "Intercapillary Lesions."

53. White, "Natural Course."

54. AB to EPJ, 30 March 1948, JDCA.

55. EB to EPJ, 1 October 1949, JDCA.

56. HFR to AB, 17 November 1951, JDCA. Root reported to Arnold the following clinical information: a blood pressure of 140/78 mg Hg; fasting blood sugar 85 mg/dl, nonprotein nitrogen 32 mg/dl; urine sugar 5.5 percent (that is, 5.5. mg/dl), urine albumin 20 mg percent (that is, 20 mg/dl); X-ray examinations normal; and Grade 4 diabetic retinitis.

57. EB to EPJ, 10 March 1954, JDCA.

58. AB to EPJ, 15 March 1954, JDCA.

59. EPJ to EB, 16 March 1954, and EPJ to AB, 18 March 1954, JDCA.

60. AB to HFR, 7 November 1954, JDCA.

61. Inpatient medical chart, 28 April 1955, and HFR to LMD, 10 May 1955, JDCA.

62. Root, Pote, and Frehner, "Triopathy of Diabetes."

63. AB to HFR, 13 June 1955, JDCA.

64. Ibid.

65. Renée C. Fox's study of critically ill patients, conducted during the early 1950s, identified similar problems and methods of coping; see *Experiment Perilous*.

66. HFR to local cardiologist, 10 May 1955, JDCA.

67. HFR to AB, 16 June 1955, JDCA.

68. AB to HFR, 16 October 1955, JDCA.

69. Inpatient medical chart, 25 March 1956, JDCA. Cheyne-Stokes respirations are a gravely disturbed breathing pattern, while "coffee-ground vomit" indicates gastrointestinal bleeding; a Levine tube would be passed through the mouth to the stomach in an attempt to control the bleeding.

70. William A. Meissner, M.D. [pathologist], to EPJ, 28 March 1956, JDCA.

71. Frank C. Wheelock Jr. [operating surgeon who collaborated with McKittrick in surgical practice] to Allen Joslin, 3 April 1956, JDCA. These comments can be viewed as expressing and maintaining a surgical community's values and ethical positions, similar to those explored by Bosk in *Forgive and Remember*.

72. Allen Joslin to EB, 2 April 1956, JDCA.

73. EB to Allen Joslin, 11 April 1956, JDCA.

74. Joslin, "Renaissance of Control." The most blasphemous document, from Joslin's point of view, probably would have been Edward Tolstoi's *Living with Diabetes*, a book published in 1952 expressly for the lay diabetic audience, preaching looser glycemic control in order to promote a more "normal" lifestyle. For both sides of the control argument, see the editorials by Guest (pro) and Marble (con), "'Free Diet' for Diabetes."

75. The Diabetes Control and Complications Trial Research Group, "Effects of Intensive Treatment of Diabetes."

76. This argument draws on the work of Douglas, summarized in *How Institutions Think*.

77. For a discussion of these issues, see Fox, "Human Condition of Health Professionals."

Chapter Six

1. Patient to PW, 8 December 1968, White Papers (carton 2, loose papers after file 4), Schlesinger Library, Cambridge, Mass.

2. Gabbe, "Story of Two Miracles" and "Pregnancy in Women with Diabetes Mellitus." The general framework and content of this chapter appeared, in a less developed version, in Feudtner and Gabbe, "Diabetes and Pregnancy."

3. The evidence for these trends is presented in Leavitt, *Brought to Bed.*

4. For an overview, see Apple and Golden, *Mothers and Motherhood.*

5. Duncan, "On Puerperal Diabetes."

6. J. Williams, "Clinical Significance of Glycosuria."

7. DeLee, *Principles and Practice of Obstetrics,* 1st ed.

8. For representative reviews of this era, see Parsons, Randall, and Wilder, "Pregnancy and Diabetes," and Stander and Peckham, "Diabetes Mellitus and Pregnancy."

9. Joslin, "Pregnancy and Diabetes Mellitus." We would conclude that, viewed from the perspective of our current understanding of diabetes, many of the cases that Joslin presented in this review—indeed, probably all of them—were of either gestational diabetes or Type 2 adult-onset diabetes. Nevertheless, the optimistic and therapeutically aggressive position Joslin takes here is prototypical of him and greatly informs his subsequent views regarding pregnancy in women with what we would now term Type 1 juvenile-onset diabetes.

10. Barnett and Younger, *In Celebration of the Golden Anniversary.*

11. Fitz and Murphy, "Diabetes, Insulin and Pregnancy"; Joslin and White, "Diabetic Children"; White, *Diabetes in Childhood and Adolescence.*

12. DeLee, *Principles and Practice of Obstetrics.* 5th ed., 543.

13. Joslin, *Treatment of Diabetes Mellitus,* 4th ed., 861.

14. Mother to PW, 18 April 1932, JDCA.

15. PW to LMD, 12 May 1932, JDCA.

16. Titus, "Diabetes in Pregnancy."

17. LMD to EPJ, 5 December 1932, JDCA.

18. EPJ to LMD, 8 December 1932, JDCA.

19. LMD to EPJ, 6 January 1933, JDCA.

20. EPJ to LMD, 10 January 1933, JDCA.

21. Patient to EPJ, 18 April 1934, JDCA.

22. EPJ to patient, 21 April 1934, JDCA.

23. LMD to EPJ, 3 May 1934, JDCA.

24. EPJ to LMD, 7 May 1934, JDCA.

25. On her visit to Boston, Susan had been admitted to the hospital with 3.4 percent sugar in her urine, which subsequently dropped to only as low as 1.7 percent. Joslin was consoled by a twenty-four-hour urine collection that revealed only

27 grams of protein, and blood glucose levels that ranged from 210 to 240 mg/dl (EPJ to LMD, 19 May 1934, JDCA).

26. LMD to EPJ, 30 September 1934, JDCA.
27. Patient to EPJ, 29 September 1937, JDCA.
28. White, "Pregnancy Complicating Diabetes."
29. Ibid.
30. White, Titus, Joslin, and Hunt, "Prediction and Prevention."
31. Ibid.
32. Ibid.
33. O. Smith, "Diethylstilbestrol."
34. Herbst, Ulfelder, and Poskanzer, "Adenocarcinoma of the Vagina."
35. Intake sheet, 13 October 1920, JDCA.
36. Outpatient medical record, 28 March 1929, JDCA.
37. Patient to EPJ, 25 March 1938, JDCA.
38. Note to PW, June 1941, JDCA.
39. Inpatient medical record, 17 November 1945, JDCA.
40. Ibid., 24 November 1945.
41. Outpatient chart notes, 8 and 26 December, 1945; 7, 21, 28 January; 7, 18, 25 February 1946, JDCA.
42. Details regarding exactly what occurred to mother or child are lacking (inpatient medical record, 3 and 4 April 1946, JDCA).
43. Patient to PW, 14 July 1950, JDCA.
44. PW "to whom it may concern," 16 November 1944, JDCA.
45. PW to patient, 3 May and 17 June 1948, 13 December 1951, JDCA.
46. Patient to PW, 27 August 1949, JDCA.
47. PW to patient, 5 May 1952, JDCA.
48. PW to patient's mother, 10 July 1952, JDCA.
49. White, "Pregnancy Complicating Diabetes."
50. White, Koshy, and Duckers, "Management of Pregnancy Complicating Diabetes."
51. White, "Diabetes in Pregnancy," in Joslin, *Treatment of Diabetes Mellitus,* 4th ed.
52. Patient to EPJ, enclosing diet card, January 1928, JDCA.
53. Patient to EPJ, 23 March 1936, JDCA.
54. EPJ to patient, 25 March 1936, JDCA.
55. Patient to EPJ, 25 May 1936, JDCA.
56. Allan Joslin to patient, 18 June 1937, JDCA.
57. Follow-up note from EPJ to patient, 23 June 1938, JDCA.
58. Pincus and White, "On the Inheritance of Diabetes."
59. Patient to EPJ, 24 January 1940, JDCA.
60. Outpatient chart, 7 February 1941, JDCA.
61. Patient to PW, 25 February 1941, JDCA.
62. PW to patient, 1 March 1941, JDCA.
63. Patient to PW, 23 June 1941, JDCA.
64. Outpatient obstetrical chart, JDCA.

65. Inpatient chart, Faulkner Hospital, 19 August 1941, JDCA.

66. Inpatient chart, New England Deaconess Hospital, and handwritten consent, 18 August 1941, JDCA.

67. Birth announcement, 29 August 1941, JDCA.

68. PW to patient, 19 September 1941, JDCA.

69. Patient to PW, 26 January 1943, JDCA.

70. Interview of M. Donna Younger, M.D., by Chris Feudtner, 1 July 1992.

71. Patient to PW, 26 January 1943, JDCA.

72. Note from patient to PW, enclosing photograph of daughter, 6 September 1943, JDCA.

73. Note from PW to patient, 10 September 1943, JDCA.

74. Follow-up note from PW to patient, 12 July 1944, JDCA.

75. Patient to EPJ, 18 September 1941, JDCA.

76. PW to patient, 26 September 1941, JDCA.

77. Follow-up notes from the clinic to the patient, 19 August 1943 and 12 July 1944, JDCA.

78. Discharge summary, 17 January 1948, JDCA. *Staphylococcus albus* has been renamed *S. epidermidis*.

79. PW to patient, 16 January 1948, JDCA.

80. Patient to PW, 29 January 1948, JDCA.

81. PW to patient, 4 February 1948, JDCA.

82. Patient to PW, 4 September 1953, JDCA.

83. Ibid., 3 February 1954.

84. Ibid., 6 September 1943.

85. PW to patient, 10 September 1943, JDCA.

86. Letters from HFR to patient, 22 August 1950, and PW to patient, 9 July 1952, JDCA.

87. A different patient to PW, 24 September 1937, JDCA.

88. Patient's husband to PW, 8 September 1954, JDCA.

89. PW to patient's husband, 16 September 1954, JDCA.

90. Gabbe, "Story of Two Miracles."

91. White, "Pregnancy Complicating Diabetes," in Joslin et al., *Treatment of Diabetes Mellitus*, 8th ed.

Chapter Seven

1. Western Union telegram from LMD to EPJ, 12 November 1915, JDCA. This telegram contained the vertical spacing markers.

2. Telegram from LMD to EPJ, 13 November 1915, JDCA. This telegram did not contain the spacing markers. I have added them so as to make the message easier to read; unavoidably, they may give the passage a clearer, more specific meaning than was intended.

3. LMD to EPJ, 14 November 1915, JDCA.

4. EPJ chart note, 21 November 1915, JDCA.

5. Telegram from LMD to EPJ, 20 November 1915, JDCA. I added the spacing markers.

6. Flowsheet from 21 November to 19 December 1915, JDCA.

7. Charles F. Painter, M.D., wrote to Joslin that he had seen "the Flowers child a day or two ago and have got him started on exercises." On a separate piece of paper, unsigned and undated, the following instructions were handwritten:

1. Hands on hips—stretch tall—breathe deep—6 (8–10)
2. Tall walk—pushing stick over head—4
3. Sitting trunk raising, against resistance—5
4. Sitting trunk circumduction, 5
5. Double arm swim—deep breathing 6 (8–10)
6. Lying joint flexion and extension against resistance—arms—hands—fingers—legs—feet—6
7. Lying leg raising. Knee bent—straighten—lower slowly—6 alternate—(straight later)
8. Stick behind shoulders—side bend—alternate 6—take in good standing position
9. Hands on wall—head bend backward—against resistance—6 (8–10)
10. Raise stick forward, upward. Breathe deep—rise on toes—6—(8–10)

Painter's letter continued, showing further divisions of labor in this boy's care: "For the guidance of your nurse I think it will be possible to find some photographed illustrations of these exercises which can be pasted on a sheet of cardboard to use as a guide for work in the average case" (Charles F. Painter to EPJ, 17 December 1915, JDCA).

Joslin may have pursued this exercise therapy based, in part, on the recent article by Frederick Allen, "Note Concerning Exercise in Treatment of Severe Diabetes."

8. Flowsheet from 21 November to 19 December 1915, and "12/18/15 Blood Sugar Average 0.14% [mg/dl]" on a small slip of paper, JDCA.

9. This Hippocratic aphorism historically referred to both acute and chronic cases; since both kinds of cases were cared for in the home, even acute cases then had a negotiated quality that is largely absent from hospital acute care today. See *Aphorisms,* section 1, number 1, in Lloyd, *Hippocratic Writings.*

10. Note on back of follow-up card from EPJ, with illegible signature, 11 January 1917, JDCA. In the quotation, I have substituted the word "Protein" for the older, essentially synonymous term "Proteids."

11. LMD to EPJ, 2 April 1917, JDCA.

12. Within medical circles there is a growing appreciation, spurred on by debate regarding informed consent, that the relationship between patient and doctor is a contextually dependent entity. For a broadly schematic account, see Emanuel and Emanuel, "Four Models of the Physician-Patient Relationship."

13. For a medically oriented overview of these challenges, see Holmes, "Diabetes in its Psychosocial Context," and Krall, Entmacher, and Drury, "Life Cycle in Diabetes."

14. Joslin, "Routine Treatment of Diabetes with Insulin," 1581.

15. Joslin, "Section VI," of *Treatment of Diabetes Mellitus,* 3rd ed.

16. Joslin, *Diabetic Manual for the Patient* (1959); quotation from p. 121 and criteria for medals on pp. 206–13.

17. Joslin, "Diabetes for the Diabetics," 143.

18. Flowsheet, 31 March to 11 April 1925, JDCA.

19. TPV to EPJ, 16 August 1928, JDCA. "Marking" was apparently a common folk belief during this period; see Ladd-Taylor, *Raising a Baby the Government Way*.

20. EPJ to TPV, 18 August 1928, JDCA.

21. TPV to EPJ, 20 March 1930, JDCA.

22. EPJ to TPV, 22 March 1930, JDCA.

23. Ibid., 27 March 1930.

24. For an overview of birthing practices in America, and specifically the transition from home to hospital births, see Leavitt, *Brought to Bed*.

25. JH, JDCA; these details are noted on a "Social and Economic Status" evaluation slip included in John's chart.

26. From patient's mother to PW, 15 April 1940, JDCA.

27. PW to patient's mother, 16 April 1940, JDCA.

28. PW to JH, 6 May 1940 and 17 October 1942, JDCA.

29. Ibid., 17 November 1942. His blood sugar was 234 mg/dl, and his urine had shown 6.2 mg/dl sugar.

30. JH to PW, 17 December 1942, JDCA.

31. Ibid., 21 December 1942.

32. PW to JH, 23 December 1942, JDCA.

33. Ibid., 29 December 1942.

34. JH to PW, 22 February 1943, JDCA. John was admitted to this college.

35. PW to JH, 3 March 1944, JDCA.

36. Titus to EPJ, 9 January 1931, JDCA.

37. [EPJ] to TPV, 12 January 1931, JDCA.

38. Ibid., 20 January 1931.

39. Titus to HFR, 30 January 1931, JDCA.

40. [HFR] to TPV, 10 February 1931, and HFR to LMD, 4 March 1931, JDCA.

41. Flowsheet, 15 to 26 May 1931; Titus to EPJ, 26 May 1931; and Priscilla White to LMD, 28 May 1931, JDCA.

42. Numbers, "Third Party," 187–89.

43. In 1932, after a half decade of research and deliberation, the Committee on the Costs of Medical Care presented a comprehensive analysis, which noted, "with a few exceptions, that as the income of families increases the volume of medical care received by individuals in these families increases. It will be observed that in some instances persons in the lowest income group obtain more care than those in the next higher income group; this is doubtless due to the availability of free care from private practitioners, hospitals, or health departments." See *Medical Care for the American People*, 5–7.

44. See Chapter 2 and Figure 2.4 for further details. This trend, although more significant and prolonged, mirrored the slight general decline in general hospital admissions during the same period; one can infer that the Depression had a greater effect on a patient's or family's decision to bypass a general practitioner

and seek a specialist such as Joslin than on a decision to seek hospital care; see Stevens, *In Sickness and in Wealth,* 140–49.

45. TPV to EPJ, 7 August 1934, JDCA.

46. EPJ to Titus, 9 August 1934, and Titus to EPJ, 13 August 1934, JDCA.

47. TPV to PW, 31 October 1934, JDCA. The X-ray treatment was presumably for an "enlarged" thymus, a procedure common during this period.

48. JH to PW, 10 April 1947, JDCA.

49. PW to JH, 18 April 1947, JDCA.

50. JH to PW, 10 July 1948, JDCA.

51. Ibid.

52. PW to JH, 19 July 1948, JDCA.

53. TPV to EPJ, 16 March 1948, JDCA.

54. EPJ to TPV, 23 March 1948, JDCA.

55. TPV to EPJ, 7 February 1952, JDCA.

56. TPV to PW, 23 February 1952, JDCA.

57. PW to TPV, 27 February 1952, JDCA.

58. TPV to PW, 18 August 1952 and 23 July 1954 (dates received by White), JDCA.

59. TPV to EPJ, 12 November 1955, JDCA.

60. Ibid., 25 June 1957.

61. EPJ to TPV, 3 July 1957, JDCA.

62. PW to JH, 31 August 1949 (reporting the results of a recent visit, White enthused, "This is splendid and I am delighted that you are doing so well"); JH to EPJ, 19 May 1953 ("I am feeling fine and am in good health"; in this letter he also mentions the birth of two children and makes another request for information about diabetes and diabetic research); JH to EPJ, 13 March 1960 ("As in my previous reports, my health has been excellent—"); all from JDCA.

63. JH to EPJ, 13 March 1960, JDCA.

64. EPJ to JH, 18 March 1960, JDCA.

65. Corbin and Strauss, "Managing Chronic Illness at Home."

66. Autopsy report, JDCA. Pituitary stalk resection was an experimental, radical attempt at halting the progression of diabetic retinopathy. Used for several years in the early 1960s before being proved useless, the procedure was based on a single case report. See Poulsen, "Diabetes and Anterior Pituitary Insufficiency."

67. "Workman that Needeth Not to be Ashamed." The quotations are taken from the congratulatory letters of (in order) Charles H. Best, Joseph Pierre Hoet, Bernardo A. Houssay, and George Packer Berry.

Chapter Eight

1. Much of the argument that I make in this chapter is directly related to the movement within medicine called "patient-centered care" (or family-centered care, although these are not necessarily the same thing). For an overview, see the seminal collection of papers edited by Gerteis, Edgman-Levitan, Daley, and Delbanco, *Through the Patient's Eyes.*

2. Joslin, *Treatment of Diabetes Mellitus,* 3rd ed., v–vi.

3. The choice of the word "redeemed" for a biblically minded man like Joslin could not have been without overtones of a deeper faith when confronted by suffering: "For I know that my redeemer liveth" (Job 19:25).

4. EPJ to deceased patient's brother, 25 September 1926, JDCA. The phrase "the insulin" is his wording.

5. The most recent study of life expectancy for patients with Type 1 diabetes living in America found that 79.6 percent of the patients were alive thirty years after diagnosis, with strong evidence that patients diagnosed more recently have a longer life expectancy; see Nishimura et al., "Mortality Trends in Type 1 Diabetes."

6. My statement regarding the two- or threefold greater risk of death is meant to roughly convey the estimate from the study by Nishimura et al., cited above: the cohort of patients diagnosed with Type 1 diabetes between 1975 and 1979 had a standardized mortality ratio of 281; given the temporal trend toward greater longevity that they found among their cohorts, the current risk is almost certainly less than this figure. For a recent study of the persistent short-term risks posed by Type 1 diabetes, see Rewers et al., "Predictors of Acute Complications." In the same issue of *JAMA,* another study quantifies the risk of the long-term sequelae. See Karter et al., "Ethnic Disparities."

7. Thomas, "On the Science and Technology of Medicine."

8. Dubos, *Mirage of Health.*

9. Joslin, "Shattuck Lecture," 852. The passage that Joslin quotes (which I italicized) is from Proverbs 13:12; he inserted the word "long."

10. Intake sheet, 30 July 1915, and subsequent chart entries, JDCA.

11. Inpatient flow sheets, 1915 to 1921, JDCA.

12. Maria Hanka to EPJ, 5 March 1920, JDCA.

13. Patient's father to EPJ, 31 October 1920, JDCA.

14. Patient's mother to EPJ, 3 June 1922, JDCA.

15. Joslin, "Shattuck Lecture," 847. In this part of his lecture, Joslin was reading from a text prepared by Horace Gray, who assisted Joslin in caring for his pediatric patients; Joslin acknowledged Gray's contribution in a footnote.

16. Ibid., 847–48. According to current height and weight percentiles, Maria would have been of remarkably short stature and low weight, well below the fifth percentile for both. She was, however, proportional in her reduction of stature and weight, with a Body Mass Index of 16.1. By current standards, as published in 2000 by the National Center for Health Statistics in collaboration with the National Center for Chronic Disease Prevention and Health Promotion, this BMI value corresponds to between the 25th and 50th percentile for a girl almost 10 years of age. The point here is that Maria, despite long-standing diabetes, was growth stunted but not emaciated.

Joslin, who used the rhetorical tactic of the inspirational patient throughout his career, had recently addressed the pessimism of his medical colleagues regarding young diabetics in his article "Today's Problem in Diabetes." As Joslin asked in the pages of the *Journal of the American Medical Association,* "Is treatment of diabetes worth while?" Statistics showed that diabetics were living longer using the new dietary methods, he noted, but "the real reason why I think it is worth while to continue to treat diabetics despite 900 deaths is this: For about two years I have had under my care a physician's daughter and a workman's son, each with diabetes and each an only child." Joslin described how the parents of these young patients had watched previous children die and "realize only too well the situation. . . . Previous experience taught them to care only for comfort, not for life." But by following the precepts of modern treatment, strict though they be, he continued, the parents had not only "obtained some measure of comfort for their children, which they sought, but with the bright news which comes from Toronto a hope for life, which they hardly dared to anticipate."

17. See the beginning of Chapter 4 for details regarding Mudge's case.

18. EPJ to patient's mother, 2 September 1922, JDCA.

19. Fragment of letter from patient's mother to EPJ, undated, JDCA.

20. Ecclesiastes 9:11.

21. The recent book by Foner, *Who Owns History?*, helped bring into sharper focus these thoughts regarding the relationship of the past to the present.

22. A brief account of how Lee Ducat organized the Juvenile Diabetes Foundation—which is almost the stuff of legends in certain segments of the diabetes community—can be found in the American Diabetes Association, *Journey and the Dream*, 152–53. For more on the Juvenile Diabetes Foundation, its views and activities, see their internet website at <http://www.jdf.org> (accessed 25 July 2002).

23. Blakeslee, "Program to Cut Risks of Diabetes."

24. Cassell, *Nature of Suffering;* Callahan, *Troubled Dream of Life;* Aronowitz, *Making Sense of Illness;* and Rosenberg, "Tyranny of Diagnosis," all consider aspects of these tensions in a thoughtful manner.

25. The contrast between disease-specific care pathways and individualized clinical decision-making tailored to a specific patient represents another inextinguishable tension, one that plays out in efforts to improve the quality of care by minimizing practice variation. Although the report of the Committee on Quality of Health Care in America, *Crossing the Quality Chasm,* called for effective and efficient evidence-based care of specific diseases, as well as patient-centered care, reconciling these aims nonetheless presents substantial challenges. For a more in-depth look at the history of care protocols in diabetes history, and the tension it embodies, see Feudtner, "Pathways to Health." For more on the current-day manifestations of these issues, see Feudtner, "Patients' Stories and Clinical Care."

26. For more on the rise of informed consent as a new medical modus operandi and as legal doctrine in the period stretching from the late 1940s to the early 1970s that includes the Nuremberg Code, the Declaration of Helsinki, the reports by Henry K. Beecher, and the cases of *Salgo, Natanson,* and *Canterbury,* see Faden and Beauchamp, *History and Theory of Informed Consent.*

27. My thoughts regarding complicated medical decisions and how we might improve our decision-making processes has been greatly influenced by a wonderful book on decision-making by Hammond, Keeney, and Raiffa, *Smart Choices.* This book developed from ideas more completely explored in two other works: Keeney, *Value-Focused Thinking,* and Keeney and Raiffa, *Decisions with Multiple Objectives.*

28. Joslin, "Has the Treatment of Diabetes Mellitus Improved?"

29. My approach to medical decision-making has been substantially influenced not only by Hammond, Kenney, and Raiffa in *Smart Choices* but also by my involvement in pediatric palliative and end-of-life care. For those readers seeking more detailed guidance about confronting a major illness, I recommend Lynn and Harrold, *Handbook for Mortals*.

30. Christakis, *Death Foretold*.

BIBLIOGRAPHY

Manuscript and Archival Collections
Boston, Massachusetts
    Countway Library Rare Book Department, Historical Collection, Harvard
        Medical School
            E. P. Joslin Papers, 1906–62
    Joslin Diabetes Center Historical Archive
Cambridge, Massachusetts
    Schlesinger Library, Radcliffe College
            Priscilla White Papers
Chicago, Illinois
    Northwestern University Memorial Hospital Archives
            Joseph B. DeLee Papers
            Passavent Memorial Hospital Records (Arthur Colwell)
    Rush-Presbyterian–St. Luke's Medical Center Archives
            Faculty Members Biographical Files, 1837–1942
            Rollin Turner Woodyatt Papers
    University of Chicago Library, Department of Special Collections
            Morris Fishbein Papers
            James B. Herrick Papers
            Presidents' Papers
Cincinnati, Ohio
    Cincinnati Medical Heritage Center, University of Cincinnati Medical Center
            Cecil Striker Papers
New York, New York
    Medical Archives of the New York Hospital–Cornell Medical Center
            Henricus J. Stander Papers, 1927–48
Philadelphia, Pennsylvania
    American Philosophical Society Library
            Cyril Norman Hugh Long Papers
            Eugene L. Opie Papers
            Elmer J. Sveringhaus Papers, 1920–45
    Center for the Study of the History of Nursing, School of Nursing, University
        of Pennsylvania
    Historical Collection of the Pennsylvania Hospital
    Historical Collections of the Library of the College of Physicians of
        Philadelphia

Toronto, Canada
    Thomas Fisher Rare Book Library, University of Toronto
        Frederick Banting Papers
        Charles Herbert Best Papers

Published Sources

Abel, John. "Crystallized Insulin." *Proceedings of the National Academy of Sciences* 12 (1926): 132.

Ackerknecht, Erwin H. *Malaria in the Upper Mississippi Valley, 1760–1900.* Baltimore: Johns Hopkins University Press, 1945.

———. "Metabolism from Liebig to the Present." *Ciba Symposia* 6 (June 1944): 1825–33.

———. "A Plea for a 'Behaviorist' Approach in Writing the History of Medicine." *Journal of the History of Medicine and Allied Sciences* 22 (1967): 211–14.

———. *A Short History of Medicine.* Rev. ed. Baltimore: Johns Hopkins University Press, 1982.

———. *Therapeutics from the Primitives to the 20th Century. With an Appendix: History of Dietetics.* New York: Hafner Press, 1973.

Aging in America: Trends and Projections, 1991 Edition. Department of Health and Human Services Publ. no. (FCoA) 91–28001. Prepared by the U.S. Senate Special Committee on Aging, the American Association of Retired Persons, the Federal Council on the Aging, and the U.S. Administration on Aging. [Washington, D.C.]: U.S. Department of Health and Human Services, 1991.

Alexander, Jeffrey C., and Steven Seidman, eds. *Culture and Society: Contemporary Debates.* New York: Cambridge University Press, 1990.

Allen, Frank N. "The Writings of Thomas Willis, M.D.: Diabetes Three Hundred Years Ago." *Diabetes* 2 (January 1953): 74–78.

Allen, Frederick M. "Arnoldo Cantani, Pioneer of Modern Diabetes Treatment." *Diabetes* 1 (1952): 63–65.

———. "Investigative and Scientific Phases of the Diabetic Question." *Journal of the American Medical Association* 66 (1916): 1525–32.

———. "Methods and Results of Diabetic Treatment." *New England Journal of Medicine* 203 (4 December 1930): 1133–39.

———. "Note Concerning Exercise in Treatment of Severe Diabetes." *Boston Medical and Surgical Journal* 173 (1915): 743–44.

———. "The Present Outlook of Diabetic Treatment." *Transactions of the Association of American Physicians* 32 (1917): 138–48.

———. "Prolonged Fasting in Diabetes." *Transactions of the Association of American Physicians* 30 (1915): 323–29.

———. "Studies Concerning Diabetes." *Journal of the American Medical Association* 63 (1914): 939.

———. *Studies Concerning Glycosuria and Diabetes.* Boston, Mass.: W. M. Leonard, 1913.

———. "The Treatment of Diabetes." *Boston Medical and Surgical Journal* 172 (1915): 241–47.

———. *Treatment of Kidney Disease and High Blood Pressure*. Morristown, N.J.:
The Physiatric Institute, 1925.

———, ed. *Journal of Metabolic Research* 2 (1922).

Allen, Frederick M., and James W. Sherrill. "Clinical Observations with Insulin.
1. The Use of Insulin in Diabetic Treatment." *Journal of Metabolic Research*
2 (1922): 803–985.

Allen, Frederick M., Edgar Stillman, and Reginald Fitz. *Total Dietary Regulation in
the Treatment of Diabetes*. New York: The Rockefeller Institute for Medical
Research, 1919.

American Association for the History of Medicine. "Report of the Committee on
Ethical Codes: Ethical Codes Concerning Historical Research." *Bulletin of the
History of Medicine* 65 (1991): 565–70.

American Diabetes Association. *The Journey and the Dream: A History of the American
Diabetes Association*. [Maclean, Va.]: American Diabetes Association, 1990.

*American Medical Directory: A Register of Legally Qualified Physicians of the United
States*. 11th ed. Chicago: American Medical Association Press, 1929.

Apple, Rima D., and Janet Golden, eds. *Mothers and Motherhood: Readings in
American History*. Columbus: Ohio State University Press, 1997.

Aretaeus. "Cure of Diabetes." In *Therapeutics of Chronic Diseases, Book II*, 485–86.
Edited and translated by Francis Adams, in *The Extant Works of Aretaeus, the
Cappodocian*. London: for the Sydenham Society, 1856.

———. "On Diabetes." In *On the Causes and Symptoms of Chronic Diseases, Book II*,
338–40. Edited and translated by Francis Adams, in *The Extant Works of
Aretaeus, the Cappodocian*. London: for the Sydenham Society, 1856.

Aries, Philippe. *The Hour of Our Death*. Translated by Helen Weaver. New York:
Oxford University Press, 1981.

Aronowitz, Robert A. *Making Sense of Illness: Science, Society, and Disease*. New York:
Cambridge University Press, 1998.

Atwater, W. O., and A. P. Bryant. *The Chemical Composition of American Food
Materials, Bulletin No. 28*. Rev. ed. Washington, D.C.: U.S. Department of
Agriculture, Office of Experiment Stations, 1906.

Bang, Ivar. *Der Blutzucker*. Wiesbaden: Verlag von J. F. Begmann, 1913.

Barach, Joseph H. "Historical Facts in Diabetes." *Annals of Medical History*
10 (1928): 387–401.

Barnett, Donald M. *Elliott P. Joslin, M.D.: A Centennial Portrait*. Boston, Mass.:
Joslin Diabetes Center, 1998.

Barnett, Donald M., and M. Donna Younger. *In Celebration of the Golden
Anniversary of Association of Dr. Priscilla White with Joslin Clinic and New England
Deaconess Hospital*. Boston, Mass.: Joslin Diabetes Center, 1974.

Bartecchi, Carl E., Thomas D. MacKenzie, and Robert W. Schrier. "The Human
Costs of Tobacco Use." *New England Journal of Medicine* 330 (1994): 907–12,
975–80.

Bates, Barbara. *Bargaining for Life: A Social History of Tuberculosis, 1876–1938*.
Philadelphia: University of Pennsylvania Press, 1992.

Bates, Donald G. "Sydenham and the Medical Meaning of 'Method.'" *Bulletin of the History of Medicine* 51 (1977): 324–38.

Becker, Howard S. *Art Worlds.* Berkeley: University of California Press, 1982.

Becker, Howard S., and Michal M. McCall, eds. *Symbolic Interaction and Cultural Studies.* Chicago: University of Chicago Press, 1990.

Benedict, Francis G., and Elliott P. Joslin. *Metabolism in Diabetes Mellitus.* Washington, D.C.: Carnegie Institution of Washington, 1910.

———. *A Study of Metabolism in Severe Diabetes.* Washington, D.C.: Carnegie Institution of Washington, 1912.

Benedict, Stanley R. "The Detection and Estimation of Glucose in Urine." *Journal of the American Medical Association* 57 (1911): 1193–94.

———. "A Method for the Estimation of Reducing Sugars." *Journal of Biological Chemistry* 9 (1911): 57–59.

Beneliol, Jeanne Quint. "Childhood Diabetes: The Commonplace in Living Becomes Uncommon." In *Chronic Illness and the Quality of Life,* edited by Anselm L. Strauss and Barney G. Glaser, 89–98. St. Louis: C. V. Mosby Co., 1975.

Berkelman, Ruth L. "Emerging Infectious Diseases in the United States, 1993." *Journal of Infectious Diseases* 170 (1994): 272–77.

Blakeslee, Sandra. "Program to Cut Risks of Diabetes Surprisingly Fails to Lure Patients." *New York Times,* 28 February 1994, A1 and B8.

Bliss, Michael. *Banting: A Biography.* Toronto: University of Toronto Press, 1984.

———. *The Discovery of Insulin.* Chicago: University of Chicago Press, 1982.

———. "Rewriting Medical History: Charles Best and the Banting and Best Myth." *Journal of the History of Medicine and Allied Sciences* 48 (1993): 253–74.

Blotner, Harry. "Coronary Disease in Diabetes Mellitus." *New England Journal of Medicine* 203 (1930): 709–13.

———. "The Use of Insulin in an Out-Patient Department." *New England Journal of Medicine* 200 (1929): 491–94.

Bluebond-Langner, Myra. *In the Shadow of Illness: Parents and Siblings of the Chronically Ill Child.* Princeton, N.J.: Princeton University Press, 1996.

———. *The Private Worlds of Dying Children.* Princeton, N.J.: Princeton University Press, 1978.

Bosk, Charles L. *Forgive and Remember: Managing Medical Failure.* Chicago: University of Chicago Press, 1979.

Brandt, Allan M. *No Magic Bullet: A Social History of Venereal Disease in the United States since 1880.* New York: Oxford University Press, 1987.

Brosco, Jeffrey P. "Sin or Folly: Child and Community Health in Philadelphia, 1900–1930." Ph.D. diss., University of Pennsylvania, 1994.

Brown, Theodore M. "Physiology and the Mechanical Philosophy in Mid-Seventeenth-Century England." *Bulletin of the History of Medicine* 51 (1977): 25–54.

Burke, Peter. *History and Social Theory.* Ithaca, N.Y.: Cornell University Press, 1992.

Burnhan, John C. *Bad Habits: Drinking, Smoking, Taking Drugs, Gambling, Sexual*

Misbehavior, and Swearing in American History. New York: New York University Press, 1993.

Cabot, Richard C. "The Doctor and the Community." *American Medicine* 8 (1904): 731–32.

————. "The Use of Truth and Falsehood in Medicine: An Experimental Study." *American Medicine* 5 (1903): 344–49.

Callahan, Daniel. *The Troubled Dream of Life: Living with Mortality*. New York: Simon & Schuster, 1993.

Cassell, Eric J. *The Nature of Suffering and the Goals of Medicine*. New York: Oxford University Press, 1991.

Chafe, William H. *The American Woman: Her Changing Social, Economic, and Political Roles, 1920–1970*. New York: Oxford University Press, 1972.

Charmaz, Kathy. *Good Days, Bad Days: The Self in Chronic Illness and Time*. New Brunswick, N.J.: Rutgers University Press, 1991.

Charon, Rita. "Narrative Medicine: A Model for Empathy, Reflection, Profession, and Trust." *Journal of the American Medical Association* 286 (2001): 1897–1902.

Chevreul, Michel E. "Note sur le sucre de diabetes." *Annuales de Chimie* 95 (1815): 319–20.

Christakis, Nicholas A. *Death Foretold: Prophecy and Prognosis in Medical Care*. Chicago: University of Chicago Press, 1999.

Clarke, Adele E. "Women's Health: Life-Cycle Issues." In *Women, Health, and Medicine in America: A Historical Handbook,* edited by Rima D. Apple, 3–39. New Brunswick, New Jersey: Rutgers University Press, 1990.

Clinical Section of the Suffolk District Medical Society. "The Treatment of Diabetes." *Boston Medical and Surgical Journal* 135 (1896): 245–47.

Coles, Robert. *The Call of Stories: Teaching and the Moral Imagination*. Boston: Houghton Mifflin Co., 1989.

Collins, Joseph. "Diabetes, Dread Disease, Yields to New Gland Cure." *New York Times,* 6 May 1923, 12.

Committee on Quality of Health Care in America, Institute of Medicine. *Crossing the Quality Chasm: A New Health System for the 21st Century*. Washington, D.C.: National Academy Press, 2001.

Corbin, Juliet, and Anselm Strauss. "Managing Chronic Illness at Home: Three Lines of Work." In *The Sociology of Health and Illness: Critical Perspectives*. 3rd ed., edited by Peter Conrad and Rochelle Kern, 122–35. New York: St. Martin's Press, 1990.

Cott, Nancy F. *The Grounding of Modern Feminism*. New Haven, Conn.: Yale University Press, 1987.

Cowan, Ruth Schwartz. *More Work for Mother: The Ironies of Household Technology from the Open Hearth to the Microwave*. New York: Basic Books, 1983.

Crosby, Alfred W. *America's Forgotten Pandemic: The Influenza of 1918*. New York: Cambridge University Press, 1989.

————. *The Columbian Exchange: Biological and Cultural Consequences of 1492*. Westport, Conn.: Greenwood Press, 1972.

Cullen, William. "Chapter XII: Of the Diabetes." *First Lines of Practice of Physic.* Vol. 4. Edinburgh: C. Elliot, 1786.

—————. *Synopsis and Nosology, Being an Arrangement and Definition of Diseases.* 1769. Reprint, Hartford, Conn.: 1793.

Cunningham, Andrew. "Thomas Sydenham: Epidemics, Experiment, and the 'Good Old Cause.'" In *The Medical Revolution of the Seventeenth Century,* edited by Roger French and Andrew Wear, 164–90. New York: Cambridge University Press, 1989.

Darnton, Robert. *The Great Cat Massacre and Other Episodes in French Cultural History.* New York: Vintage, 1984.

Dartmouth Medical School, the Center for the Evaluative Clinical Sciences. *The Dartmouth Atlas of Health Care, 1998.* Chicago: American Hospital Publ., 1998.

Davidson, Mayer B. "The Continually Changing 'Natural History' of Diabetes Mellitus." *Journal of Chronic Disease* 34 (1981): 5–10.

Davis, Natalie Zemon. *The Return of Martin Guerre.* Cambridge, Mass.: Harvard University Press, 1983.

DeLee, Joseph B. *The Principles and Practice of Obstetrics.* 1st ed. Philadelphia, Pa.: W. B. Saunders, 1913.

—————. *The Principles and Practice of Obstetrics.* 4th ed. Philadelphia, Pa.: W. B. Saunders, 1924.

—————. *The Principles and Practice of Obstetrics.* 5th ed. Philadelphia, Pa.: W. B. Saunders, 1928.

Demos, John. *Past, Present, and Personal: The Family in the Life Course in American History.* New York: Oxford University Press, 1986.

The Diabetes Control and Complications Trial Research Group. "The Effects of Intensive Treatment of Diabetes on the Development and Progression of Long-Term Complications in Insulin-Dependent Diabetes Mellitus." *New England Journal of Medicine* 329 (1993): 977–86.

Dobson, Matthew. "Experiments and Observations on the Urine of a Diabetic." In *Medical Observations and Inquiries,* 298–316. London: T. Cadell, 1776.

Douglas, Mary. *How Institutions Think.* Syracuse, N.Y.: Syracuse University Press, 1986.

Dubos, René. *Mirage of Health: Utopias, Progress, and Biological Change.* 1959. Reprint, New Brunswick, N.J.: Rutgers University Press, 1987.

Dubos, René, and Jean Dubos. *The White Plague: Tuberculosis, Man, and Society.* 1952. Reprint, New Brunswick, N.J.: Rutgers University Press, 1987.

Duncan, Matthews J. "On Puerperal Diabetes." *Transactions of the Obstetrical Society, London* 24 (1882): 256–85.

Dutton, Diana B. *Worse than the Disease: Pitfalls of Medical Progress.* New York: Cambridge University Press, 1988.

Dwyer, Ellen. *Homes for the Mad: Life Inside Two Nineteenth-Century Asylums.* New Brunswick, N.J.: Rutgers University Press, 1987.

Eisenberg, John M. *Doctors' Decisions and the Cost of Medical Care: The Reasons for*

Doctors' Practice Patterns and Ways to Change Them. Ann Arbor, Mich.: Health Administration Press Perspectives, 1986.

Eisenberg, Leon. "Science in Medicine: Too Much or Too Little and Too Limited in Scope?" *American Journal of Medicine* 84 (1988): 483–91.

"Elliott P. Joslin, M.D., Sc.D. [obituary]." *British Medical Journal* (1962): 729–30.

"Elliott Proctor Joslin, M.D., 1869–1962 [obituary]." *New England Journal of Medicine* 266 (1962): 415–16.

Emanuel, Ezekiel J., and Linda L. Emanuel. "Four Models of the Physician-Patient Relationship." *Journal of the American Medical Association* 267 (1992): 2221–26.

Engel, George L. "The Need for a New Medical Model: A Challenge for Biomedicine." *Science* 196 (1977): 129–36.

Epstein, Albert A. "An Accurate Microchemical Method of Estimating Sugar in the Blood." *Journal of the American Medical Association* 63 (1914): 1667–68.

Erikson, Eric H. *The Life Cycle Completed: A Review.* New York: W. W. Norton, 1982.

Ettling, John. *The Germ of Laziness: Rockefeller Philanthropy and Public Health in the New South.* Cambridge, Mass.: Harvard University Press, 1981.

"Ex-Secretary Lansing, Ill from Diabetes, Improves under Treatment with Insulin." *New York Times,* 28 June 1993, 1.

Faber, Knud. *Nosography: The Evolution of Clinical Medicine in Modern Times.* 2nd ed. New York: Paul B. Hoeber, Inc., 1930.

Faden, Ruth R., and Tom L. Beauchamp. *A History and Theory of Informed Consent.* New York: Oxford University Press, 1986.

Feudtner, Chris. "A Disease in Motion: Diabetes History and the New Paradigm of Transmuted Disease." *Perspectives in Biology and Medicine* 39 (Winter 1996): 158–70.

———. "'Minds the Dead have Ravished': Shell Shock, History, and the Ecology of Disease-Systems." *History of Science* 31 (1993): 377–420.

———. "Pathway to Health: Juvenile Diabetes Mellitus and the Origins of Managerial Medicine." In *The Formative Years: Childhood Health and Health Care, 1880–2000,* edited by Alexandra Stern and Howard Markel, 208–32. Ann Arbor: University of Michigan Press, 2002.

———. "Patients' Stories and Clinical Care: Uniting the Unique and the Universal?" *Journal of General Internal Medicine* 13 (1998): 846–49.

———. "The Predicament of Dangerous Safety: Living with 'Juvenile' Diabetes in 20th Century America." *Western Journal of Medicine* (July 2000): 64–67.

———. "To Live a Normal Life: History and Health Behavior." *Journal of the American Medical Association* 271 (1994): 82–83.

———. "The Want of Control: Ideas, Innovations, and Ideals in the Modern Management of Diabetes Mellitus." *Bulletin of the History of Medicine* 69 (1995): 66–90.

Feudtner, Chris, and Steven G. Gabbe. "Diabetes and Pregnancy: Four Motifs of Modern Medical History." *Clinical Obstetrics and Gynecology* 43 (March 2000): 4–16.

Finlay, Mark R. "Quackery and Cookery: Justus von Liebig's Extract of Meat and the Theory of Nutrition in the Victorian Age." *Bulletin of the History of Medicine* 66 (1992): 404–18.

Fitz, Reginald H., and Elliott P. Joslin. "Diabetes Mellitus at the Massachusetts General Hospital from 1824 to 1898. A Study of the Medical Records." *Journal of the American Medical Association* 31 (1898): 165–71.

Fitz, Reginald, and William P. Murphy. "Diabetes, Insulin and Pregnancy." *Boston Medical and Surgical Journal* 193 (1925): 1092–94.

Flint, Austin. *A Treatise on the Principles and Practice of Medicine*. Philadelphia: Henry C. Lea, 1866.

Foner, Eric. *Who Owns History? Rethinking the Past in a Changing World*. New York: Hill and Wang, 2002.

———, ed. *The New American History*. Philadelphia, Pa.: Temple University Press, 1990.

Foster, Nellis B. "The Dietetic Treatment of Diabetes Mellitus." *American Journal of the Medical Sciences* 141 (1911): 167–85.

Foucault, Michel. *The Birth of the Clinic: An Archaeology of Medical Perception*. Translated by Alan M. Sheridan. London: Tavistock Publ., 1973.

Fox, Renée C. *Experiment Perilous: Physicians and Patients Facing the Unknown*. 1959. Reprint, Philadelphia: University of Pennsylvania Press, 1974.

———. "The Human Condition of Health Professionals." In *Essays in Medical Sociology: Journeys into the Field*. 2nd ed., rev. and enl. New Brunswick, N.J.: Transaction Books, 1988.

Fox, Renée C., and Judith P. Swazey. *The Courage to Fail: A Social View of Organ Transplants and Dialysis*. 2nd ed. Chicago: University of Chicago Press, 1978.

———. *Spare Parts: Organ Replacement in American Society*. New York: Oxford University Press, 1992.

Frank, Ludwig L. "Diabetes Mellitus in the Texts of Old Hindu Medicine (Charaka, Susruta, Vagbhata)." *American Journal of Gastroenterology* 27 (1957): 76–95.

Fussell, Paul. *Wartime: Understanding and Behavior in the Second World War*. New York: Oxford University Press, 1989.

Gabbe, Steven G. "Pregnancy in Women with Diabetes Mellitus: The Beginning." *Clinics in Perinatology* 20 (1993): 507–15.

———. "A Story of Two Miracles: The Impact of the Discovery of Insulin on Pregnancy in Women with Diabetes Mellitus." *Obstetrics and Gynecology* 79 (1992): 295–99.

Garland, G. M. "Treatment of Diabetes: Comments of Dr. Garland from the Clinical Section of the Suffolk District Medical Society Meeting." *Boston Medical and Surgical Journal* 135 (1896): 245–47.

Geertz, Clifford. *The Interpretation of Cultures*. New York: Basic Books, 1973.

———. *Local Knowledge: Further Essays in Interpretive Anthropology*. New York: Basic Books, 1983.

Geiss, Linda S., et al. "Surveillance for Diabetes Mellitus—United States, 1980–1989." *Morbidity and Mortality Weekly Report* 42, no. SS-2 (1993): 1–20.

Gerber, Linda M., and Douglas E. Crews. "Evolutionary Perspectives on Chronic

Degenerative Diseases." In *Evolutionary Medicine,* edited by Wenda R. Trevathan, E. O. Smith, and James J. McKenna, 443–69. New York: Oxford University Press, 1999.

Gerhardt, Uta, and Marianne Brieskorn-Zinke. "The Normalization of Hemodialysis at Home." In *The Adoption and Social Consequences of Medical Technologies,* edited by Julius A. Roth and Sheryl Burt Ruzek, 271–317. Published in the series, *Research in the Sociology of Health Care* 4 (1986).

Gerteis, Margaret, Susan Edgman-Levitan, Jennifer Daley, and Thomas L. Delbanco, eds. *Through the Patient's Eyes: Understanding and Promoting Patient-Centered Care.* San Francisco, Calif.: Jossey-Bass Publishers, 1993.

Geyelin, H. Rawle, George Harrop, Majorie F. Murray, and Eugenia Corwin. "The Use of Insulin in Juvenile Diabetes." *Journal of Metabolic Research* 2 (1922): 767–91.

Giacometti, Luigi, and Margaret Barss. "Paul Langerhans: A Tribute." *Archives of Dermatology* 100 (1969): 770–72.

Glory Enough for All. Television Mini-series. Gemstone Productions. Toronto: 1988.

Goffman, Erving. *Asylums: Essays on the Social Situation of Mental Patients and Other Inmates.* New York: Anchor Books, 1961.

———. *The Presentation of Self in Everyday Life.* New York: Anchor Books, 1959.

Goodall, Harry W. "Papers on Diabetes Mellitus, with Discussion: Section of Medicine, Massachusetts Medical Society [Dr. Goodall's comments]." *Boston Medical and Surgical Journal* 175 (1916): 156.

Goodall, Harry W., and Elliott P. Joslin. "The Clinical Value of the Estimation of Ammonia in Diabetes." *Medical Papers Dedicated to Reginald Heber Fitz* (Reprinted from *Boston Medical and Surgical Journal* 158, no. 19, [1908]) (1908): 164–83.

Graff, Harvey J., ed. *Growing up in America: Historical Experiences.* Detroit: Wayne State University Press, 1987.

Grey, Margaret, and Frances W. Thurber. "Adaption to Chronic Illness in Childhood: Diabetes Mellitus." *Journal of Pediatric Nursing* 6 (1991): 302–9.

Grob, Gerald N. *From Asylum to Community: Mental Health Policy in Modern America.* Princeton: Princeton University Press, 1991.

———. "The Social History of Medicine and Disease in America: Problems and Possibilities." *Journal of Social History* 10 (June 1977): 391–409.

Guest, George M. "'Free Diet' for Diabetes, Pro [editorial]." *Diabetes* 1 (1952): 487–88.

Haber, Carole. *Beyond Sixty-Five: The Dilemma of Old Age in America's Past.* New York: Cambridge University Press, 1983.

Hagedorn, H. C., B. Norman Jensen, N. B. Krarup, and I. Wodstrup. "Protamine Insulinate." *Journal of the American Medical Association* 106 (1936): 177–80.

Hall, Stephen S. *Invisible Frontiers: The Race to Synthesize a Human Gene.* New York: Atlantic Monthly Press, 1987.

Halpern, Sydney A. *American Pediatrics: The Social Dynamics of Professionalism, 1880–1980.* Berkeley: University of California Press, 1988.

Hammond, G. Denman. "Late Adverse Effects of Treatment among Patients Cured of Cancer during Childhood." *CA—A Cancer Journal for Clinicians* 42 (1992): 261–62.

Hammond, John S., Ralph L. Keeney, and Howard Raiffa. *Smart Choices: A Practical Guide to Making Better Decisions.* Boston, Mass.: Harvard Business School Press, 1999.

Hannon, R. R., and William S. McCann. "A Graphic Method for the Calculation of Diabetic Diets in the Proper Ketogenic-Antiketogenic Ratio." *Johns Hopkins Hospital Bulletin* 33 (1922): 128–29.

Harden, Victoria A. *Rocky Mountain Spotted Fever: History of a Twentieth-Century Disease.* Baltimore: Johns Hopkins University Press, 1990.

Harrington, Charles. "The Value of So-Called Diabetic Foods." *Boston Medical and Surgical Journal* 118 (1888): 286–88.

Harris, Seale. *Banting's Miracle: The Story of the Discovery of Insulin.* Philadelphia: J. B. Lippincott Company, 1946.

Harrison's Principles of Internal Medicine. 15th ed. Edited by Eugene Brauwald, Anthony Fauci, Dennis Kasper, Stephen Hauser, Dan L. Longo, and J. Larry Jameson. New York: McGraw Hill Professional, 2001.

Heimer, Carol A., and Lisa R. Staffen. *For the Sake of the Children: The Social Organization of Responsibility in the Hospital and the Home.* Chicago: University of Chicago Press, 1998.

Henderson, Alfred R. "Frederick M. Allen, M.D., and the Physiatric Institute of Morristown, N.J. (1920–1938)." *Academy Medicine of New Jersey Bulletin* 16 (1970): 40–49.

Herbst, Arthur L., Howard Ulfelder, and David C. Poskanzer. "Adenocarcinoma of the Vagina: Association of Maternal Stilbesterol Therapy with Tumor Appearance in Young Women." *New England Journal of Medicine* 284 (1971): 878–81.

Herrick, James B. "The Oatmeal Diet in the Treatment of Diabetes Mellitus." *Journal of the American Medical Association* 50 (1908): 861–65.

Heyn, Louis G. "Abstract of Discussion: Comments Following Paper by Elliott P. Joslin, 'My Experience with Diabetic Patients Living Ten or More Years,' at the Section on Practice of Medicine of the American Medical Association Meeting." *Journal of the American Medical Association* 59 (1912): 935–36.

Hoffman, Beatrix. *The Wages of Sickness: The Politics of Health Insurance in Progressive America.* Chapel Hill: University of North Carolina Press, 2001.

Holmes, David M. "Diabetes in Its Psychosocial Context." In *Joslin's Diabetes Mellitus.* 12th ed., edited by Alexander Marble et al., 882–906. Philadelphia: Lea and Febiger, 1985.

Holmes, Frederic Lawrence. *Between Biology and Medicine: The Formation of Intermediary Metabolism.* Berkeley: Office for History of Science and Technology, University of California, 1992.

Holmes, William H. "Simplification of Woodyatt Method for Calculating the Optimal Diabetic Diet." *Journal of the American Medical Association* 78 (1922): 22–23.

Holt, Anna C. *Elliott Proctor Joslin: A Memoir, 1869–1962.* Worcester, Mass.: Asa
    Bartlett Press, 1969.
Hornor, Albert A. "Definition and Detection of Acidosis in Diabetes Mellitus."
    Boston Medical and Surgical Journal 175 (1916): 148–52.
Houssay, B. A. "The Discovery of Pancreatic Diabetes: The Role of Oscar
    Minkowski." *Diabetes* 1 (1952): 112–16.
Howell, Joel D. *Technology in the Hospital: Transforming Patient Care in the Early
    Twentieth Century.* Baltimore: Johns Hopkins University Press, 1995.
Hudson, Robert P. *Disease and Its Control: The Shaping of Modern Thought.*
    Westport, Conn.: Greenwood Press, 1983.
Hunt, Lynn, ed. *The New Cultural History.* Berkeley: University of California Press,
    1989.
"Incidence of Treatment for End-Stage Renal Disease Attributed to Diabetes
    Mellitus—United States, 1980–1989." *Morbidity and Mortality Weekly Report* 41
    (1992): 834–37.
Iseman, Michael D. "Evolution of Drug-Resistant Tuberculosis: A Tale of Two
    Species." *Proceedings of the National Academy of Sciences U.S.A.* 91 (1994):
    2428–29.
Jain, Lucky, and D. Vidyasagar. "Iatrogenic Disorders in Modern Neonatology."
    Clinics in Perinatology 16 (1989): 255–73.
Janeway, Theodore C. "The Dietetic Treatment of Diabetes." *American Journal of
    the Medical Sciences* 137 (1909): 313–29.
Janney, N. W. "Treatment of Diabetes from the General Practitioner's
    Standpoint." *Journal of the American Medical Association* 70 (1918): 1282–87.
Jewson, Norman. "The Disappearance of the Sick-man from Medical Cosmology,
    1770–1880." *Sociology* 10 (1977): 225–44.
John, Henry J. "Methods of Precision in the Diagnosis of Diabetes: A New
    Instrument." *Journal of the American Medical Association* 78 (1922): 103–5.
Jones, Daniel Fiske, Leland S. McKittrick, and Howard F. Root. "Abdominal
    Surgery in Diabetes." *Journal of the American Medical Association* 85 (1925):
    809–12.
Jones, Daniel Fiske, Leland S. McKittrick, and D. L. Sisco. "Surgical Treatment
    of Gallbladder Disease in Diabetics." *Boston Medical and Surgical Journal* 191
    (1924): 709.
Joslin, Elliott P. "Abolishing Diabetic Coma." *Journal of the American Medical
    Association* 93 (1929): 33.
———. "Apollinaire Bouchardat, 1806–1886." *Diabetes* 1 (1952): 490–91.
———. "The Causes of Death in Diabetes." *American Journal of the Medical Sciences*
    151 (1916): 313–21.
———. "The Changing Diabetic Clientele." *Transactions of the Association of
    American Physicians* 39 (1924): 304–7.
———. "Cost of Hospital Care [unsigned editorial]." *New England Journal of
    Medicine* 237 (1947): 461–62.
———. "Diabetes for the Diabetics." *Diabetes* 5 (1956): 137–46.

————. "Diabetic Coma [unsigned editorial]." *New England Journal of Medicine* 201 (1929): 1007–8.

————. *A Diabetic Manual for the Mutual Use of Doctor and Patient.* 1st ed. Philadelphia: Lea and Febiger, 1918.

————. *A Diabetic Manual for the Mutual Use of Doctor and Patient.* 2nd ed. Philadelphia: Lea and Febiger, 1919.

————. *A Diabetic Manual for the Mutual Use of Doctor and Patient.* 3rd ed. Philadelphia: Lea and Febiger, 1924.

————. *A Diabetic Manual for the Mutual Use of Doctor and Patient.* 4th ed. Philadelphia: Lea and Febiger, 1929.

————. *A Diabetic Manual for the Mutual Use of Doctor and Patient.* 5th ed. Philadelphia: Lea and Febiger, 1934.

————. *A Diabetic Manual for the Mutual Use of Doctor and Patient.* 6th ed. Philadelphia: Lea and Febiger, 1937.

————. *A Diabetic Manual for the Mutual Use of Doctor and Patient.* 7th ed. Philadelphia: Lea and Febiger, 1941.

————. *A Diabetic Manual for the Doctor and Patient.* 8th ed. Philadelphia: Lea and Febiger, 1948.

————. *A Diabetic Manual for the Doctor and Patient.* 9th ed. Philadelphia: Lea and Febiger, 1953.

————. *A Diabetic Manual for the Patient.* 10th ed. Philadelphia: Lea and Febiger, 1959.

————. "Diabetic Standards." *American Journal of the Medical Sciences* 145 (1913): 474–86.

————. "A Half-Century's Experience in Diabetes Mellitus." *British Medical Journal* 1 (1950): 1095–98.

————. "Has the Treatment of Diabetes Mellitus Improved? [unsigned editorial]." *Boston Medical and Surgical Journal* 139 (1898): 176–77.

————. "Heroin." *Boston Medical and Surgical Journal* 140 (1899): 429.

————. "Ideals in the Treatment of Diabetes and Methods for their Realization." *New England Journal of Medicine* 198 (1928): 379–82.

————. "The Improvement in the Treatment of Diabetes Mellitus." *Boston Medical and Surgical Journal* 153 (1905): 11–15.

————. "Insulin in the Routine Treatment of Diabetes." *Journal of the American Medical Association* 80 (1923): 1726.

————. *Joslin's Diabetes Mellitus.* 13th ed. Edited by C. Ronald Kahn and Gordon C. Weir. Malvern, Pa.: Lea and Febiger, 1994.

————. *Joslin's Diabetes Mellitus.* 14th ed. Edited by C. Ronald Kahn, George L. King, Robert J. Smith, Alan M. Jacobson, Gordon C. Weir, and Alan C. Moses. Philadelphia: Lippincott Williams & Wilkins, 2003.

————. "Metabolism in Diabetic Coma, with Especial Reference to Acid Intoxication." *Journal of Medical Research* 1 (1901): 306–30.

————. "My Experience with Diabetic Patients Living Ten or More Years." *Journal of the American Medical Association* 59 (1912): 933–36.

———. "Pancreatic Diabetes [unsigned editorial]." *Boston Medical and Surgical Journal* 131 (1894): 592–93.

———. "The Pathology of Diabetes." *Boston Medical and Surgical Journal* 132 (1895): 114–15.

———. "Pathology of Diabetes Mellitus." *Boston Medical and Surgical Journal* 130 (1894): 309–11, 330–34.

———. "Pregnancy and Diabetes Mellitus." *Boston Medical and Surgical Journal* 173 (1915): 841–49.

———. "Present-Day Treatment and Prognosis in Diabetes." *American Journal of the Medical Sciences* 150 (1915): 485–96.

———. "Recent Progress in Therapeutics." *Boston Medical and Surgical Journal* 141 (1899): 521–25.

———. "A Renaissance of the Control of Diabetes [guest editorial]." *Journal of the American Medical Association* 156 (1954): 1584–85.

———. "The Routine Treatment of Diabetes with Insulin." *Journal of the American Medical Association* 80 (1923): 1581–83.

———. "The Shattuck Lecture: The Treatment of Diabetes Mellitus." *Boston Medical and Surgical Journal* 186 (1922): 833–52.

———. "Today's Problem in Diabetes in Light of Nine Hundred and Thirty Fatal Cases." *Journal of the American Medical Association* 78 (1922): 1506–10.

———. *The Treatment of Diabetes Mellitus, with Observations upon the Disease Based upon One Thousand Cases.* 1st ed. Philadelphia: Lea and Febiger, 1916.

———. *The Treatment of Diabetes Mellitus, with Observations upon the Disease Based upon Thirteen Hundred Cases.* 2nd ed. Philadelphia: Lea and Febiger, 1917.

———. *The Treatment of Diabetes Mellitus, with Observations upon the Disease Based upon Three Thousand Cases.* 3rd ed. Philadelphia: Lea and Febiger, 1923.

———. *The Treatment of Diabetes Mellitus.* 4th ed. Philadelphia: Lea and Febiger, 1928.

———. *The Treatment of Diabetes Mellitus.* 5th ed. Philadelphia: Lea and Febiger, 1935.

———. *The Treatment of Diabetes Mellitus.* 6th ed. Philadelphia: Lea and Febiger, 1937.

Joslin, Elliott P., F. Gorham Brigham, and Albert A. Horner. "An Analysis of Fourteen Cases of Diabetes Mellitus Unsuccessfully Treated by Fasting." *Boston Medical and Surgical Journal* 174 (1916): 371–78; 425–29.

Joslin, Elliott P., and Harry W. Goodall. "A Diabetic Chart." *Boston Medical and Surgical Journal* 158 (1908): 248–51.

Joslin, Elliott P., Horace Gray, and Howard F. Root. "Insulin in Hospital and Home." *Journal of Metabolic Research* 2 (1922): 651–99.

Joslin, Elliott P., Howard F. Root, Alexander Marble, Priscilla White, Allan P. Joslin, and George W. Lynch. "Protamine Insulin." *New England Journal of Medicine* 214 (1936): 1079–85.

Joslin, Elliott P., Howard F. Root, Priscilla White, and Alexander Marble. *The Treatment of Diabetes Mellitus.* 7th ed. Philadelphia: Lea and Febiger, 1940.

Joslin, Elliott P., Howard F. Root, Priscilla White, Alexander Marble, and

C. Cabell Bailey. *The Treatment of Diabetes Mellitus.* 8th ed. Philadelphia: Lea and Febiger, 1946.

Joslin, Elliott P., Howard F. Root, Priscilla White, and Alexander Marble. *The Treatment of Diabetes Mellitus.* 9th ed. Philadelphia: Lea and Febiger, 1952.

———. *The Treatment of Diabetes Mellitus.* 10th ed. Philadelphia: Lea and Febiger, 1959.

Joslin, Elliott P., and Priscilla White. "Diabetic Children." *Journal of the American Medical Association* 92 (1929): 143–46.

Joslin Diabetes Manual. By the physicians of the Joslin Diabetes Center. 12th ed. Philadelphia: Lea and Febiger, 1989.

Kahn, C. Ronald, with Richard Kitch, Terri-Lyn Bellman, and Patricia Griffiths, compilers. *The Joslin Diabetes Center, 1898–1988: A History of the First 90 Years Through Its Publications.* Annotated by Alexander Marble, George Cahill Jr., Robert Spiro, Kenneth E. Quickel Jr., and C. Ronald Kahn. Boston, Mass.: Joslin Diabetes Center, 1988.

Karter, Andrew J., Assiamira Ferrara, Jennifer Y. Liu, Howard H. Moffet, Lynn M. Ackerson, and Joe V. Selby. "Ethnic Disparities in Diabetic Complications in an Insured Population." *Journal of the American Medical Association* 287 (2002): 2519–27.

Katz, Michael B. *In the Shadow of the Poorhouse: A Social History of Welfare in America.* New York: Basic Books, 1986.

Keegan, John. *The Face of Battle: A Study of Agincourt, Waterloo, and the Somme.* New York: Viking Press, 1976.

Keeney, Ralph L. *Value-Focused Thinking: A Path to Creative Decisionmaking.* Cambridge, Mass.: Harvard University Press, 1992.

Keeney, Ralph L., and Howard Raiffa. *Decisions with Multiple Objectives: Preferences and Value Tradeoffs.* New York: John Wiley & Sons, 1976.

Kimmelstiel, Paul, and Clifford Wilson. "Intercapillary Lesions in the Glomeruli of the Kidney." *American Journal Pathology* 12 (1936): 83–98.

King, Lester S. "Classification." In *Medical Thinking: A Historical Preface,* 105–27. Princeton, N.J.: Princeton University Press, 1982.

———. "Empiricism, Rationalism, and Diabetes." *Journal of the American Medical Association* 187 (1964): 521–26.

Kleinman, Arthur. *The Illness Narratives: Suffering, Healing, and the Human Condition.* New York: Basic Books, Inc., 1988.

Knowles, John H., ed. *Doing Better and Feeling Worse: Health in the United States.* New York: W. W. Norton & Company, 1977.

Krall, Leo P., Paul S. Entmacher, and Thomas F. Drury. "Life Cycle in Diabetes: Socioeconomic Aspects." In *Joslin's Diabetes Mellitus.* 12th ed., edited by Alexander Marble et al., 907–36. Philadelphia: Lea and Febiger, 1985.

Krall, Leo P., Rachmiel Levine, and Donald Barnett. "The History of Diabetes." In *Joslin's Diabetes Mellitus.* 13th ed., edited by Ronald C. Kahn and Gordon C. Weir. Malvern, Pa.: Lea and Febiger, 1994.

Krolewski, Andrzej S., James H. Warram, A. Richard Christlieb, Edward J.

Busick, and C. Ronald Kahn. "The Changing Natural History of Nephropathy in Type I Diabetes." *American Journal of Medicine* 78 (May 1985): 785–94.

Krolewski, Andrzej S., James H. Warram, Paola Valsania, Blaise C. Martin, Lori M. B. Laffel, and A. Richard Christlieb. "Evolving Natural History of Coronary Artery Disease in Diabetes Mellitus." *American Journal of Medicine* 90 (1991): 2A/56s–2A/60s.

Kuebler-Ross, Elizabeth. *On Death and Dying.* New York: Macmillan Publ. Co., 1969.

Kunin, Calvin M. "Resistance to Antimicrobial Drugs—A Worldwide Calamity." *Annals of Internal Medicine* 118 (1993): 557–61.

Kurtz, Z., C. S. Peckham, and A. E. Ades. "Changing Prevalence of Juvenile-Onset Diabetes Mellitus." *Lancet* 2 (1988): 88–90.

Kussmaul, Adolf. "Zur Lehre von Diabetes Mellitus." *Deutsches Archiv für Klinische Medizin* 14 (1874): 1–46.

Lacey, A. H. "The Unit of Insulin." *Diabetes* 16 (1967): 198–200.

Ladd-Taylor, Molly. *Raising a Baby the Government Way: Mother's Letters to the Children's Bureau, 1915–1932.* New Brunswick, N.J.: Rutgers University Press, 1986.

Lane, Joan. "'The Doctor Scolds Me': The Diaries and Correspondence of Patients in Eighteenth-Century England." In *Patients and Practitioners: Lay Perceptions of Medicine in Pre-Industrial Society,* edited by Roy Porter, 205–48. New York: Cambridge University Press, 1985.

LaPorte, R. E., H. A Fishbein., A. L. Drash, L. H. Kuller, B. B. Schneider, and D. K. Orcha. "The Pittsburgh Insulin-Dependent Diabetes Mellitus (IDDM) Registry. The Incidence of Insulin-Dependent Diabetes Mellitus in Allegheny County, Pennsylvania (1965–1976)." *Diabetes* 30 (1981): 279–84.

Leavitt, Judith Walzer. *Brought to Bed: Childbearing in America, 1750–1950.* New York: Oxford University Press, 1986.

———. *Typhoid Mary: Captive to the Public's Health.* Boston, Mass.: Beacon Press, 1996.

Lederberg, Joshua, Robert E. Shope, and Stanley C. Oaks Jr., eds. *Emerging Infections: Microbial Threats to Health in the United States.* Washington, D.C.: National Academy Press, 1992.

Leopold, Ellen. *A Darker Ribbon: Breast Cancer, Women, and Their Doctors in the Twentieth Century.* Boston, Mass.: Beacon Press, 1999.

Lerner, Barron H. *Contagion and Confinement: Controlling Tuberculosis along the Skid Road.* Baltimore: Johns Hopkins University Press, 1998.

Leuchtenburg, William E. *The Perils of Prosperity, 1914–1932.* Chicago: University of Chicago Press, 1958.

Lewis, Robert C., and Stanley R. Benedict. "A Method for the Estimation of Sugar in Small Quantities of Blood." *Journal of Biological Chemistry* 20 (1915): 61–72.

Lloyd, G. E. R. *Hippocratic Writings.* Edited by G. E. R. Lloyd and translated by J. Chadwick and W. N. Mann. 1950. New York: Penguin Books, 1978.

Lusk, Graham. *Elements of the Science of Nutrition*. Philadelphia: W. B. Saunders Co., 1906.

———. "Metabolism in Diabetes." *Archives of Internal Medicine* 3 (1909): 1–22.

Lynn, Joanne, and Joan Harrold. *Handbook for Mortals: Guidance for People Facing Serious Illness*. New York: Oxford University Press, 1999.

MacDonald, Michael. *Mystical Bedlam: Madness, Anxiety, and Healing in Seventeenth-Century England*. New York: Cambridge University Press, 1981.

Major, Ralph H. "The Treatment of Diabetes Mellitus with Insulin." *Journal of the American Medical Association* 80 (1923): 1597–1600.

Marble, Alexander. "'Free Diet' for Diabetes, Con [editorial]." *Diabetes* 1 (1952): 488–89.

Marchland, Roland. *Advertising the American Dream: Making Way for Modernity, 1920–1940*. Berkeley: University of California Press, 1985.

Marsh, Phil L., L. H. Newburgh, and L. E. Holly. "The Nitrogen Requirement Form Maintenance in Diabetes Mellitus." *Archives of Internal Medicine* 29 (1922): 97–130.

Martin, Edward. "Leg Ulcers." *University Medicine Magazine [University Pennsylvania]* 1 (1888): 332–57.

McCollum, Elmer V. *A History of Nutrition: The Sequence of Ideas in Nutrition Investigations*. 92–99. Boston: Houghton Mifflin, 1957.

McCormick, Marie C. "Survival of Very Tiny Babies—Good News and Bad News." *New England Journal of Medicine* 331 (1994): 802–3.

McKeown, Thomas. *The Origins of Human Disease*. Cambridge, Mass.: Basil Blackwell, 1988.

———. *The Role of Medicine: Dream, Mirage, or Nemesis?* Princeton, N.J.: Princeton University Press, 1979.

McKittrick, Leland S., and Howard F. Root. *Diabetic Surgery*. Philadelphia: Lea and Febiger, 1929.

McLoughlin, G. *A Short History of the First Liverpool Infirmary, 1749–1824*. London: Phillimore, 1978.

McNeill, William H. *Plagues and Peoples*. New York: Anchor Books, 1976.

Mechanic, David. "Chapter Nine: Illness Behavior." In *Medical Sociology*, 249–89. 1968. Reprint, New York: Free Press, 1978.

Meckel, Richard A. *Save the Babies: American Public Health Reform and the Prevention of Infant Mortality, 1850–1929*. Baltimore: Johns Hopkins University Press, 1990.

Medical Care for the American People: The Final Report of the Committee on the Costs of Medical Care. 1932. Reprint, Washington, D.C.: U.S. Department of Health, Education, and Welfare, 1970.

Medvei, Victor Cornelius. *The History of Clinical Endocrinology: A Comprehensive Account of Endocrinology from Earliest Times to the Present Day*. Pearl River, N.Y.: Parthenon Publ. Group, 1993.

Meek, Dr. Frederick M. "Eulogy for Dr. Elliott P. Joslin." *The Pulse: New England Deaconess Hospital* (March 1962): 4.

Melosh, Barbara. *"The Physician's Hand": Work, Culture, and Conflict in American Nursing.* Philadelphia: Temple University Press, 1982.

Mosenthal, Herman O., Samuel W. Clausen, and Alma Hiller. "The Effect of Diet on Blood Sugar in Diabetes Mellitus." *Archives of Internal Medicine* 21 (1918): 93–108.

Murnaghan, Jane H., and Paul Talalay. "H. H. Dale's Account of the Standardization of Insulin." *Bulletin of the History of Medicine* 66 (1992): 440–50.

———. "John Jacob Abel and the Crystalization of Insulin." *Perspectives in Biology and Medicine* 10 (1967): 334–80.

Naunyn, Bernhard. "Excerpts from Autobiograph." In *400 Years of a Doctor's Life,* edited by George Rosen and Beate Caspari-Rosen, 188–91. New York: Henry Schuman, 1947.

Newburgh, L. H., and P. L. Marsh. "Further Observations on the Use of a High Fat Diet in the Treatment of Diabetes Mellitus." *Archives of Internal Medicine* 31 (1923): 455–90.

———. "The Use of a High Fat Diet in the Treatment of Diabetes Mellitus." *Archives of Internal Medicine* 26 (1920): 647–62.

———. "The Use of a High Fat Diet in the Treatment of Diabetes Mellitus. Second Paper: Blood Sugar." *Archives of Internal Medicine* 27 (1921): 699–705.

Nishimura, Rimei, Ronald E. LaPorte, Janice S. Dorman, Naoko Tajima, Dorothy Becker, and Trevor J. Orchard. "Mortality Trends in Type 1 Diabetes: The Allegheny County (Pennsylvania) Registry 1965–1999." *Diabetes Care* 24 (May 2001): 823–27.

Noorden, Carl von. "The Oats Cure in Severe Cases of Diabetes Mellitus." *Post-Graduate* 19 (1904): 408–14.

Nothman, Martin M. "The History of the Discovery of Pancreatic Diabetes." *Bulletin of the History of Medicine* 28 (1954): 272–74.

Numbers, Ronald L. *Almost Persuaded: American Physicians and Compulsory Health Insurance, 1912–1920.* Baltimore: Johns Hopkins University Press, 1978.

———. "The Third Party: Health Insurance in America." In *The Therapeutic Revolution: Essays in the Social History of American Medicine,* edited by Morris J. Vogel and Charles E. Rosenberg, 177–200. Philadelphia: University of Pennsylvania Press, 1979.

"Of What Shall Diabetics Die? [unsigned editorial]." *New England Journal of Medicine* 210 (1934): 43.

O'Hara, Dwight. "A Chart for the Rapid Estimation of Woodyatt's Optimal Diabetic Diet." *Journal of the American Medical Association* 78 (1922): 1124.

Olser, William. "Constitutional Diseases: VII. Diabetes Mellitus." In *The Principles and Practice of Medicine.* New York: D. Appleton and Company, 1892.

Omran, Abdel R. "The Epidemiologic Transition: A Theory of the Epidemiology of Population Change." *Milbank Memorial Fund Quarterly* 49 (1971): 509–38.

Opie, Eugene L. "The Relationship of Diabetes Mellitus to Lesions of the Pancreas. Hyaline Degeneration of the Islands of Langerhans." *Journal of Experimental Medicine* 5 (1900): 527–40.

Papaspyros, Nikos Spyros. *The History of Diabetes Mellitus.* 2nd ed. London: Robert Stockwell, 1964.

Parsons, Eloise, Lawrence M. Randall, and Russell M. Wilder. "Pregnancy and Diabetes." *Medical Clinics of North America* (1926): 679–88.

Parsons, Talcott. "Illness and the Role of the Physician: A Sociological Perspective." In *Personality in Nature, Society, and Culture.* 2nd Rev. ed., edited by Clyde Kluckhorn, Henry A. Murray, and David M. Schneider, 609–17. New York: Knopf, 1953.

———. "The Sick Role and the Role of the Physician Reconsidered." *Milbank Memorial Fund Quarterly* 53 (1975): 257–78.

———. *The Social System.* Glencoe, Ill.: The Free Press, 1951.

Pasko, Thomas, and Bradley Seidman. *Physician Characteristics and Distribution in the U.S.* 2002–3 ed. Chicago: American Medical Association, Division of Survey and Data Resources, 2002.

Patterson, James T. *The Dread Disease: Cancer and Modern American Culture.* Cambridge, Mass.: Harvard University Press, 1987.

Peery, Thomas M. "The New and Old Diseases: A Study of Mortality Trends in the United States, 1900–1969." *American Journal of Clinical Pathology* 63 (1975): 453–74.

Peitzman, Steven J. "From Dropsy to Bright's Disease to End-Stage Renal Disease." *The Milbank Quarterly* 67, suppl. 1 (1989): 16–32.

Peterson, Genevieve. "The Social Aspects of Diabetes: A Study of Sixty Cases." *New England Journal of Medicine* 211 (1934): 397–402.

Pfaff, Franz. "Treatment of Diabetes Mellitus." *Boston Medical and Surgical Journal* 135 (1896): 234–36.

Pincus, G., and Priscilla White. "On the Inheritance of Diabetes: An Analysis of 675 Family Histories." *American Journal of the Medical Sciences* 186 (1933): 1–4.

Poit, Peter, and Monir Q. Islam. "Sexually Transmitted Diseases in the 1990s: Global Epidemiology and Challenges for Control." *Sexually Transmitted Diseases* 21 (1994): S7–S13.

Pollack, Herbert. "Stanley Rossiter Benedict, Creator of Laboratory Tests for Glycosuria." *Diabetes* 2 (1953): 420–21.

Porter, Dorothy, and Roy Porter. *Patient's Progress: Doctors and Doctoring in Eighteenth-Century England.* Stanford: Stanford University Press, 1989.

Porter, Roy. "Gout: Framing and Fantasizing Disease." *Bulletin of the History of Medicine* 68 (1994): 1–28.

———. "The Patient's View: Doing Medical History from Below." *Theory & Society* 14 (1985): 175–98.

Poulsen, J. E. "Diabetes and Anterior Pituitary Insufficiency: Final Course and Postmortem Study of a Diabetic Patient with Sheehan's Syndrome." *Diabetes* 15 (1966): 73–77.

Presley, James Wright. "A History of Diabetes Mellitus in the United States, 1880–1990." Ph.D. diss., University of Texas at Austin, 1991.

Prout, William. *On the Nature and Treatment of Stomach and Urinary Diseases: Being an Inquiry into the Connexion [sic] of Diabetes, Calculus, and Other Affections of the*

Kidney and Bladder, with Indigestion. 3rd, much enl. ed. London: John
  Churchill, 1840.
The Pulse: New England Deaconess Hospital [Newsletter]. March 1962.
The Research Laboratories of Eli Lilly and Company. *Treatment of Diabetes
  Mellitus: A Method of Diet Calculation and the Use of Insulin.* Indianapolis, Ind.:
  Eli Lilly and Company, 1926.
Reverby, Susan M. *Ordered to Care: The Dilemma of American Nursing, 1850–1945.*
  New York: Cambridge University Press, 1987.
Reverby, Susan, and David Rosner. "Beyond 'the Great Doctors.'" In *Health Care
  in America: Essays in Social History,* edited by Susan Reverby and David Rosner,
  3–16. Philadelphia: Temple University Press, 1979.
Rewers, Arleta, H. Peter Chase, Todd Mackenzie, Philip Walravens, Mark
  Roback, Marian Rewers, Richard F. Hamman, and Georgeanna Klingensmith.
  "Predictors of Acute Complications in Children with Type 1 Diabetes." *Journal
  of the American Medical Association* 287 (2002): 2511–18.
Riesman, David, with Nathan Glazer and Reuel Denney. *The Lonely Crowd: A Study
  of the Changing American Character.* 1950. Abridged ed., New Haven, Conn.:
  Yale University Press, 1969.
Risse, Guenter B. *Hospital Life in Enlightenment Scotland: Care and Teaching at the
  Royal Infirmary of Edinburgh.* New York: Cambridge University Press, 1986.
Risse, Guenter B., and John Harley Warner. "Reconstructing Clinical Activities:
  Patient Records in Medical History." *Social History of Medicine* 4 (1992):
  183–205.
Ritholz, Marilyn D., and Alan M. Jacobson. "Living with Hypoglycemia." *Journal
  of General Internal Medicine* 13 (1998): 799–804.
Rogers, Orville F., Jr. "Observations on the Blood Sugar in Diabetes Mellitus."
  Boston Medical and Surgical Journal 175 (1916): 152–56.
Rollo, John. *An Account of Two Cases of the Diabetes Mellitus: With Remarks, as They
  Arose during the Progress of the Cure.* London: T. Gillet for Charles Dilly, 1897.
———. *Cases of the Diabetes Mellitus, with the Results of the Trials of Certain Acids, and
  other Substances, in the Cure of the Lues Venerea.* 2nd ed. London: T. Gillet for
  Charles Dilly, 1798.
———. *Observations on the Acute Dysentery, with the Design of Illustrating its Causes
  and Treatment.* London: Charles Dilly, 1786.
———. *Observations on the Diseases which Appeared in the Army on St. Lucia, in 1778
  and 1779.* London: Charles Dilly, 1781.
Root, Howard F. "The Association of Diabetes and Tuberculosis." *New England
  Journal of Medicine* 210 (1934): 1–13; 78–92; 127–47; 192–206.
———. "Dr. Elliott P. Joslin, 1869–1962." *The Pulse: New England Deaconess
  Hospital* (March 1962): 1–3.
Root, Howard F., William H. Pote, and Hans Frehner. "Triopathy of Diabetes:
  Sequence of Neuropathy, Retinopathy, and Nephropathy in One Hundred
  Fifty-Five Patients." *Archives of Internal Medicine* 94 (1954): 931–41.
Root, Howard F., and Mark H. Rogers. "Diabetic Neuritis with Paralysis." *New
  England Journal of Medicine* 202 (29 May 1930): 1049–53.

Root, Howard F., Priscilla White, Alexander Marble, and Elmer H. Stotz. "Clinical Experience with Protamine Insulinate." *Journal of the American Medical Association* 106 (1936): 180–83.

Rose, Peter I., ed. *Socialization and the Life Cycle.* New York: St. Martin's Press, 1979.

Rosen, George. *Fees and Fee Bills: Some Economic Aspects of Medical Practice in Nineteenth-Century America.* Baltimore: Johns Hopkins University Press, 1946.

———. *Preventive Medicine in the United States, 1900–1975: Trends and Interpretations.* New York: Prodist, 1977.

———. *The Structure of American Medical Practice, 1875–1941.* Edited by Charles E. Rosenberg. Philadelphia: University of Pennsylvania Press, 1983.

Rosenberg, Charles E. *The Care of Strangers: The Rise of America's Hospital System.* New York: Basic Books, 1987.

———. *The Cholera Years: The United States in 1832, 1849, and 1866.* 1962. Reprint, Chicago: University of Chicago Press, 1987.

———. *Explaining Epidemics and Other Studies in the History of Medicine.* New York: Cambridge University Press, 1992.

———. "Making It in Urban Medicine: A Career in the Age of Scientific Medicine." *Bulletin of the History of Medicine* 64 (1990): 163–86.

———. "Social Class and Medical Care in Nineteenth-Century America: The Rise and Fall of the Dispensary." *Journal of the History of Medicine* 29 (1974): 32–54.

———. "The Therapeutic Revolution: Medicine, Meaning, and Social Change in Nineteenth-Century Medicine." In *Explaining Epidemics and Other Studies in the History of Medicine.* New York: Cambridge University Press, 1992.

———. *The Trial of the Assassin Guiteau: Psychiatry and Law in the Gilded Age.* Chicago: University of Chicago Press, 1968.

———. "The Tyranny of Diagnosis: Specific Entities and Individual Experience." *The Milbank Quarterly* 80 (2002): 237–60.

Rosenberg, Charles E., and Carroll Smith-Rosenberg. "Piety and Social Action: Some Origins of the American Public Health Movement." In *No Other Gods: On Science and American Social Thought,* 109–22. Baltimore: Johns Hopkins University Press, 1976.

Rothman, Shiela M. *Living in the Shadow of Death: Tuberculosis and the Social Experience of Illness in American History.* New York: Basic Books, 1994.

Santiago, Denise Marie. "Two Groups Put Up $40 Million to Broaden Diabetes Research." *Philadelphia Inquirer,* 9 April 1995, A19.

Schadewaldt, Hans. "The History of Diabetes Mellitus." In *Diabetes: Its Medical and Cultural History. Outlines, Texts, Bibliography,* edited by Dietrich von Engelhardt, 85–86. New York: Springer-Verlag, 1989.

"The Shattuck Lecture [unsigned editorial]." *Boston Medical and Surgical Journal* 186 (1922): 857.

Shorter, Edward. *Bedside Manners: The Troubled History of Doctors and Patients.* New York: Simon and Schuster, 1985.

Shryock, Richard Harrison. *The Development of Modern Medicine: An Interpretation of*

the Social and Scientific Factors Involved. 1936. Reprint, Madison: University of
     Wisconsin Press, 1974.
Sicherman, Barbara. "The New Mission of the Doctor: Redefining Health and
     Health Care in the Progressive Era, 1900–1917." In *Nourishing the Humanistic
     in Medicine: Interactions with the Social Sciences,* edited by William R. Rogers and
     David Bernard, 95–124. Pittsburgh, Pa.: University of Pittsburgh Press, 1979.
Sigerist, Henry E. *Early Greek, Hindu, and Persian Medicine.* Vol. 2 of *A History of
     Medicine.* New York: Oxford University Press, 1961.
——. *The Great Doctors: A Biographical History of Medicine.* New York: W. W.
     Norton, 1933.
——. *Primitive and Archaic Medicine.* Vol. 1 of *A History of Medicine.* New York:
     Oxford University Press, 1951.
Sinding, Christiane. "Making the Unit of Insulin: Standards, Clinical Work, and
     Industry, 1920–1925." *Bulletin of the History of Medicine* 76 (2002): 231–70.
Smith, John Maynard, David J. P. Barker, Caleb E. Finch, Sharon L. R. Kardia,
     S. Boyd Eaton, Thomas B. L. Kirkwood, Ed LeGrand, Randolph M. Nesse,
     George C. Williams, and Linda Partridge. "The Evolution of Non-Infectious
     and Degenerative Disease." In *Evolution in Health and Disease,* edited by
     Stephen C. Stearns, 267–72. New York: Oxford University Press, 1999.
Smith, O[live] Watkins. "Diethylstilbestrol in the Prevention and Treatment of
     Complications of Pregnancy." *American Journal of Obstetrics and Gynecology* 56
     (1948): 821–34.
Spence, Jonathan D. *The Death of Woman Wang.* New York: Penguin, 1978.
Stander, H. J., and C. H. Peckham. "Diabetes Mellitus and Pregnancy." *American
     Journal of Obstetrics and Gynecology* 14 (1927): 313–21.
Starr, Paul. *The Social Transformation of American Medicine: The Rise of a Sovereign
     Profession and the Making of a Vast Industry.* New York: Basic Books, 1982.
Stern, Alexandra, and Howard Markel, eds. *The Formative Years: Childhood Health
     and Health Care, 1880–2000.* Ann Arbor: University of Michigan Press, 2002.
Stevens, Rosemary. *In Sickness and in Wealth: American Hospitals in the Twentieth
     Century.* New York: Basic Books, 1989.
Strauss, Anselm, Shizuko Fagerhaugh, Barbara Suczek, and Carolyn Wiener.
     Social Organization of Medical Work. Chicago: University of Chicago, 1985.
Street, John Phillips. "Diabetic Foods Offered for Sale in the United States:
     A Preliminary Report." *Journal of the American Medical Association* 60 (1913):
     2037–39.
Strouse, Solomon. "Control Methods in the Treatment of Diabetes Mellitus."
     Journal of the American Medical Association 75 (1920): 97–100.
"Surgery and Diabetes [unsigned editorial]." *Boston Medical and Surgical Journal*
     193 (1925): 842.
Sydenham, Thomas. Preface to the Third Edition of *The Works of Thomas
     Sydenham, M.D.* Edited by R. G. Latham and translated from the Latin edition
     of Dr. Greenhill. London: The Sydenham Society, 1848.
——. "Processus Integri: Chapter XXXVII.—On Diabetes." In *The Works of*

Thomas Sydenham, M.D. Edited by R. G. Latham and translated from the Latin edition of Dr. Greenhill. London: Printed for the Sydenham Society, 1850.

Szasz, T. S., and M. H. Hollender. "The Basic Models of the Doctor-Patient Relationship." *Archives of Internal Medicine* 97 (1956): 585–92.

Taylor, F. K. *The Concepts of Illness, Disease, and Morbus.* New York: Cambridge University Press, 1979.

Temkin, Owsei. *The Falling Sickness: A History of Epilepsy from the Greeks to the Beginnings of Modern Neurology.* 1945. Reprint, Baltimore: Johns Hopkins University Press, 1971.

———. "The Scientific Approach to Disease: Specific Entity and Individual Sickness." In *The Double Face of Janus and Other Essays in the History of Medicine,* 441–55. Baltimore: Johns Hopkins University Press, 1977.

Tentler, Leslie Woodcock. *Wage-Earning Women: Industrial Work and Family Life in the United States, 1900–1930.* New York: Oxford University Press, 1979.

Thomas, Lewis. "On the Science and Technology of Medicine." In *Doing Better and Feeling Worse: Health in the United States,* edited by John H. Knowles, 35–46. New York: W. W. Norton & Company, 1977.

"Thomas Willis." In *Dictionary of National Biography.* Vol. 21. Edited by Sidney Lee, 496–97. New York: The Macmillan Co., 1909.

Titus, Raymond S. "Diabetes in Pregnancy from the Obstetrical Point of View." *American Journal of Obstetrics and Gynecology* 33 (1937): 386–92.

Tolstoi, Edward. *Living with Diabetes.* New York: Crown Publ., 1952.

———. "Treatment of Diabetes Mellitus: The Controversy of the Past Decade." *Cincinnati Journal of Medicine* 30 (1949): 1–7.

Tompkins, Walter A. *Continuing Quest: Dr. William David Sansum's Crusade against Diabetes.* Santa Barbara, Calif.: Schauer Printing Co., 1977.

Townsend, Charles W. "Diabetes Mellitus in Children." *Boston Medical and Surgical Journal* 140 (1899): 445–46.

Tracy, Sarah W. "George Draper and American Constitutional Medicine, 1916–1946." *Bulletin of the History of Medicine* 66 (1992): 53–89.

Ulrich, Laurel Thatcher. *A Midwife's Tale: The Life of Martha Ballard, Based on Her Diary, 1785–1812.* New York: Knopf, 1990.

U.S. Bureau of the Census. *Historical Statistics of the United States, Colonial Times to 1970.* Electronic edition on CD-ROM. Edited by Susan Carter, Scott Gartner, Michael Haines, Alan Olmstead, Richard Sutch, and Gavin Wright. New York: Cambridge University Press, 1997.

U.S. Preventive Services Task Force. *Guide to Clinical Preventive Services: Report of the U.S. Preventive Services Task Force.* Baltimore: Williams & Wilkins, 1996.

Van Maanen, John. *Tales of the Field: On Writing Ethnography.* Chicago: University of Chicago Press, 1988.

Von Engelhardt, Dietrich, ed. *Diabetes: Its Medical and Cultural History: Outlines, Texts, Bibliography.* New York: Springer-Verlag, 1989.

Von Mering, J., and O. Minkowski. "Diabetes Mellitus nach Pankreas Extirpation." *Archiv für experimentelle Pathologie und Pharmakologie* 26 (1889): 371–87.

———. "Diabetes mellitus nach Pankreasexstirpation." *Centralblatt für Klinische Medicin* 10 (1889): 393–94.

Wagener, Henry P., Thomas J. Story Dry, and Russell M. Wilder. "Retinitis in Diabetes." *New England Journal of Medicine* 211 (1934): 1131–37.

Wagener, Henry P., and Russell M. Wilder. "The Retinitis of Diabetes Mellitus." *Journal of the American Medical Association* 76 (1921): 515.

Wailoo, Keith. "'A Disease Sui Generis': The Origins of Sickle Cell Anemia and the Emergence of Modern Clinical Research, 1904–1924." *Bulletin of the History of Medicine* 65 (1991): 185–208.

———. *Drawing Blood: Technology and Disease Identity in Twentieth-Century America.* Baltimore: Johns Hopkins University Press, 1997.

———. *Dying in the City of Blues: Sickle Cell Anemia and the Politics of Race and Health.* Chapel Hill: University of North Carolina Press, 2001.

Wakefield, Homer. "Some Common Errors in the Treatment of Diabetes." *Medical Record* 80 (1911): 571–73.

Walker, Joan B. *Chronicle of a Diabetic Service.* London: British Diabetic Association, 1989.

Warner, John Harley. "Ideals of Science and Their Discontents in Late-Nineteenth-Century American Medicine." *Isis* 82 (1991): 454–78.

———. *The Therapeutic Perspective: Medical Practice, Knowledge, and Identity in America, 1820–1885.* Cambridge, Mass.: Harvard University Press, 1986.

Watson, Thomas. "Lecture LXXVII: Suppression of the urine. Diabetes . . . Diuresis." In *Lectures on the Principles and Practice of Physic; Delivered at King's College, London.* 3rd American ed., edited by D. Francis Condie, 866–77. Philadelphia: Lea and Blanchard, 1847.

Weindling, Paul. "From Infectious to Chronic Diseases: Changing Patterns of Sickness in the Nineteenth and Twentieth Centuries." In *Medicine in Society: Historical Essays,* edited by Andrew Wear, 303–16. New York: Cambridge University Press, 1992.

White, Priscilla. "Diabetes Complicating Pregnancy." *American Journal of Obstetrics and Gynecology* 33 (1937): 380–85.

———. *Diabetes in Childhood and Adolescence.* Philadelphia, Pa.: Lea and Febiger, 1932.

———. "Diabetes in Pregnancy." In *The Treatment of Diabetes Mellitus.* 4th ed., edited by Elliott P. Joslin. Philadelphia: Lea and Febiger, 1928.

———. "Diabetes Mellitus in Pregnancy." *Clinics in Perinatology* 1 (1974): 331–47.

———. "Natural Course and Prognosis of Juvenile Diabetes." *Diabetes* 5 (November 1956): 445–50.

———. "Pregnancy Complicating Diabetes." *Surgery, Gynecology, Obstetrics* 61 (1935): 324–32.

———. "Pregnancy Complicating Diabetes." In *The Treatment of Diabetes Mellitus.* 8th ed., edited by Elliott P. Joslin, Howard F. Root, Priscilla White, Alexander Marble, and C. Cabell Bailey. Philadelphia: Lea and Febiger, 1946.

———. "Pregnancy Complicating Diabetes." *American Journal of Medicine* 7 (1949): 609–16.

White, Priscilla, and Hazel Hunt. "Cholesterol of the Blood of Diabetic
  Children." *New England Journal of Medicine* 202 (1930): 607–16.
White, Priscilla, Philip Koshy, and Janine Duckers. "The Management of
  Pregnancy Complicating Diabetes and of Children of Diabetic Mothers."
  Medical Clinics of North America (1953): 1481–96.
White, Priscilla, Raymond S. Titus, Elliott P. Joslin, and Hazel Hunt. "Prediction
  and Prevention of Late Pregnancy Accidents in Diabetes." *American Journal of
  the Medical Sciences* 198 (1939): 482–92.
Wiener, C., Strauss A., S. Fagerhaugh, and Barbara Suczek. "Trajectories,
  Biographies, and the Evolving Medical Scene: Labor and Delivery and the
  Intensive Care Nursery." *Sociology of Health and Illness* 1 (1979): 261–83.
Wilder, Russell M. "'Optimal' Diets for Diabetic Patients." *Journal of the American
  Medical Association* 83 (1924): 733–36.
Williams, J. Whitridge. "The Clinical Significance of Glycosuria in Pregnant
  Women." *American Journal of the Medical Sciences* 137 (1909): 1–26.
Williams, John R. "A Clinical Study of the Effects of Insulin in Severe Diabetes."
  Journal of Metabolic Research 2 (1922): 729–51.
Willis, Thomas. "Chapter IV: The Kinds and Forms of Ischuretcial Medicines, or
  Such as Help to Stop the Urine in Excess." In Part 1 of *Pharmaceutic Rationalis;
  or, An Exercitation of the Operations of Medicines in Humane Bodies. Shewing the
  Signs, Causes, and Cures of Most Distempters Incident Thereunto.* Translated from
  the Latin by S. Pordage, in *Dr. Willis's Practice of Physick, Being all the Medical
  Works of that Renowned and Famous Physicians, Contained within.* London:
  T. Dring, C. Harper, and J. Leigh, 1681.
———. "Section IV, Chapter III: Of the Too Much Evacuation by Urine, and Its
  Remedy; and Especially of the Diabetes or Pissing Evil, Whose Theory and
  Method of Curing, Is Inquired Into." In Part I of *Pharmaceutic Rationalis; or, An
  Exercitation of the Operations of Medicines in Humane Bodies. Shewing the Signs,
  Causes, and Cures of Most Distempters Incident Thereunto.* Translated from the
  Latin by S. Pordage, in *Dr. Willis's Practice of Physick, Being all the Medical Works
  of that Renowned and Famous Physician, Contained within.* London: T. Dring,
  C. Harper, and J. Leigh, 1681.
Woodyatt, Rollin T. "Bernhard Naunyn." *Diabetes* 1 (1952): 240–41.
———. "Objects and Methods of Diet Adjustment in Diabetes." *Archives of
  Internal Medicine* 28 (1921): 125–41.
———. "Objects and Methods of Diet Adjustment in Diabetes." *Transactions of the
  Association of American Physicians* 36 (1921): 269–92.
"A Workman that Needeth Not to be Ashamed [letters submitted by Charles H.
  Best, Joseph Pierre Hoet, Bernardo A. Houssay, R. D. Lawrence, Russell M.
  Wilder, J. M. Hayman, George Packer Berry, Chester S. Keefer, and John
  Lister]." *New England Journal of Medicine* 261 (1959): 455–60.
Wrenshall, G. A., G. Hetenyi, and W. R. Feasby. *The Story of Insulin: Forty Years of
  Success against Diabetes.* Edited by Abraham Marcus. London: The Bodley
  Head, 1962.

Young, F. G. "Claude Bernard and the Discovery of Glycogen: A Century of Retrospect." *British Medical Journal* 1 (1957): 1431–37.

Zelizer, Viviana A. *Pricing the Priceless Child: The Changing Social Value of Children.* New York: Basic Books, 1985.

ACKNOWLEDGMENTS

A work of history depends upon sources. The patients and physicians who recorded their experiences and thoughts are the sine qua non of this book, and their efforts warrant my principal acknowledgment.

Over the past decade and a half, while laboring on this project in an intermittent and rather peripatetic manner, I benefited greatly from the advice and support of Lester Baker, Charles Rosenberg, Renée Fox, Rosemary Stevens, Roger Smith, John Brook, Jan Golinski, Stephen Pumfrey—and more recently, Fred Rivara, Richard Shugerman, Jeff Wright, John Neff, and Tom Koepsell. The colleagueship and friendship of Keith Wailoo, Jeff Brosco, Dimitri Christakis, Nicholas Christakis, Bert Garrett, Steve Gruber, Shari Rudavski, and Peter Schwartz have been priceless. Lyn Bassett, Marisa Gallo, Paul Seckinger, Doug Keen, and Asaf Rotem each provided important aid along the way. Steve Gabbe was an enthusiastic collaborator on an earlier version of Chapter 6. In the history of medicine and science community, Robbie Aronowitz, Barbara Bates, Leon Eisenberg, Janet Golden, Joel Howell, Rob Kohler, Barron Learner, Susan Lindee, Ken Ludmerer, Howard Markel, Steve Martin, Russell Maulitz, Steve Peitzman, and Janet Tighe have been extremely helpful. At the University of North Carolina Press, the steadfast encouragement and patience of Studies in Social Medicine editors Alan Brandt and Larry Churchill, and especially of Sian Hunter, kept me moving toward the finish line.

I conducted the majority of my primary source research at the Joslin Diabetes Center, where I would not have been able to proceed without the generous assistance of Jim and Susan Warram, Andrzej Krolewski, Lori Laffel, Don Barnett, and Donna Younger. I am also grateful for the assistance given me by Susan Rishworth at the J. Bay Jacobs, M.D., Library of the American College of Obstetricians and Gynecologists in Washington, D.C.; and by the staffs at the other archives that I visited, including the American Philosophical Society in Philadelphia; the Center for the Study of the History of Nursing, School of Nursing, University of Pennsylvania in Philadelphia; the Clendening History of Medicine Library, University of Kansas Medical Center in Kansas City, Kansas; the Cincinnati Medical Heritage Center, University of Cincinnati Medical Center in Cincinnati; the Countway Library Rare Book Department, Harvard Medical School in Boston; the Fisher Library, University of Toronto in Toronto; the History of Medicine Division, National Library of Medicine in Bethesda; the Medical Archives of the New York Hospital–Cornell Medical Center in New York City; Northwestern University Memorial Hospital Archives in Chicago; the Historical Collection of Pennsylvania Hospital in Philadelphia; the Rush-Presbyterian–St. Luke's Medical Center Archives in Chicago; the Schlesinger Library, Radcliffe College in Cambridge, Massachusetts; and the University of Chicago Library, Department of Special Collections in Chicago. I particularly want to thank the staff of the Library of the College of Physicians of Philadelphia in Philadelphia for their friendly service.

Over the years, I have received funding support from several organizations: the National Library of Medicine (publication grant 1G13LM07157); the Agency for Healthcare Research and Quality, for the dissertation work (grant number HS07476-01) and currently for a career development award (KO8 HS 00002); the Rotary International Foundation; the Measey Foundation; the Combined Degree Program of the University of Pennsylvania School of Medicine; a National Research Service Award Fellowship from the Agency for Healthcare Research and Quality, administered through the Leonard Davis Institute of the University of Pennsylvania; the Paupukkeewis Fund; the Logan Clendening Travelling Fellowship; the ACOG-Ortho Fellowship in the History of American Obstetrics and Gynecology; and the Wood Fellowship of the College of Physicians of Philadelphia.

Finally, for their unflagging enthusiasm and belief in the worthiness of this project, I thank Betty and Charlie Feudtner, Beth Feudtner, Mark and Kim Feudtner, Mildred Feudtner, and—most of all—my wife, Lynda Bascelli, and our son, Jack.

INDEX

betes mellitus, xxi, 3; and dietary therapy, 49; and pancreatic gland extract, 51, 89; and insulin therapy, 55, 90; and diabetic management, 68; and hypoglycemic reactions, 105; and diabetic control, 130, 212; and postpregnancy complications, 164

Blood tests, 13, 15, 91

Blood vessel damage, 39, 109, 191, 212

Blue Cross, 72

Bradley, Robert F., 83–86

Breast cancer, 214

Bright's disease, 174

Burns, Arnold (pseudonym), 121–23, 133–43, 144, 145

Cancer: and disease transmutation, xvi, 23, 203, 214; and therapeutic success, 9; history of, 11; and causes of death, 21; and monitoring, 95

Causes of death, 10, 20, 21, 24–25, 40, 42, 138

Cesarean section, 151, 154, 155, 156, 157, 163, 178, 179

Chittenden, Russell H., 45

Cholera, 21

Cholesterol levels, 27

Chorionic gonadotropin, 158

Chronic illness: and goals of care, xiii, 213, 216–17, 218; Type 1 diabetes mellitus as, xv, xvi, 4; and diabetes transmutation, xv, xvi, 10, 17, 23, 25, 37, 43, 66, 111; and acute exacerbations, xvi, 78, 91, 135; and medical intervention's consequences, 10; and causes of death, 21; and illness transformation, 26, 27, 44, 214; and responsibility, 66, 182, 192; and diabetic language, 67; and normal life, 81, 212, 233 (n. 50); and patient-oriented accounts, 87–88; work of, 91; and therapeutic success, 195; and technological innovation, 209

Circulatory problems, 65

Cognitive deficits, 203

Collip, James B., 6, 36, 50, 51, 133

Coma: and Type 2 diabetes mellitus, xxi; and Type 1 diabetes mellitus, xxi, 3; and death, xxi, 6, 24, 48, 109, 130, 131, 136, 172; and patient records and letters, 13, 46; and insulin therapy, 36, 39, 208; and diabetic control, 65, 124, 131, 135–36, 138, 140, 174, 237–38 (n. 38), 238 (n. 41); and diabetic management, 68; and surgery, 69; and pregnancy, 76, 150, 157; symptoms of, 107; and daily living with diabetes, 107–9; Joslin's campaign to abolish diabetic, 135

Complications: and natural history of disease, 43

Complications of diabetes. See Sequelae of diabetes

Congenital defects, 10, 214

Congestive heart failure, 110, 139, 165

Connaught Laboratories, 53

Constitutional treatments, 46, 229 (n. 17)

Control, 28, 29, 214–20. See also Diabetic control

Coronary artery disease, 27

Cultural beliefs: and medical care, xiv, 28; and diabetes history, xv, xvii; and illness transformation, 26–28, 44; and normalcy, 81; and pregnancy, 147, 166; and logic of innovation, 167, 168; and responsibility, 173; and therapeutic success, 192; and death, 219

Daily living with diabetes: insulin discovery in context of, 10; work of, 10, 15, 44, 54, 91, 118–19, 167, 169, 202–3, 211; and medical changes, 11, 79–80; and patient records and letters, 15, 78–79, 93–95; and illness transformation, 25–28, 212–

13; and dietary therapy, 63, 91, 93, 97–100, 211; and hypoglycemic reactions, 63, 104–7; and diabetic language, 63–68, 77–81; and feelings of good health, 80–81; and patient-oriented accounts, 87–88, 118–19, 208; and insulin injections, 91, 100–104, 119, 202, 211; and urine tests, 92, 95–96, 119, 211; and diabetic specialist visits, 92–93; and blood glucose monitors, 95, 119, 211; and monitoring work, 95–97, 216; and symptom work, 104–10; and patient/doctor relationships, 111–14, 119; and identity work, 114–17, 119; and patient attitudes, 115, 120

Dane, Bernadette (pseudonym), 150, 161–66

Death: and coma, xxi, 6, 24, 48, 109, 130, 131, 136, 172; causes of, 10, 20, 21, 24–25, 40, 42, 138; infant mortality, 10, 76, 149, 150, 154, 155, 157, 158, 177, 178, 183, 215; pregnancy and, 147, 149, 150, 152, 154; and cultural beliefs, 219

DeLee, Joseph B., 74, 150, 152

Dementia, 21

Depression, 95

Diabetes: meaning of, 4. *See also* Type 1 diabetes mellitus; Type 2 diabetes mellitus

Diabetes Control and Complications Trial (DCCT), 212

Diabetes education: and Type 1 diabetes mellitus, 3; and diabetic management, 65, 91; and insulin injections, 101–2; Joslin and, 121, 132, 193; and responsibility, 177, 181

Diabetes history: and Type 1 diabetes mellitus, xiv–xvi; and patient-oriented accounts, xv, xvi–xvii, 25, 27, 28, 220; and diabetics' accounts, xvi–xvii; and current view of diabetes, xviii–xxii; and technology ethos, 4–12; and life expectancy, 6, 13, 18–19; and Joslin's records and letters, 12–17; and diabetes transmutation, 17–25, 36–48; and transformed illness phenomenon, 25–28; implications of, 29; and therapeutic failure, 187

Diabetes transmutation: and chronic illness, xv, xvi, 10, 17, 23, 25, 37, 43, 66, 111; and sequelae or complications of diabetes, 10, 23, 24–25, 43, 122, 138; and diabetes history, 17–25, 36–48; and medical therapeutics, 21, 23, 26, 37, 38, 39, 60, 63, 209, 210; and life expectancy, 23–25, 43; and insulin, 25, 36–37; and dietary therapy, 37, 48–49; cycles of, 38, 39, 40, 41; and Joslin, 38, 60–61; and illness transformation, 43–44, 203, 204, 209, 212; and insulin therapy, 50–54; and social change, 56–60; and pregnancy, 146

Diabetic care: Joslin's philosophy of, 16, 17, 35, 79, 98, 133, 193, 235 (n. 16); philosophy of Joslin Diabetes Center, 16, 78–79; as specialty, 57; evolution of, 63–65; varieties of, 66; and quality of life, 167; and diabetic transmutation, 209; and pharmaceuticals, 210. *See also* Diabetic control; Diabetic management

Diabetic control: and Type 1 diabetes mellitus as chronic illness, 4; and diabetic world, 28, 29; and pregnancy, 29, 76, 157, 162, 238 (n. 41); and diabetes transmutation, 37; and illness transformation, 44; and dietary therapy, 48–49, 124–25, 126, 127–32, 137, 140, 143, 161–62, 174, 201, 205; and diabetic language, 65, 67, 74; and coma, 65, 124, 131, 135–36, 138, 140,

174, 237–38 (n. 38), 238 (n. 41);
and sequelae or complications of
diabetes, 65–66, 122, 135, 137–
43, 174, 175; and self-control, 66,
124, 125, 127, 130, 190; and moral
character, 66, 174, 192, 194; and
family or parents, 122, 123, 124,
125, 126, 129, 130–31, 133; and
medical therapeutics, 122, 127–28,
131, 137, 144, 158, 236 (n. 4); and
diabetic management, 122, 143–45,
212; and pre-insulin period, 123–
31; and urine tests, 125, 126, 129,
130–31, 136, 140, 162; and insulin
therapy, 132–37, 162, 174, 207,
237 (nn. 25, 26); and technological
innovation, 210; and reductive vs.
holistic thinking, 213

Diabetic language: and daily living
with diabetes, 63–68, 77–81; and
diabetic control, 65, 67, 74; and
human development, 67

Diabetic management: and diabetic
world, 28, 29; and illness transformation, 44; and dietary therapy,
54, 55, 62, 65, 68; and insulin therapy, 54–56, 68–69, 79, 121–22; and
social changes, 59–60, 122–23; and
physicians' role, 65, 66–67, 231
(n. 7); and diabetic language, 65,
74; and diabetes education, 65, 91;
and daily living with diabetes, 91;
and diabetic control, 122, 143–45,
212; and pregnancy, 147, 148, 152,
154–61, 167; and responsibility,
186–87

*Diabetic Manual for the Mutual Use of
Doctor and Patient* (Joslin): and daily
living with diabetes, 92, 93, 96; and
dietary therapy, 98; and insulin
injections, 101; and identification
card, 107; and acidosis, 108; and
ideal patient attitudes, 115; and
identity work, 115, 117; continued
publication of, 193

Diabetic mothers. *See* Pregnancy
Diabetic specialists, 65, 90, 91, 92–
93
Diabetic triopathy, 139–40
Diabetic variations, 39–40, 41
Diabetic world: Joslin's place in, 16,
33, 193–95; and illness transformation, 27–28, 211; and responsibility,
28, 29; and diabetic language,
63–64; and Rainsford's cartoons,
94–95; and sense of self, 176–81;
maturing in, 182–87
Dialysis. *See* Renal dialysis
Diarrhea, 21
Dickonson, Peter, 5
Dietary therapy: Type 2 diabetes
mellitus, xxi, xxii; Type 1 diabetes
mellitus, xxii; history of, 6, 48–49,
50, 97–98, 99; and Joslin, 12–13,
17, 31, 45, 47, 48–49, 89, 90, 98,
128, 131–32, 171, 174; and diabetes
transmutation, 37, 48–49; and
diabetic control, 48–49, 124–25,
126, 127–32, 137, 140, 143, 161–
62, 174, 201, 205; and diabetic
management, 54, 55, 62, 65, 68;
and daily living with diabetes, 63,
91, 93, 97–100, 119; and diabetic
language, 68; and sequelae or complications of diabetes, 85–86; and
judgments about patient conduct,
97; food category pocket card, 98;
and insulin injections, 102, 133;
and pregnancy, 151, 155, 156, 157;
and responsibility, 179, 180–81,
205–7
Diethylstilbestrol (DES), 23, 158, 163
Dietitians, 27, 91
Disease diminishment, 21
Disease emergence, 21
Disease reemergence, 21
Disease substitution, 21, 219
Disease transmutation: and cancer,
xvi, 23, 203, 214; and disease diminishment or substitution, 21;

management, 68; and pregnancy, 75–76, 150, 157, 164–65; yeast infections, 110; and diabetic control, 131, 238 (n. 41); and workplace discrimination, 186; and immunosuppression, 203; and immunizations, 215

Influenza, 21

Informed consent, 215, 247 (n. 26)

Insulin: and Type 1 diabetes mellitus, xviii, xx, xxi, xxii, 3–4, 6–8, 121–22, 216; discovery of, xviii, 4, 6–11, 15, 17, 18–19, 50, 120, 146, 200; and metabolism, xx; and Type 2 diabetes mellitus, xxi, xxii; and patient records and letters, 13; and life expectancy, 13, 18–19, 26, 56–57; and diabetes transmutation, 25, 36–37; longer-acting varieties of, 26, 55, 137, 161; supply of, 54; standardization of, 54–55, 89, 102, 230 (n. 42)

Insulin-dependent diabetes. *See* Type 1 diabetes mellitus

Insulin injections: and Type 1 diabetes mellitus, xviii, xxi, 3–4; and Type 2 diabetes mellitus, xxii; and patient records and letters, 15; and daily living with diabetes, 91, 100–104, 119, 202, 211; and exercise, 102, 133; and hypoglycemic reactions, 104–7; and diabetic control, 212

Insulin shock. *See* Hypoglycemic reactions

Insulin therapy: and therapeutic success, 6, 7–10, 52–53, 54, 90–91, 195, 202, 203, 204, 205; development of, 11, 36, 50–55, 89–91, 132, 201, 205; and chronic illness, 27; short-term consequences of, 38–39; and hypoglycemic reactions, 39, 54, 162, 202, 212, 216; allergies to, 53; and diabetic management, 54–56, 68–69, 79, 121–22; and

Joslin, 55, 87, 89, 90–91, 100, 121–22, 132–33, 174, 202, 205, 207, 237 (n. 25); and daily living with diabetes, 63, 100; and diabetic language, 64–65; expenses of, 69, 134, 237 (n. 31); and metabolism, 132, 187, 192–93; and diabetic control, 132–37, 162, 174, 207, 237 (nn. 25, 26); and pregnancy, 155, 157; and responsibility, 173, 174–76, 182; and technological innovation, 210

Islets of Langerhans, xix, xxii, 50–51, 132

Jenner, Robin (pseudonym), 150, 158–60

Joslin, Allen (Elliot P.'s father), 34

Joslin, Allen P. (Elliot P.'s son), 93, 142, 161

Joslin, Elizabeth Denny, 92–93, 205

Joslin, Elliott, Jr., 93

Joslin, Elliott P.: and dietary therapy, 12–13, 17, 31, 45, 47, 48–49, 89, 90, 98, 128, 131–32, 171, 174; patient records and letters of, 12–17, 47, 78, 204–7, 246–47 (n. 16); view of patient/doctor relationships, 13–14, 57–58, 133–35, 215; diabetic care philosophy of, 16, 17, 35, 79, 98, 133, 193, 235 (n. 16); and insulin discovery, 17; and patient life expectancy, 18–19, 21, 57, 226 (n. 31); career of, 33–36, 44–47, 60, 193–95, 228 (n. 15); and diabetes transmutation, 38, 60–61; and causes of death of juvenile diabetics, 40; and insulin therapy, 55, 87, 89, 90–91, 100, 121–22, 132–33, 174, 202, 205, 207, 237 (n. 25); and self-control, 66, 121; and medical judgment shifts, 68–69; and medical billing issues, 69, 71, 112, 134–35, 237 (n. 36); on pregnancy, 74, 150–52, 155–56, 178, 240 (n. 9); and sequelae or

living with diabetes, 91, 108; and diabetic control, 124, 125, 127–29, 130; and dietary therapy, 182; and patient-centered care, 199

Opiates, 46
Opie, Eugene, 50, 132
Oral glucose tolerance test, 26
Oral hypoglycemic agents, 26, 65, 91
Organotherapy, 51, 132
Organ transplantation, 37, 84, 85, 203, 208, 209, 210, 211
Osler, William, 33
Outpatient clinics, 65, 91
Ovarian cancer, 214

Pancreas: and Type 1 diabetes mellitus, xviii, xix, xx; and diabetes history, 26; and discovery of insulin, 50; and transplantation of pancreatic tissue, 210
Pancreatic extract, 7–8, 46, 50–53, 89, 130, 207
Pancreatic theory of diabetes, 50–53, 132
Papyrus Ebers, 4
Paracelsus, 199
Parents. *See* Family or parents
Paternalism, 71, 194
Patient-centered care, priorities of, 199, 213
Patient/doctor relationships: and Joslin, 13–14, 57–58, 133–35, 215; and diabetes transmutation, 57; and life expectancy, 57; and responsibility, 66–67, 173, 179, 180, 181, 185, 189–92, 231 (n. 9); and Priscilla White, 77, 79, 121, 133, 137, 162–64, 166, 237 (n. 27); and pregnancy, 77, 161–64; and diabetic control, 79, 123, 126–28; and later stages of life, 82, 187; and judgments about patient conduct, 97, 176; and patient records and letters, 111, 112–14, 180; and medi-

cal expenses, 111–12, 134–35, 137, 163, 182–84; and daily living with diabetes, 111–14, 119
Patient image: and biomedical view of disease, xv–xvi; and patient records and letters, 15, 113–14; and sense of self, 64, 81, 138, 176–81; and identity work, 114–17, 119, 123, 176–81, 187; and sequelae or complications of diabetes, 141; and pregnancy, 147
Patient-oriented accounts: and diabetes history, xv, xvi–xvii, 25, 27, 28, 220; and narration, 86–88, 234 (n. 60); and daily living with diabetes, 87–88, 118–19, 208; and responsibility, 169; and therapeutic success, 195; and contradiction of medical therapeutics, 204
Patient records and letters: and diabetes history, 12–17; of Joslin, 12–17, 47, 78, 204–7, 246–47 (n. 16); and family or parents, 14, 15, 78–79, 82, 83–86; and daily living with diabetes, 15, 78–79, 93–95; and illness transformation, 44; and diabetic management, 54, 55, 123; and diabetic language, 63, 68; and acute exacerbations, 78, 91; and patient/doctor relationships, 111, 112–14, 180; and diabetic control, 125–26; and vision problems, 140, 159
Patient rights, 215
Paulesco, Nicolas, 51
Pediatric endocrinology, 57
Penicillin, 24, 85, 164
People care, xiv, 220
Personal responsibility. *See* Responsibility
Pharmaceuticals: and chronic illness, xiii; and Type 2 diabetes mellitus, xxi, xxii; and metabiosis, 40; and diabetic management, 65; and diabetic care, 210. *See also* Insulin
Physical examinations, 14, 75, 140

insulin therapy, 173, 174–76, 182; and authority, 174, 175, 177, 181, 185; and sequelae or complications of diabetes, 175–76, 185, 191, 212; and identity work, 176–81, 187; and dietary therapy, 179, 180–81, 205–7; and diabetic management, 186–87; and incomplete control, 214

Retinal photocoagulation, 210

Retinopathy: as complication of diabetes, 83, 110, 138–40, 188, 190, 202, 235–36 (n. 28); and pituitary gland, 192, 245 (n. 66)

Ritalin, 215

Rollo, John, 6, 50, 98, 99, 224 (n. 7)

Root, Howard F., 80, 87, 90, 138, 139–41, 190, 207

Ryder, Teddy, 200–201

Sansum, William David, 51

Scientific knowledge: and biomedical model, xv–xvi; and diabetes history, xvii, 26. *See also* Technological innovation

Scott, E. L., 51

Screening programs, 211

Self, sense of, 64, 81, 138, 176–81. *See also* Patient image

Self-care. *See* Daily living with diabetes

Self-control: and diabetic language, 64; in Joslin philosophy, 66, 121; and diabetic control, 66, 124, 125, 127, 130, 190; and identity work, 117

Sequelae of diabetes: and medical therapeutics, xxii, 132; limb amputations, 9, 10, 36, 109, 141, 142, 202; blindness, 9, 10, 36, 110, 190–91, 202; kidney damage, 9, 27, 39, 46, 82, 83–85, 138, 139, 140; and diabetes transmutation, 10, 23, 24–25, 43, 122, 138; heart attack, 10, 24, 139, 190, 202; renal failure, 10, 36, 82, 83, 110, 138, 202; and ill-

ness transformation, 26, 27; nerve damage, 27, 109–10, 139, 202; long-term, 39, 43, 64, 65, 82, 83, 84, 110; blood vessel damage, 39, 109, 191; and employment, 59, 83, 84, 85, 107, 138–39, 140, 141; and diabetic control, 65–66, 122, 135, 137–43, 174, 175; and surgery, 69; and pregnancy, 75–77; and later stages of life, 81–86, 187; retinopathy, 83, 110, 138–40, 188, 190, 202, 235–36 (n. 28); and dietary therapy, 85–86; and daily living with diabetes, 91; gangrene, 109, 141, 174; and technological innovation, 138; and urine tests, 138, 159; and moral character, 140; and patient image, 141; and family/parents, 141–42; postpregnancy, 164–66, 167; neuritis, 174; and responsibility, 175–76, 185, 191, 212; ketoacidosis, 202

Shoes, 65, 91, 131–32

Sickle cell disease, 11

Smith, George Van S., 158

Smith, Olive Watkins, 158

Social changes: and diabetic management, 59–60, 122–23; and diabetics, 59–60, 211; and pregnancy, 147, 166; and technological innovation, 168

Social history, 77–78

Social policy, 21

Social workers, 27, 91, 179

Starvation metabolism, xxi

Starvation therapy, 48, 49, 98, 151, 171, 176, 201

Sterilization, 157, 163

Stroke, 10, 48, 83, 138, 141

Sulfa antimicrobials, 24, 76

Surgical procedures, 40, 60, 68–69, 111. *See also* Cesarean section

Swine flue, 23

Syphilis, 21

Syringes: changes in, 26; and diabetic

proliferative retinopathy, 64, 159; and retinopathy, 83, 110, 138–40, 188, 190, 192, 202, 235–36 (n. 28), 245 (n. 66); and patient records and letters, 140, 159

Von Mering, Joseph, 50, 132

Vulnerability, xxii, 68

Walden, George, 54

Watson, Thomas, 169

White, Priscilla: and pregnancy, 76, 133, 146, 152–54, 157, 160–61, 167, 179; and patient/doctor relationship, 77, 79, 121, 133, 137, 162–64, 166, 237 (n. 27); personal life of, 87; on prevention of coma, 135–36; and Type 1 diabetes mellitus, 152; and diabetic control, 161–62; and medical expenses, 163; view

of postpregnancy sequelae or complications, 164–66; view of patient responsibility, 179–80, 181, 185

Williams, J. Whitridge, 150

Williams, John R., 48–49, 52, 53

Willis, Thomas, 5

Wilson, Alvin (pseudonym), 12–13

Wilson, Clifford, 82, 138

Woodyatt, Rollin T., 51, 136

Workplace discrimination, 27, 185–86. *See also* Employment

World War I, 71

World War II, 59, 72, 81, 111

Wound healing, 69

Yeast infections, 110

Zuelzer, Georg Ludwig, 51

STUDIES IN SOCIAL MEDICINE

Nancy M. P. King, Gail E. Henderson, and Jane Stein, eds., *Beyond Regulations: Ethics in Human Subjects Research* (1999).

Laurie Zoloth, *Health Care and the Ethics of Encounter: A Jewish Discussion of Social Justice* (1999).

Susan M. Reverby, ed. *Tuskegee's Truths: Rethinking the Tuskegee Syphilis Study* (2000).

Beatrix Hoffman, *Wages of Sickness: The Politics of Health Insurance in Progressive America* (2000).

Margarete Sandelowski, *Devices and Desires: Gender, Technology, and American Nursing* (2000).

Keith Wailoo, *Dying in the City of the Blues: Sickle Cell Anemia and the Politics of Race and Health* (2001).

Judith Andre, *Bioethics as Practice* (2002).

Chris Feudtner, *Bittersweet: Diabetes, Insulin, and the Transformation of Illness* (2003)

FEUDTNER@
email.chop.edu